AN ILLUSTRATED COLOUR TEXT

CLINICAL HISTORY TAKING AND EXAMINATION

To Mozart, who received less attention
than he deserved whilst this book was
being prepared!

AN ILLUSTRATED COLOUR TEXT

CLINICAL HISTORY TAKING AND EXAMINATION

PHILIP D. WELSBY FRCP (Ed)
Consultant Physician (Communicable Diseases),
The City Hospital,
Royal Infirmary and Associated Hospitals Trust,
Edinburgh, UK

Illustrated by IAN RAMSDEN

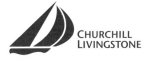
CHURCHILL
LIVINGSTONE

NEW YORK, EDINBURGH, LONDON, MADRID, MELBOURNE, SAN FRANCISCO, TOKYO 1996

CHURCHILL LIVINGSTONE
Medical Division of Pearson Professional Limited

Distributed in the United States of America by Churchill Livingstone Inc., 650 Avenue of the Americas, New York, N.Y. 10011 and by associated companies, branches and representatives throughout the world.

First published 1996

ISBN 0-443-04328-0

British Library of Cataloguing in Publication Data
A catalogue record for this book is available from the British Library.

Library of Congress Cataloging in Publication Data
A catalogue record for this book is available from the Library of Congress.

For Churchill Livingstone

Publisher: Timothy Horne
Project Editor: Jim Killgore
Design: Sarah Cape
Electronic page make-up: Pat Miller, Fionna Robson, Sarah Cape, Oxprint
Pre-Press Desktop operators: David Thomson, Kate Wallshaw, Gerard Heyburn
Design and production management: Sarah Cape
Project controller: Nancy Arnott, Kay Hunston, Debra Barrie

PREFACE

This book is based upon teaching of medical students and contains information and practical advice on clinical aspects of history taking and examination.

The only excuse for another book on history taking and examination must be that the approach adopted is different from most other books. This is a single author book written unashamedly from a general point of view by a non-academic, avoiding medical jargon as much as is possible. Specialist explanations and classification systems have been modified when simplicity seemed more appropriate for students.

I have restricted information to that which I judge a recently qualified doctor might be expected to know.

Some knowledge of preclinical sciences is assumed. Details of anatomy and physiology are included when such knowledge is essential to understand the mode of production of symptoms and signs associated with various conditions.

The temptation to pontificate pretentiously about the doctor-patient relationship has been resisted, but two generalisations are relevant. Firstly, always treat patients as you would wish yourself or your relatives to be treated. Secondly, always be aware of the privileged position you have. Because we see patients in all manner of stressful situations we can gain more insights into human nature in a day than some people can obtain in a lifetime.

Edinburgh   P.D.W.
1996

ACKNOWLEDGEMENTS

The author wishes to thank a number of colleagues for allowing use of the following illustrations:

- Arthritis and Rheumatism Council, Fig. 3, page 112
- Dr R. Emond: Fig. 1, page 14; Fig. 8, page 125
- Professor A Emery: Fig. 1, page 104
- Dr B Frier: Fig. 3, page 73
- Dr P Hayes: Fig. 1, page 70
- Dr M Jones: Fig. 2, page 73
- Professor G Nuki: Fig. 4, page 118
- Dr P Padfield: Fig. 2, page 10
- Dr K Swa: Fig. 8, page 11; Fig. 1, page 80; Fig. 2, page 80; Fig. 3, page 80; Fig. 5, page 81; Fig. 6, page 81
- Dr A Wightman: Fig. 4, page 112.

CONTENTS

BASIC PRINCIPLES

SYSTEMS

SPECIAL TOPICS

BASIC
PRINCIPLES

HISTORY TAKING (I)

INTRODUCTION

The purpose of doctoring is to provide patients with correct treatment: to do this it is usually necessary to take a history and perform an examination. The importance of the history cannot be overestimated. Studies performed with hospital out-patients show that diagnoses are made from the history in the vast majority of patients. Examination only provides significant unexpected findings in a minority.

GENERAL APPROACH

Always respect the patient's privacy and confidentiality when taking a history or presenting the findings. Ensure that you or your patient cannot be overheard and that no one else (except a chaperone if appropriate) can see the examination taking place. Similarly do not discuss patients with colleagues in public.

Try to see things from the patient's point of view. Some patients may irritate or annoy, but it is essential for doctors to exhibit a neutral position whenever possible (whatever their private thoughts may be). Remember that there may be an understandable medical or situational reason why some patients provoke irritation or annoyance. Always introduce yourself and greet patients appropriately in a friendly relaxed fashion and *never* forget the patient's name.

The history you take should tell a clear story. Unfortunately, few patients are competent story tellers and the doctor has to assist the patient so that accurate interpretations can be made.

With complex histories, the first symptom often identifies the site of the initiating pathology.

After introducing yourself to the patient, the best opening gambit in my opinion is to ask 'What can I do for you?'. This starts by showing goodwill and an attempt to be helpful. The reply also tells you what the patient expects, and gives him/her the chance to have the first word. It often enables more direct but open-ended follow-on questions such as 'What exactly is the problem?' and 'Could you tell me how this developed?'.

Unless the problem is predictably simple (as for routine surgical admissions), in most instances it is probably best to write down only the important occurrences and their timing so that you can spend most of the time concentrating on what the patient has to say. Complex histories can rarely be written directly into the notes as the patient tells the story.

QUESTIONING TECHNIQUE

Any question you may ask should be simple, clear and couched in terms that the patient will understand. Try to avoid medical jargon, but be careful that the translation of what the patient says into medical jargon is accurate. Patients often use medical terms incorrectly and often use diagnostic terms when descriptive terms would be more helpful.

Relevant questions can be asked as the patient tells the story. It may be best to let the patient continue uninterrupted, or to interpose questions sparingly. A structure can also be imposed with multiple questions. A useful ploy when a patient is hopelessly polysymptomatic or garrulous is to confess that *you* are having difficulty in focusing on the problems. Ask the patient to help by recounting the main problems within 1 minute.

If a patient is so talkative that interruptions to ask questions may be perceived as rudeness by the patient it is useful to interrupt with a 'Yes but ... 'when the patient takes a breath at the end of a sentence.

Avoid asking too many *leading questions* as some patients instinctively like to agree with the doctor's suggestions. However, leading questions are useful:

- *When it helps the patient's self-expression.* In such circumstances it is useful to provide several possible replies. This technique is also useful to avoid asking direct yes or no questions that might be embarrassing to the patient if the reply is positive, or embarrassing for the doctor to have asked if the reply is a forthright negative. For example, it may be appropriate to ask 'Are you single, married, separated or divorced?' rather than asking about each in turn.

- *When you are consciously helping the patient to 'confess' historical points that might not be otherwise volunteered.* Again provision of a menu of replies minimizes the chance of false positive responses.

- *When asking questions that are aimed to elicit a negative reply* (excluding the possibility that the patient is trying to please by replying 'yes'). A reply 'Never' to 'When did you last cough up blood?' excludes haemoptysis.

- *When suspecting poor compliance with drug therapy.* A more truthful reply will be obtained by asking 'Do you find it easy to remember to take each dose?'.

False prompt questions can be asked which are specifically designed to get the patient to volunteer an important historical point. Points that a patient volunteers are likely to be uninfluenced by a patient's desire to please. For example, if a patient with rheumatoid arthritis volunteers that 'The stiffness is worse in the morning' in reply to a question 'Is the stiffness worse in the evening?', then the doctor can be certain that the stiffness is worse in the morning.

Direct questions are useful, especially if asked in such a fashion that an answer has to be yes or no (for example 'Did you or did you not have loss of consciousness?'). At some stage during the history taking it may be useful to ask the patient what they think is wrong. The replies are usually interesting — and may be correct. But more importantly, false or irrational fears can thereby be revealed and allayed rapidly.

The basic main headings for questions that should be asked routinely are illustrated in Figure 1.

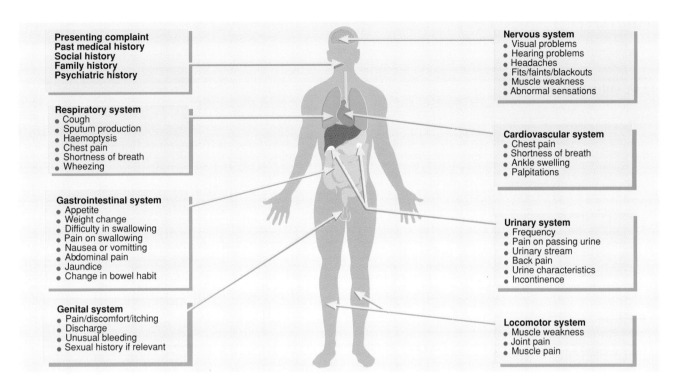

Fig. 1 **Routine questions in history taking.** The basic 'stem' questions should be asked routinely. Write up the history starting with the history of the presenting complaint and then follow on with relevant systematic questions, and conclude with the routine questions. It follows that the sequence of the writing-up will vary in individual patients. A problem orientated approach is not used here because this method of patient evaluation has not found widespread acceptance despite its immense logical appeal.

PRESENTING COMPLAINTS

The presenting complaints should be clearly defined as soon as possible. For each presenting complaint the timing of onset, the mode of evolution, the severity, the results of previous investigations and the effects of treatment may all be relevant.

A decision has to be made at an early stage of history taking as to whether the presenting complaints are obviously integrated into a simple sequence or whether they are separate and have to be dealt with independently during the subsequent history taking. A degree of flexibility is required, as it may later become apparent that initially disparate complaints were, in fact, related.

CHARACTERISTICS OF PAIN

Pains associated with specific organs or conditions are detailed in the relevant chapters. Pains which are not obviously arising from a particular organ or structure should be described according to their characteristics, of which there are nine main categories:

- *The site.*
- *The character.* Patients often need to be given a menu of adjectives from which to choose. Was the pain burning, sharp, stabbing or crushing in nature? Was it superficial 'bright' pain or 'deep' pain?
- *The mode of onset.* Was the onset abrupt or gradual?

- *The progression.* What was the duration of the pain: continuous or intermittent? If the latter, what was the frequency of occurrence and nature?
- *The radiation.* Where did it move to?
- *The relationship to any other bodily function or position.*
- *The modifying factors.* Did anything make the pain better or make it worse?
- *The treatment given (if any).* Ask for details and if the treatment helped.
- *The depth of the pain.* Is the pain a superficial or internal (deep) pain? This question is frequently omitted and is often of great help in differential diagnosis.

History taking (I)
- Diagnoses are usually made from the history.
- Ensure that your conversations with patients cannot be overheard.
- Never forget the patient's name.
- Avoid asking leading qestions.
- Defne the presenting complaint(s) as soon as possible.

HISTORY TAKING (II)

PAST MEDICAL HISTORY

Previous illnesses
Questions traditionally cover rheumatic fever, diabetes and tuberculosis, but in most patients it is more relevant to ask about any heart, lung, gut, waterworks or nervous diseases (nervous diseases usefully cover neurological and mental disorders).

Previous treatments
Details of previous operations, hospitalizations or significant accidents should be elicited.

Previous medication
Ask about any medicines the patient is taking, including self-medication, and then ascertain whether or not they are, in fact, taking them. Studies have revealed that only about a third of general practice patients take medicines as prescribed. It is useful to ask patients if they find it difficult to take their medicines; this enables them to confess to poor compliance. Always ask women (if in the appropriate age group) whether they are on the oral contraceptive pill. Most women do not consider the pill to be a medicine.

Allergies or drug reactions
Patients should be asked about allergies or reactions to anything, including medicines.

FAMILY HISTORY

Inquire if the patient is single, married, separated or divorced. If separated or divorced, it may be relevant to ask when and why. Ask if the patient has had any children. A tactful approach with a woman patient is to ask how many times she has been pregnant, and then how many children she has. This will bring the line of questioning to possible spontaneous abortions, miscarriages, still births, terminations, and deaths in childhood. Figure 1 details the conventional symbols used in constructing a family tree.

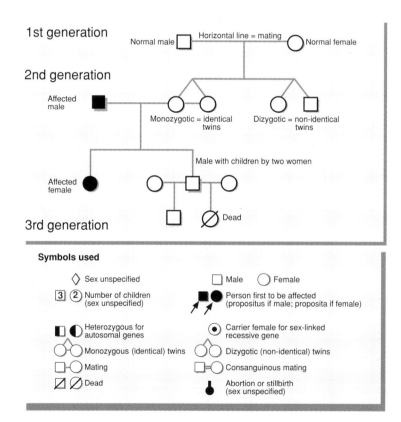

Fig. 1 **Conventional symbols used in constructing a family tree.**

SOCIAL HISTORY

Assessment of a patient's appearance, manner and content of general conversation will provide some social background, but more specific questions may have to be asked where relevant. Be careful: there is sometimes a fine line between gratuitous nosiness and medically justified curiosity, and the patient's placement of this line may differ from yours.

Employment
There is increasing evidence that unemployment predisposes to physical illness as well as mental stress. In addition, certain occupations can be associated with specific disorders.

Ask the patient 'Do you have a job at the moment?'. If the answer is 'Yes', ascertain what the job entails and how long the patient has spent in that job. If the answer is 'No', find out what, if any, training the patient has received. With older teenagers this may pose a problem as some are embarrassed about their unemployed (or unemployable) status, whilst others are still at school. A useful question to ask such patients is 'What do you do with yourself most days?'. Ask if the patient has any financial worries or related stress (doctors may be able to ensure that patients are receiving all possible benefits).

Housing

Inquire where the patient lives and whether there are any associated financial or social problems with their housing circumstances.

Hobbies

Certain hobbies carry medical risks. For example, bird fanciers may have psittacosis or bird fanciers' lung. Ask about any particular interest or hobby: 'What do you do in your spare time?'.

Recent travel abroad

Travel, especially in tropical countries, may be relevant to illness. Incubation periods can be used to include or exclude various infectious illnesses (Table 1).

Table 1. **Diseases which can be acquired abroad: incubation periods**

Disease	Minimum incubation period	Maximum incubation period	Average incubation period
Brucellosis	7 days	Uncertain	
Kala azar	10 days	2 years	2–4 months
Hepatitis A	28 days	42 days	35 days
Hepatitis B	6 weeks	6 months	
Falciparum malaria	8 days	25 days*	12 days
Vivax malaria	8 days	27 days*	14 days
Typhoid fever	7 days	21 days	8–14 days
Yellow fever	3 days	15 days	3–6 days

*In non-immunes (longer in immunes or those who received inadequate prophylaxis)

Stress

Stress may contribute to, or indeed be the only reason for, a patient's presentation. A useful approach if there is a suspicion of burdensome stress is to ask 'Are there any (other) problems you should tell me about?'.

Alcohol intake

The patient's occupation, demeanor or breath might be suggestive of alcohol problems. The smell of alcohol is usually easily detectable, but heavy drinkers who have stopped drinking just before seeing the doctor often have a sweet acetaldehyde breath.

You may ask the patient:

- Do you ever feel that you should cut down on your drinking?
- Do others annoy you by criticism of your drinking?
- Do you ever feel guilty about your drinking?
- Do you have to have a drink in the morning (to steady the nerves or get rid of a hangover)?

A useful gambit to help patients confess a higher intake than they might realize is to ask 'What is your favourite drink?'. One can then ask if the patient drinks an excessive amount as defined in Figure 2. For example, ask 'Do you drink half a bottle of whisky a day?'. An instant (surprised) 'No' is a reasonable guide to a much smaller intake, but a 'Yes' answer or any hesitation whilst calculating before replying has obvious implications!

Drug abuse

Asking some people about drug abuse is essential but runs the risk of causing offence to non-abusers. A useful ploy is to ask outright: 'What drugs do you take?'. Drug abusers usually give a truthful reply, but if non-abusers are offended one can instantly defuse the situation by saying 'I mean medical drugs such as heart tablets.'

Sexual activity

Sexually transmitted diseases (STD) are not uncommon. At STD clinics there is one new attendance for each 96 people in the population each year! Especially since the advent of human immunodeficiency virus (HIV) infection, STDs may contribute to illnesses in many organ systems. Nevertheless, only ask about sexual activity if it might be relevant to the illness.

Apologize for having to ask such private questions and explain why it is medically appropriate for you to ask. Then ask if the patient is sexually active. Males who are sexually active, but who might be homosexual (and currently as a group at higher than average risk of HIV infection), can be asked if they are exclusively heterosexual. This line of questioning causes no offence to those who might take offence at the suggestion of homosexuality.

Asking about previous STDs also requires tact. A useful approach is to ask if there have been any infections affecting 'down below' in males or of 'the front passage' in females. If women are affronted by this suggestion add 'like thrush', an infection which does not necessarily have a STD connotation. In either sex if the answer is 'Yes', ask 'was it something you might have caught from someone else?'.

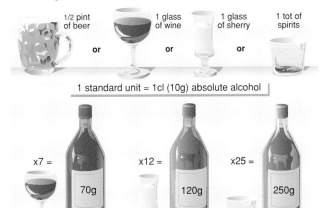

Fig. 2 **Assessing alcohol intake.** The 'standard' unit used in the UK is one centilitre (approximately 10 g) of absolute alcohol. This is equivalent to a half-pint of average-strength beer, a glass of wine, a small glass of sherry or a single tot of spirits. Cirrhosis may be present with a daily intake of six pints of beer, a bottle of wine or a third of a bottle of spirits. Even lower levels may cause cirrhosis in some patients (women are more susceptible than men).

History taking (II)

- There is a fine line between gratuitous nosiness and medically justified curiosity.
- Febrile patients should be asked if they have been abroad.
- Alcohol overuse is rarely volunteered.
- Sexually transmitted diseases are more common than we think.

GENERAL EXAMINATION (I)—Sequence, General Observations and Nails

Examinations are best conducted with the patient lying on a bed or couch (the respiratory system can be usefully examined with the patient standing). The patient's height and weight should be recorded at the initial consultation.

SEQUENCE OF EXAMINATION

In practice, the best order of examination should begin with a careful appraisal of the whole patient and his/her presentation. This can then be followed by an examination of the hands, upper limbs, neck, head, chest, abdomen and lower limbs, with a secondary reappraisal if the nervous and locomotor system require detailed examination (Fig. 1).

The equipment required to conduct a non-specialized examination generally comprises a spatula, cotton wool (for testing sensation), a torch, a stethoscope, an ophthalmoscope/auriscope, a sphygmomanometer and a disposable paperclip for pinprick appreciation (using a disposable paperclip reduces risk of spread of infection from patient to patient).

In several situations it is essential to explain to the patient what you want to do and the reason why. Whenever possible it is advisable to have a chaperone present when examining members of the opposite sex.

Students often neglect important clues by confining their inspections to the patient. The patient's mode of arrival and deportment may reveal many relevant considerations. In hospital practice, observation of the temperature chart, sputum pot contents and lockertop articles may all provide much useful information.

The next section will detail the clinical signs which may be found on examination in the sequence suggested in Figure 1, beginning with relevant general observations.

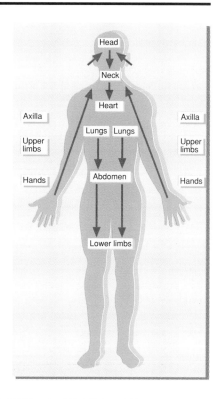

Fig. 1 **The suggested order of clinical examination.**

GENERAL OBSERVATIONS

Abnormal swellings

Swellings of various organs are detailed in the relevant sections. Swellings which are not obviously arising from a particular organ or structure should be described according to eight main characteristics (Fig. 2):

- *Size.*
- *Shape.* Lymph node swellings tend to have a smooth surface.
- *Tenderness.* Most, but not all, inflammatory swellings are tender.
- *Consistency.* Most acute inflammatory swellings are not rock-hard, although they may be tense. Rock-hard swellings should be considered malignant until proved otherwise.
- *Mobility or attachment.*
- *Pulsatile nature.* If intrinsically pulsatile, the swelling itself will expand in at least two dimensions, but if the pulsation is transmitted from under-lying structures then it will pulsate in one dimension only.

- *Indentability.* Only attempt to assess indentability if it is certain that there is no possibility of an underlying lesion that may burst, such as an aneurysm.
- *Translucency.* A swelling which transilluminates suggests an accumulation of clear fluid.

Pallor

Pallor is a rather subjective assessment which suggests anaemia. It is best assessed by examination of the lips and tongue, or by gentle eversion of the palpebral conjunctiva: the colour will be paler or more pink than red in colour. Pallor may also be caused by peripheral vasoconstriction.

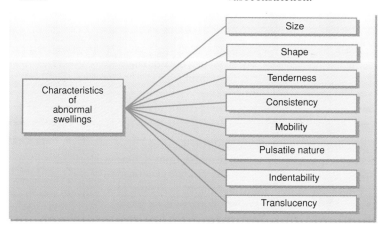

Fig. 2 **The characteristics of abnormal swellings.**

Plethora

Plethora is a weatherbeaten facial appearance resulting from a combination of excessive redness caused by a supranormal concentration of haemoglobin (polycythaemia) combined with a cyanotic tinge. Cyanosis is detailed on page 42.

Fever

The normal temperature as measured in the axilla is 37 degrees centigrade or just below. Rectal temperatures can be up to one degree higher. There are four main categories of fever (Fig. 3):

- *Continued fever* is a continuously elevated temperature usually fluctuating by less than 1 degree C.
- *Remittent fever* comprises temperature elevation for all or most of the day with a difference between maximum and minimum of 1 degree C.
- *Intermittent fever* comprises temperature peaks with return to normal.
- *Undulant fever* comprises periods of fever (usually lasting for days) separated by afebrile periods (usually lasting for a week or more).

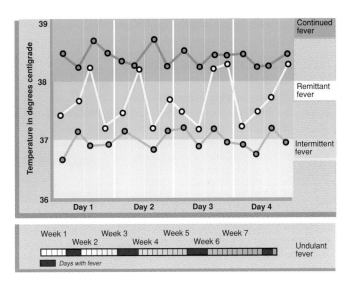

Fig. 3 **The patterns of fever.**

THE NAILS

The nails may show a number of general signs. Nails can become yellow and thickened but smooth as part of a 'yellow nail syndrome' which includes chronic oedema, pleural fluid accumulation, sinus infection or thyroid disease. In renal failure the proximal half of the nails may become white in contrast to the reddish brown of the distal half. Long duration therapy with certain drugs may affect the nail. Notably zidovudine (AZT) may cause incredibly white nails and chloroquine may impart a bluish black appearance.

Beau's lines

Episodes of illness or malnutrition can result in transverse lines or depressions caused by defective nail growth (Fig. 4). As the average life of a fingernail is 6 months, it is possible to date recent illness(es) by observing the situation of the lines.

Fungal infection

Fungal infection may cause the nails to become dull and yellow or brown, thickened, pitted and brittle. The nail may separate from the nailbed (onycholysis).

Koilonychia

In koilonychia the nails become flat or concave, thin and brittle. The condition is associated with chronic iron deficiency anaemia.

Leukonychia

In leukonychia the nails become white, approaching the whiteness of the halfmoon at the nail base. Causes include a low blood albumin or severe anaemia.

Nailbed splinter haemorrhages and pitting

Trauma is the commmonest cause of splinter haemorrhages. These are linear longitudinal haemorrhages caused by microbleeding from small blood vessels (Fig. 5). In the absence of trauma, the cause should be assumed to be infective endocarditis.

Nail pitting should suggest psoriasis, a skin disease.

Onycholosis

Onycholosis is the separation of the free edge of the nail from the nailbed. Excessive manicuring and psoriasis are common causes.

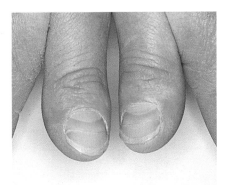

Fig. 4 **Beau's lines.**

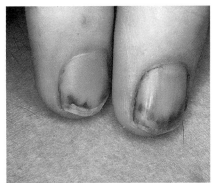

Fig. 5 **Splinter haemorhages.**

General examination (I)

- Never omit a generalised appraisal even if the patient's abnormality appears localised.
- Examine the patient in a routine defined sequence to avoid omissions.
- Chaperones should be used whenever possible if examining members of the opposite sex.

GENERAL EXAMINATION (II)—Hands

EXAMINATION

Look for abnormal resting posture, tremor or flap (p. 141), skeletal deformity or muscle wasting, and abnormalities of hand size, shape or colour. *Feel* for abnormal temperature or sensation (p. 90). Have the patient *move* the fingers to see if there is abnormal movement of joints, specific muscles, or functional groups of muscles (p. 106).

COMMON CONDITIONS

Acromegaly

In acromegaly the hands are large and spade-like, with a coarse skin texture. The condition is caused by excessive growth hormone production.

Arachnodactyly

Long thin fingers, or arachnodactyly, may be a feature of Marfan's syndrome, a disorder of connective tissue (Fig. 1). Other features include tallness, a fingertip to fingertip span greater than height, dislocation of the ocular lens, a high arched palate and heart lesions (commonly coarctation of the aorta or atrial septal defect).

Achondroplasia

Achondroplasia is characterized by small and thickened hands, with fingers of almost uniform length. Other features include dwarfism, the trunk being of normal size but with short limbs. It is caused by defective cartilage formation.

Down's syndrome

In Down's syndrome the palm has a well-marked transverse crease. Other features include a crease between the great toe and adjacent toe, mental and physical retardation, microcephaly, slanted eyes, a large tongue and congenital heart defects (in about one-third of those affected).

Claw hand

The term claw hand implies hyper-extension of some or all of the meta-carpophalangeal joints, with flexion of the interphalangeal joints. Unilateral claw hand may be caused by ulnar nerve lesions, but bilateral claw hands suggest disorders such as syringomyelia (a spinal cord disease) or leprosy (a disease which damages peripheral nerves).

Clubbing

Clubbing is an increased longitudinal and transverse curvature of the nail, often with

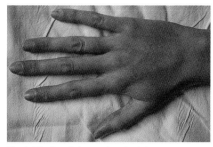
Fig. 2 **Drumstick Clubbing.**

an associated loss of the angle between the proximal nail and the nail bed (Fig. 2). If well-marked, there is swelling of the soft tissue of the pulp of the finger leading to a drumstick appearance. The oedematous swelling of the nailbed is best tested by using both index fingers to press each side of the midline of the involved nailbed. A sense of fluctuation felt by one finger on exertion of pressure by the other consti-tutes fluctuation. An isolated increased curvature of the nails (beaking) may be a normal finding. Usually all fingers are affected to a greater or lesser extent by clubbing, although subclavian artery aneurysms are reputed to be a cause of unilateral clubbing.

Clubbing may be congenital (and of no diagnostic significance) and may become more marked with increasing age. Any recent development of clubbing is highly significant, as the causes include carcinoma of the lung, certain other intrathoracic tumours, chronic suppurative lung disease, congenital cyanotic heart disease, infective endocarditis, fibrosing alveolitis, chronic malabsorption, inflam-matory bowel disease and cirrhosis. Chronic bronchitis or emphysema rarely, if ever, cause clubbing.

Hypertrophic pulmonary osteo-arthropathy is often found in associa-tion with clubbing and is usually caused by underlying carcinoma of the lung. There is pain and tenderness around the wrists.

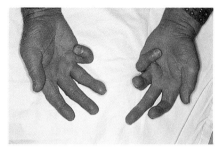
Fig. 1 **The hands in arachnodactyly.**

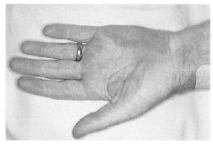
Fig. 3 **Dupuytren's contracture.**

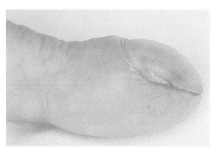
Fig. 4 **Palmar erythema.**

Dactylitis

Dactylitis is a vague non-diagnostic term denoting inflammation of a finger or fingers which leads to diffuse or bumpy finger swelling. Causes include tubercu-losis or gout.

Dupuytren's contracture

Dupuytren's contracture (Fig. 3) is characterized by fibrosis of the palmar fascia or tendons which draw the fingers (especially the ring and middle fingers) into flexion. Contractures are usually present on both hands, with a degree of asymmetry. There is no obvious cause in most patients, but in some there is associ-ated cirrhosis, alcoholism, certain occu-pations (vibrating tool use) or epilepsy.

Gout

Gout is a metabolic disorder of uric acid metabolism in which calcium biurate is deposited in various tissues. Chronic gout causes chalky deposits (tophi), which may ulcerate through overlying skin.

Nodules

Subcutaneous nodules, if associated with arthritis, are usually a marker of seroposi-tive rheumatoid arthritis. Nodules may be mistaken for lymph nodes and may be attached to underlying tissue (if attached to muscle sheaths or tendons they are usually called ganglia). Less common causes of subcutaneous nodular swellings include fat deposits, xanthomas or calcium deposits.

Heberden's nodes

Heberden's nodes are bony prominences (osteophytes) at the sides of the terminal interphalangeal joints or, less commonly, at the proximal interphalangeal joints (Bouchard's nodes). Both may be found in generalized osteoarthritis.

Palmar erythema

Palmar erythema (Fig. 4) is a persistent bilateral reddening of the palms which, unlike simple vasodilatation, is more marked around the peripheries of the palm. Whilst such erythema may have no apparent cause, there is an association with liver disease (either acute or chronic), pregnancy, rheumatoid arthritis and thyrotoxicosis.

Raynaud's phenomenon

Raynaud's phenomenon is usually a bilateral condition caused by hyperreactivity of blood vessels which go into paroxysms of prolonged spasm, often in response to cold. The fingers go white, then blue, with associated pain (see p. 118). Causes include scleroderma or systemic lupus erythematosus (SLE) both of which are collagen–vascular disorders.

Rheumatoid arthritis (Fig. 5)

The differentiation between early rheumatoid arthritis and osteoarthritis is detailed on page 113. The hand in early rheumatoid arthritis may show muscle wasting, metacarpophalangeal joint swelling, proximal interphalangeal joint swelling (perhaps leading to a spindled appearance), flexor tendon synovitis leading to trigger finger and effusions. Later changes include subluxation of metacarpophalangeal joints, ulnar deviation of the fingers, button hole deformities, swan neck deformities, Z deformities, and tendon thinning with possible ruptures.

Sarcoidosis

Infiltration of hand tissue with sarcoid tissue (a granulomatous disorder of unknown causation) may produce lupus pernio, a chronic purple discoloration of the skin which, unlike Raynaud's phenomenon, is unaffected by cold.

Scleroderma

In scleroderma the skin becomes fibrotic leading to fibrous contraction of hand skin (which in consequence cannot be pinched up). Finger movements are restricted and the skin may have a shiny glazed appearance. Subcutaneous calcium deposits may be associated.

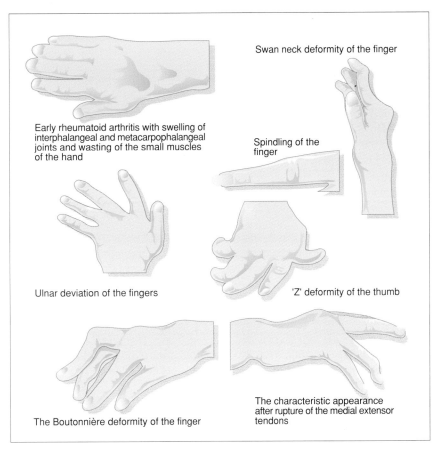

Fig. 5 **Common types of rheumatoid arthritis.**

Thyroid dysfunction

An overactive thyroid gland (thyrotoxicosis) may cause increased circulation with blood vessel dilatation leading to warm sweaty palms, possibly with palmar erythema. In contrast, an underactive thyroid (myxoedema) may cause the hands to be cool, dry and rough in texture.

Muscle wasting

Causes of muscle wasting include motor neurone disease (a progressive dysfunction of lower motor neurones) syringomyelia, ulnar or median nerve palsy, poliomyelitis, C8 or T1 nerve root lesions, peripheral neuritis or neuropathy.

Smoking

Tar discolors fingers, usually of the dominant hand. Nicotine is colourless and does not cause stains.

Lifestyle

Skin thickening suggest a manual occupation, and weatherbeaten hands an outdoor occupation. Miners may have implanted coal dust beneath the skin. Rude or crude tattoos on the hands (or elsewhere) may suggest a mildly psychopathic tendency to self-abuse and disregard for society, which is often associated with other abuses including drug addiction.

General examination (II)—hands

- Unilateral claw hand suggests an ulnar nerve lesion.
- Dupuytren's contracture presents with no obvious cause in most patients.
- Subcutaneous nodes associated with arthritis are usually a marker of seropostive rheumatoid arthritis.
- Thyrotoxicosis may lead to warm, sweaty palms; myxoedema may cause rough, dry hands.
- Raynaud's phenomenon, hyperreactivity of the blood vessels often in response to cold, may be a sign of scleroderma or SLE.
- Heberden's nodes may be found in generalized osteoarthritis.

GENERAL EXAMINATION (III)—Head, Face and Eyes

THE HEAD

Generalized enlargement of the head may be caused by congenital hydrocephalus or by Paget's disease. Normally, the shape of the head is related to the relative size of individual parts of the skull. Premature fusion of the skull bones, *craniostenosis*, causes abnormally shaped heads and, if congenital, causes prominence of the frontal bones or *bossing*. Sebaceous cysts or, less commonly, neoplasms may cause focal swellings, and palpable bony overgrowths are occasionally found over meningiomas.

THE FACE

The appearance of the face may be immediately suggestive of various disorders. In Parkinson's disease, the facial expression may be fixed with a lack of movement and expression, unblinking eyes and a slightly opened mouth (Fig. 1). Drooling occurs in severe cases because the striated muscles of swallowing are also stiff, and swallowing of saliva thereby impaired. The skin is often greasy. In severe hypothyroidism the skin is dry and puffy with alopecia of eyebrows and scalp (Fig. 2). In acromegaly (Fig. 3) there is protrusion of the jaw, and soft tissue overgrowth leads to coarsening of the facial features. In Down's syndrome (mongolism) the eyes are slanted and there is accentuation of the fold of skin (epicanthal fold) bordering the inner angle of the eye. The bridge of the nose is flattened and the mouth is often open with a large protruding tongue.

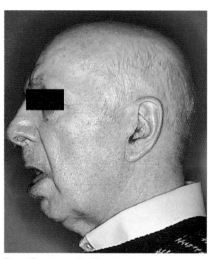

Fig. 1 **The face in Parkinson's disease.**

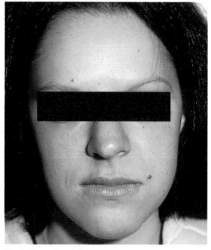

Fig. 2 **Hypothyroidism.**

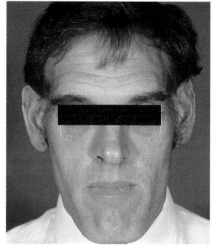

Fig. 3 **The characteristic facial features of acromegaly.**

THE EYES

The basic external anatomy of the eye is shown in Figure 4. The neurological aspects of eye examination are detailed on pages 76–83.

As part of the general examination look for evidence of the following:

- *Blepharitis:* chronic infection of the lid edge with thickening and redness of the lid margin.
- *Chemosis:* oedma of the eyelids.
- *Ectropion:* eversion of the eyelid.
- *Entropion:* inversion of the eyelid with the eyelashes often irritating the eye.
- *Orbital cellulitis:* inflammation of the orbit and periorbital tissue, usually of bacterial aetiology.
- *Phlyctenular conjunctivitis:* discrete nodular areas of inflammation at the limbus, the cornea or conjunctiva; usually a reaction to various allergic stimuli, notably active tuberculosis.
- *Pingueculae:* fatty triangles with the base at the cornea and the apex pointing to the inner or outer canthus.
- *Pterygium:* fibrosis of the same area as pingueculae.
- *Stye formation:* a staphylococcal abscess of the glands of the eyelid margin (Fig. 5).
- *Subconjunctival haemorrhages:* caused by bleeding from the poorly supported conjunctival blood vessels.
- *Xanthelasma:* fatty deposits in the skin around the eye which are often markers of hyperlipidaemia (Fig. 6).

Iridocyclitis

Iridocyclitis is inflammation of the iris and ciliary body, the causes of which include viral infection, tuberculosis, sarcoidosis and collagen–vascular diseases including rheumatoid arthritis. Symptoms of iridocyclitis include pain, intolerance of light (photophobia), lacrimation and

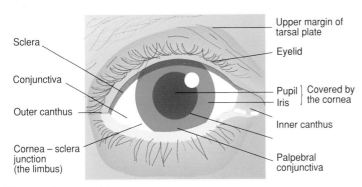

Fig. 4 **The external anatomy of the eye.**

Labels: Sclera, Conjunctiva, Outer canthus, Cornea – sclera junction (the limbus), Upper margin of tarsal plate, Eyelid, Pupil / Iris } Covered by the cornea, Inner canthus, Palpebral conjunctiva

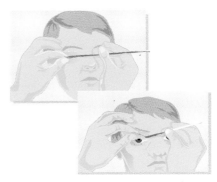

Fig. 7 **Eversion of the tarsal plate to reveal a foreign body.**

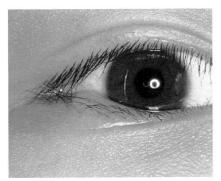

Fig. 5 **A stye.**

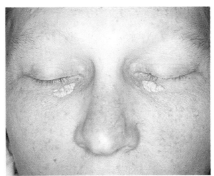

Fig. 6 **Xanthelasma.**

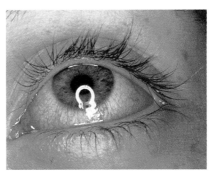

Fig. 8 **Cortical cataract seen against red reflex.**

blurred vision. There is also prominence of the small blood vessels surrounding the cornea, the iris is dull and swollen, the pupil may be small and irregular, and the fluid in the anterior chamber may be turbid (a *hypopyon*).

Foreign bodies

Non-penetrating foreign bodies may be seen on the eye or underneath the eyelids. To exclude foreign bodies underneath the upper eyelid, the upper margin of the tarsal plate can be everted by placing a probe across the top of the upper eyelid and, by grasping the eye margin and eyelashes, flipping the tarsal plate inside out to reveal the mucosal surface (Fig. 7).

Cataracts

Cataracts are areas of reduced transparency in the lens. Common causes include senile degeneration, diabetes or steroid therapy. The major symptom is of progressive, painless loss of vision. Mature cataracts are grey opacities in the lens, but other cataracts may stand out as defects in the red reflex when a light is shone directly into the eye (Fig. 8).

Acute conjunctivitis

Acute conjunctivitis (Fig. 9) is inflammation of the conjunctiva (the delicate membrane lining the eyelids and covering

the eyeball). There may be photophobia, excessive tear production and, if bacterial in nature, a purulent sticky discharge which gums up the eyes, particularly during sleep. With viral or allergic conjunctivitis, the discharge is not purulent. The conjunctival blood vessels are thickened and tortuous and move with the conjunctiva. In iritis or acute glaucoma, the blood vessels are fine, straight and pass radially from the cornea to the limbus, and do not move with the conjunctiva.

Signs in the sclera and cornea

The sclera is usually white but may be yellow if the patient is jaundiced (may be missed in poor or artificial light). The cornea should be perfectly transparent. Infection, particularly herpes simplex (which requires special fluorescein staining to demonstrate), may cause dendritic

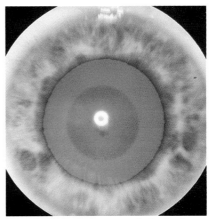

Fig. 9 **Acute conjunctivitis.**

(branching) ulcers. Foreign bodies may also cause corneal reactions and opacification. Arcus senilis is a white ring at the edge of the cornea and is usually associated with the aging process.

General examination (III)—head, face and eyes

- Generalized enlargement of the head may be due to hydrocephalus or Paget's disease.
- Coarsening of the facial features is a sign of acromegaly.
- Iridocyclitis is an inflammation of the iris and ciliary body usually caused by viral infection, tuberculosis and collagen–vascular diseases.
- Yellow sclera is a cardinal sign of jaundice.

GENERAL EXAMINATION (IV)—Mouth, Sinuses and Ears

THE MOUTH

The mouth and oral cavity (Fig. 1) should be examined systematically starting with the lips, the teeth and gums, and the hard and soft palate. Next examine the buccal mucosa and the tongue and pharynx. Ask the patient to remove any dentures before starting the examination.

The lips

Among other clinical signs the lips may show angular stomatitis with painful inflamed cracks at the corners of the mouth associated with dribbling caused by ill fitting dentures, candida infection or iron deficiency. Thickening and cracking of the lips, *cheilosis*, possibly with ulceration, is suggestive of vitamin deficiency — especially if associated with fissuring of the angles of the mouth. Herpes simplex comprises clusters of small itchy vesicles which become pustular and crust. They do not have diagnostic significance and may occur without apparent stimulus, although they may be a secondary manifestation of infection elsewhere in the body. Fissuring or nodules which do not heal should be viewed with suspicion, especially in older patients as neoplasia is a possibility.

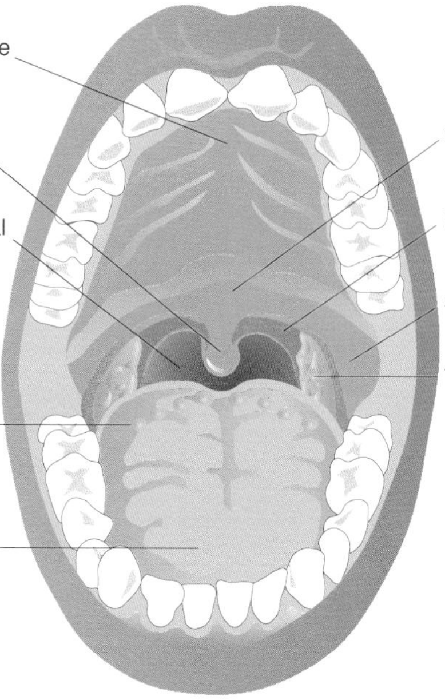

Fig. 1 **The mouth and oral cavity.**

Labels on figure: Hard palate / Uvula / Posterior pharyngeal wall / Vallate papillae / Dorsum of tongue / Soft palate / Posterior pillar / Anterior pillar / Tonsil

The teeth and gums

Look for pyorrhoea in which the gums are reddened and swollen. Pus may be visible or expressed in severe cases. Spontaneously bleeding gums may be a manifestation of uraemia, blood clotting diseases such as leukaemia, or vitamin C deficiency. Persistent intraoral ulceration may occur in acute leukaemia, agranulocytosis or as part of the cyclical orogenital ulceration of Behçet's disease. Whitish patches may be caused by thrush or leukoplakia. Gum hypertrophy is a common side-effect of longstanding phenytoin treatment.

The state of an individual's teeth often reflects his/her attitude to life — uncared for teeth often reflecting an uncaring lifestyle. Caries (cavities in the teeth), if immediately obvious, suggest a lack of dental visits. Teeth may be of abnormal colour: yellow due to smoking, dullish white caused by enamel hypoplasia if tetracyclines were given in early life, or greyish if the tooth has died.

Teeth, especially the incisors, may be notched or peg shaped in congenital syphilis.

Absent teeth or failure to wear dentures may lead to difficulty with mastication of 'tough' foods, perhaps leading to dyspepsia. The teeth are often abnormal in inherited or metabolic diseases, especially those affecting bone.

The palate

The hard palate is the bony anterior two-thirds of the palate, with the remainder constituting the soft palate. Both should be inspected for abnormalities. Small dot-like haemorrhages, palatal petechiae, occur in many throat infections but are a regular feature of glandular fever.

The buccal mucosa

Koplik's spots (Fig. 2) are like grains of salt on a background of redness and are present before the rash of measles. Oral lichen planus comprises whitish linear lacy streaks which do not ulcerate. They are often associated with skin lesions. Pigmented areas of the buccal mucosa or gums may be found in adrenal hypofunction or in heavy metal poisoning.

The tongue

The size, shape and symmetry of the tongue should be noted, both at rest and when protruded. Fungiform papillae are small reddish prominences which can be seen at

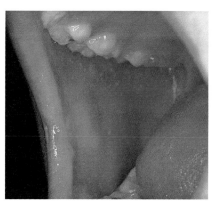

Fig. 2 **Koplik's spots in prodromal measles.**

the tip and edges of the tongue, whereas filiform papillae (the 'fur') are in rows across the tongue. Circumvallate papillae are prominent circular papillae which form a backward pointing 'V' at the back of the tongue: they are normally just out of sight.

A number of clinical signs may be noted in the tongue. *Glossitis* is a descriptive term referring to an atrophic, smooth, glazed and sore tongue. Causes include anaemia and vitamin deficiency. A *geographical tongue* is a normal finding, characterized by areas of papillae loss with the rest of the tongue being normal. The tongue may be furred if the patient is dehydrated. *Leukoplakia* is a white patch on the tongue, buccal mucosa or floor of the mouth that cannot be scraped off. Sometimes it is associated with chronic irritation or syphilis, and is often a premalignant condition. *Oral hairy leukoplakia* is a marker of HIV infection, with multiple vertical white fissures on the side of the tongue. Dilated blood vessels (telangectasia) may be found on the tongue (and elsewhere), and if also in the gut may be a source of gastrointestinal bleeding. A large tongue may be caused by acromegaly, hypothyroidism, Down's syndrome or primary amylodosis. Cyanosis may be evident.

Halitosis

Halitosis (malodourous breath) is usually caused by lack of dental care but may result from any condition which causes a sore throat. The odour of alcohol may be apparent, but as patients with an alcohol problem often abstain before seeing their doctor, there may only be a characteristic sweetish acetaldehyde-like odour. Endstage renal failure (uraemia) may give rise to a fishy odour, whereas in diabetic hyperglycaemia the smell of acetone is common. In liver failure, the breath is said to be like the belch of a cow (for those who have not had the benefit of this experience, this is like the odour of freshly cut grass which is about to rot). Lung abscesses or bronchiectasis may cause a foul halitosis

The tonsils

The tonsils lie at the back of the throat. Before the age of 10 years they are relatively large, thereafter becoming smaller. Asking the patient to say 'Ahhh' assists in visualization of the tonsils and pharynx. Do not ask the patient any questions whilst the spatula is in the mouth!

To visualize 'lowslung' tonsils, the tongue should be depressed with a spatula. To obtain good views without making the patient gag, ask him or her to relax the tongue whilst letting it lie in the floor of the mouth. A spatula should then be introduced to one side and the tongue gently pushed towards the midline with a slight withdrawing action to pull the tongue slightly forward. The tonsil on that side is then inspected, utilizing a torch. The procedure is then repeated on the other side.

THE SINUSES

The surface anatomy of the sinuses is shown in Figure 3. The skin areas over the superficially situated sinuses involved may be tender and swollen if there is sinusitis. Maxillary sinusitis may simulate toothache, which unlike uncomplicated toothache, may vary with posture (the pain of sinusitis often being a pressure-dependent closed box type of pain). Particularly in maxillary sinusitis there may be an inflamed nasal mucosa and purulent discharge. Uncomplicated nasopharyngitis tends to be predominantly a nasal illness, whereas sinusitis often presents with headache, general malaise and possibly fever.

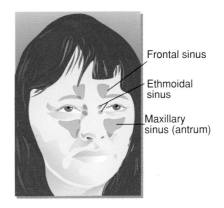

Frontal sinus

Ethmoidal sinus

Maxillary sinus (antrum)

Fig. 3 **The surface anatomy of the sinuses.**

THE EARS

Examination should include the external, middle and inner ear (Fig. 4). Chalky deposits in the earlobes are caused by long-standing gout. The auditary canal may be inflamed by infection (otitis externa). To examine the eardrum (Fig. 5) with an auriscope, the pinna should be drawn upwards and backwards to assist visualization of the tympanic membrane. Perforations, or middle ear effusions (with fluid levels behind the tympanic membrane) may be seen. With bacterial otitis media (without tympanic membrane perforation)

there will be pain, deafness, a bulging red tympanic membrane with loss of the light reflex, and prominent blood vessels. After a perforation, the pain usually diminishes and a purulent discharge may be obvious. Eustachian tube (which connects the middle ear with the throat) obstruction may cause the malleus to be rotated backwards so that the short process is more prominent. The tympanic membrane may have lost its normal pearly-grey surface, and the cone of light on illumination of the tympanic membrane may be distorted.

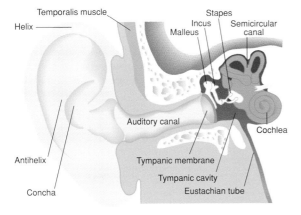

Fig. 4 **The anatomy of the ear.**

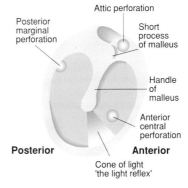

Fig. 5 **The right eardrum.**

General examination (IV)—mouth, sinuses and ears

- Examine the mouth systematically.
- Fissuring or nodules of the lips which do not heal should be treated with suspicion.
- Poor teeth often indicate poor health.
- Koplik's spots are present before a measles rash.
- Uncomplicated nasopharyngitis tends to be a nasal illness; sinusitis often presents with headache, malaise and fever.
- Draw the pinna upwards and backwards to facilitate examination of the eardrum with an auriscope.

GENERAL EXAMINATION (V)—Throat, Thyroid and Other Neck Signs

THE THROAT

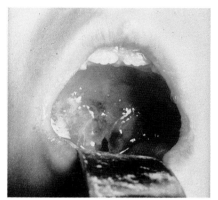

Fig.1 **The throat in diphtheria.**

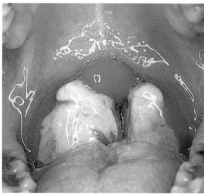

Fig. 2 **The throat in glandular fever.**

Perhaps the most common complaint requiring examination of the throat is the 'sore throat'. Because there is much overlap in appearances between various causes, this account has to deal with the various syndromes which may cause signs rather than the other way round.

Bacterial sore throats

Streptococcal infection of the throat may cause pharyngitis, tonsillitis or peritonsillar abscess formation (quinsy). Features of tonsillitis include fever and redness, congestions and oedema of the back of the throat, with small 'cheesey' exudates on the tonsils. Cervical lymph node enlargement may develop after (but only rarely before) the start of bacterial sore throats, whereas with viral sore throats, lymph node enlargement may occur first. A quinsy causes unilateral swelling with displacement of the uvula away from the midline.

Other causes of sore throat include Ludwig's and Vincent's angina. Ludwig's angina (submandibular cellulitis) is usually caused by infection with streptococci or anaerobic bacteria. There is marked pain and swelling in the submandibular area with danger of respiratory obstruction from soft tissue swelling. Vincent's angina is caused by dual infection with *Fusobacterium fusiforme* and *Borrelia vincentii*. There is pharyngitis with grey pseudomembrane formation and ulceration. Bleeding occurs on attempted removal of pseudomembrane.

Diphtheria (Fig. 1) should always be suspected in immigrants who may not have been immunized and who may have recently arrived from areas abroad where diphtheria is common. The diphtheretic membrane, if visible, is bilateral, wrinkled, sharply demarcated and firmly

adherent. It is dirty rather than white in colour, not confined to the tonsils, thick, homogeneous, surrounded by a narrow zone of inflammation and bleeds on attempted removal. Ulceration is not a feature. There is often a non-painful 'bull neck' with regional lymph node enlargement. There is a distinct risk of unpredictable and sudden respiratory obstruction as the membane may grow over or flake off and block the airway.

Viral sore throats

Viral sore throats may be indistinguishable from streptococcal sore throats. The following are the most common causes:

- *Adenovirus infection*
- *Pharyngoconjunctival fever* is a combination of conjunctivitis and pharyngitis usually caused by adenovirus infection.
- *Aphthous ulcers* comprise painful, small (about 5 mm diameter) irritating ulcers or vesicles at the front of the mouth

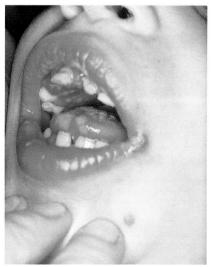

Fig. 3 **Herpes simplex gingivostomatitis.**

without extraoral spread: they are very common.

- *Chickenpox* may cause intraoral vesicles which rapidly burst leaving shallow ulcers.
- *Cytomegalovirus* may cause an exudative tonsillitis as may toxoplasmosis (a protozoan infection).
- *Glandular fever* (Epstein–Barr virus infection; Fig. 2) usually gives rise to palatal petechiae and, in classical cases, the tonsillar exudate is usually strikingly white in the early stages and confined to the tonsils. Unlike streptococcal sore throats, difficulty in swallowing is more often related to anatomical obstruction rather than to severe lancinating pain. Patients typically mouth breathe and have a nasal voice. If there is a possibility of diphtheria, the finding of non-regional lymph node enlargement or an enlarged spleen favours a diagnosis of glandular fever.
- *Hand, foot and mouth disease* is usually caused by coxsackie A16 virus. There are bright red macules or vesicles surrounded by a red halo. Lesions are on the hands, feet, and in the *front* of the mouth.
- *Herpangina* is usually caused by coxsackie A virus. There is an abrupt onset sore throat with painful dysphagia. The fauces and soft palate are red with distinct greyish patches or ulcers (a few millimetres in diameter) surrounded by red halos. These are present in the back of the mouth (unlike hand, foot and mouth disease and aphthous ulceration).
- *Herpes simplex* in young children may cause an acute gingivostomatitis (Fig. 3) with vesicles and very painful ulcers which predominantly affect the front of the mouth. Lesions outwith the oral

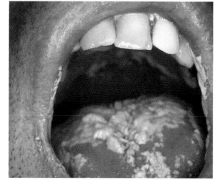

Fig. 4 **Severe oral thrush.**

cavity are common, mostly caused by dribbling of infected saliva. Such extraoral manifestations do not occur with hand, foot and mouth disease or aphthous ulcers.

- *Herpes zoster* ('shingles') may cause unilateral intraoral lesions in maxillary or mandibular shingles.
- *Rubella* may cause a mild pharyngitis, possibly with tonsillar exudates.

Sore throats caused by other conditions

Other conditions causing sore throats include *candida* ('thrush') which comprises patches of creamy white exudates that are easily pushed away leaving a reddened but non-bleeding area. The surrounding mucous membranes are inflamed. If thrush is severe (Fig. 4), always suspect HIV infection. *Kawasaki's syndrome* presents in children usually less than 2 years of age, and comprises fever with dryness and redness of the lips, tongue and oropharynx. A rash occurs later, and there is nail fold peeling, lymph node enlargement and non-pitting oedema of the hands and feet. *Stevens–Johnson syndrome* comprises erythema multiforme (p. 122) with painful oral ulcerations, and inflammation of conjunctiva and genital mucous membranes.

THE THYROID

The normal thyroid is closely affixed to the trachea and is not usually visible unless enlarged. However, by observing the patient swallowing, the thyroid may be brought into view and/or palpated. Swallowing elevates the thyroid cartilage and thus the attached thyroid gland. The thyroid isthmus connecting the two lobes lies just below the cricoid cartilage with the lobes lying along the lower half of the lateral margin of the thyroid cartilage (Fig. 5).

Correct positioning of the patient is important when examining the thyroid gland. Arrange for the patient to be sitting with the neck slightly extended so that the neck can be examined from the front side and then from the behind (Fig. 6).

Palpation of the thyroid must always be done gently. If the thyroid is enlarged (a goitre; Fig. 7), ascertain whether it is mobile. Unless there is a malignant fixation the thyroid should move along with the thyroid cartilage. Ascertain the consistency of any goitre and whether it contains several nodules (a multinodular goitre) or whether it is diffusely enlarged. Isolated swellings, especially if solitary or hard, may be caused by carcinoma or cysts, but if the hardness is diffuse a 'wooden' Reidel's thyroiditis is likely. If auscultation reveals a systolic murmur (a bruit), an abnormal circulation is present which (unless the bruit is transmitted from the major arteries nearby) is suggestive of an overactive thyroid, as in thyrotoxicosis. In females with slender necks a visible thyroid may be a normal finding.

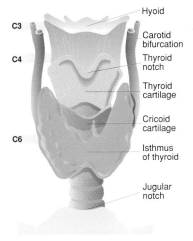

Fig. 5 **The anatomy of the thyroid gland.**

Hyoid
Carotid bifurcation
Thyroid notch
Thyroid cartilage
Cricoid cartilage
Isthmus of thyroid
Jugular notch

C3
C4
C6

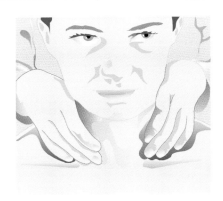

Fig. 6 **Examination of the thyroid gland from behind.**

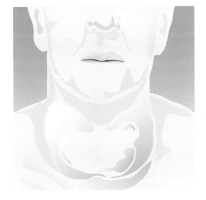

Fig. 7 **Goitre.**

OTHER NECK SIGNS

Branchial cysts
Branchial cysts are congenital malformations usually found in the upper half of the anterior neck. A small dimple may be present on the overlying skin.

Thyroglossal cysts
A persisting fetal thyroglossal duct may give rise to a single cystic midline swelling. Protrusion of the tongue pulls the cyst upwards, as the cyst is part of the duct connected with the tongue.

The parotid gland
The parotid gland lies between the descending ramus of the mandible and the anterior border of the sternomastoid. It is easy to palpate if enlarged. Parotid swelling fills in the crease behind the mandible, unlike enlarged lymph nodes which do not unless there is much associated oedema.

General examination (V) — throat, thyroid and other neck signs

- Most sore throats are viral.
- In most instances it is not possible to differentiate between viral and bacterial sore throat.
- With submandibular cellulitis (Ludwig's angina) there is a danger of respiratory obstruction.
- Diphtheria may result in unexpected respiratory obstruction.
- The thyroid is not normally visible unless enlarged.

GENERAL EXAMINATION (VI)—Lymph Nodes

THE LYMPH NODES

Lymph node examination is usefully dealt with under general examination, although each group of nodes tends to be examined as part of the relevant organs or system.

Neck lymph nodes

The neck is examined systematically for enlarged lymph nodes and other abnormalities, with palpation of the anterior and posterior triangles in turn. The anterior triangle is bordered by the sternomastoid laterally, the mandible superiorly and the midline anteriorly. The posterior triangle is bordered by the sternomastoid anteriorly, the trapezius posteriorly and the clavicle inferiorly.

The lymph nodes of the head and neck can be divided into various groups (Fig. 1a). Examine with the fingers relaxed and use a gentle 'minirotatory' movement. The tonsillar nodes lie just internal to the angle of the jaw and are often enlarged in patients who have acute throat infections. The scalenus anterior group of nodes lie on the first rib behind and just below the medial end of the clavicle, and these have to be palpated through the clavicular head of the sternomastoid. This is best achieved by asking the patient to let his/her head flop forwards and examining from behind.

Lymph nodes other than in the neck

The lymph nodes to be examined (Fig. 1b) are the epitrochlear, the axillary, the inguinal (including the femoral triangle). The epitrochlear and axillary nodes can be examined at the same time. To examine the right axilla rest the patient's right forearm along your right forearm, enabling you to abduct the patient's arm 15–25°. The fingers of your right hand can then feel for the epitrochlear node, while the fingers of your left hand can feel the anterior and medial wall of the patient's axilla. It is best to cup the fingers at the top of the axilla and to slide them down the medial wall of the axilla so that the enlarged nodes can be felt slipping upwards as your fingertips descend (Fig. 2). Then palpate the posterior wall of the axilla which is best examined from behind the patient. Repeat the above process to examine the left axilla, this time supporting the patient's left forearm on your left forearm.

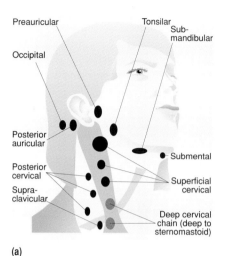

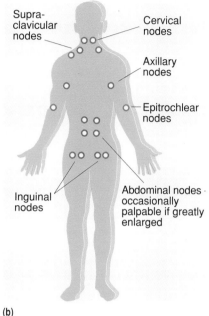

(a)

Fig. 1 **Lymph node examination** (**a**) Lymph nodes of the anterior and posterior triangles of the neck. (**b**) Lymph nodes other than in the neck to be palpated.

(b)

The inguinal lymph nodes are best examined as part of the abdominal examination (see p. 52).

If there is any doubt about the existence of small subcutaneous swellings, including lymph nodes, always ask the patient to feel and confirm their existence. Patients are better than any doctor at feeling their own superficial swellings. A normal lymph node will usually be only

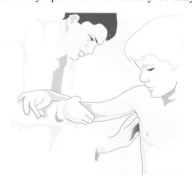

Fig. 2 **Examination of axillary lymph nodes.**

just palpable, small, smooth, non-tender, mobile and non-fluctuant.

Lymph node pathologies

Lymph nodes which are the site of acute bacterial infections may be enlarged, palpable and usually smooth, tender, fluctuant, hot and covered by reddened skin, especially if abscess formation has occurred. There may be reddened lymph channels draining into the node from a peripheral septic focus (lymphangitis). A rapid onset of generalized symmetrical lymph node enlargement tends to be of infective origin. Tuberculous lymph nodes are enlarged but are not usually warm or inflamed, hence their name cold abscesses. Malignant lymph nodes may be enlarged, palpable and smooth, although they may be also craggy, hard, non-tender and non-fluctuant. They may be fixed to surrounding tissues or may become matted together.

General examination (VI)—lymph nodes

- Normal lymph nodes are barely palpable, small, non-tender, mobile and non-fluctuant.
- Bacterially infected lymph nodes may be enlarged, palpable, tender, hot, possibly fluctuant, and covered by reddened skin.
- Malignant lymph nodes may be enlarged, and are usually smooth but may be craggy. They are usually hard, non-tender and non-fluctuant.

SYSTEMS

BASIC PRINCIPLES

STRUCTURE AND FUNCTION

The function of the cardiovascular system is to distribute blood to the tissues and to the lungs for oxygenation. To achieve this, a two-sided pump (the heart), a distribution system (the arteries) and return system (the veins) are required (Fig. 1). It is important to realize that cardiac systole (contraction) or diastole (relaxation) refers to *ventricular* systole or diastole. Both atria contract together (during ventricular diastole) and, later, both ventricles contract together during ventricular systole. When both ventricles are contracting, both atria are relaxing and vice versa.

Venous blood returns to the right atrium via the superior and inferior vena cavae. Blood then flows (with the assistance of atrial systole) through the tricuspid valve into the right ventricle during ventricular diastole. At the start of ventricular systole, the tricuspid valve shuts and the venous blood derived from the tissues is ejected into the lungs, passing through the pulmonary valve into the pulmonary arteries.

After passing through the lungs, the now oxygenated blood returns to the left atrium via the pulmonary veins. During ventricular diastole the blood passes from the left atrium through the mitral valve into the left ventricle. During ventricular systole the mitral valve shuts and blood is ejected through the aortic valve into the aorta and, thence, to the tissues of the body.

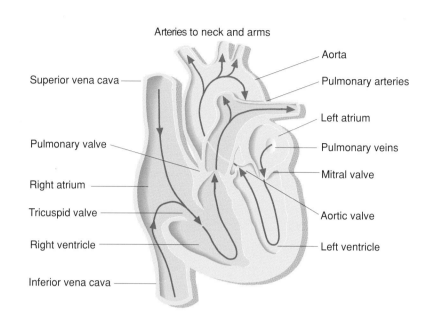

Fig.1 **Blood flow through the normal heart.** Arterial blood travels from the heart, whereas venous blood travels to the heart. This explains the seemingly paradoxical fact that the pulmonary veins contain oxygenated blood and the pulmonary arteries contain deoxygenated blood.

HEART MURMURS

Heart murmurs are smooth (rather than abrupt) musical-like sounds caused by turbulent blood flow. They occur at discrete, usually regular, points in the cardiac cycle. Heart murmur production is caused by abnormal blood flow usually through blood vessels or valves. Exercise or severe anaemia (by increasing blood flow) may cause murmurs to appear, whereas polycythaemia (by thickening the blood) may cause murmurs to disappear.

Blood vessels and valves may become either narrowed or enlarged. Heart valves may become incompetent or stenosed (in plain English leaky or narrowed). Murmurs are transmitted in the direction of abnormal blood flow.

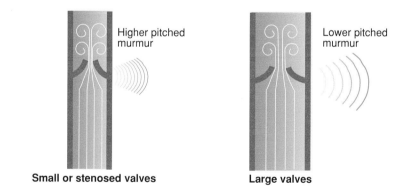

Fig.2 **The pitch of a heart murmur is related to valve size and pressure gradient.**

Just as small musical instruments produce high-pitched sounds, small heart valves (the aortic and pulmonary valves) produce high-pitched murmurs. In contrast, larger valves (the mitral and tricuspid valves) produce lower pitched murmurs (Fig. 2) just as large musical instruments produce low-pitched sounds. If the aortic or pulmonary valve are stenosed or have extra blood flowing through them, the murmurs produce crescendo and diminuendo during systole, leading to the so-called diamond-shaped ejection systolic murmurs (p.28).

EXAMINATION

Both the stethoscope diaphragm and the bell are used to listen to the heart. The stethoscope diaphragm is very tight, whereas the bell uses the patient's skin, which is usually slack. As the stethoscope's purpose is to resonate in sympathy with similarly pitched sounds the diaphragm is used to detect high-pitched murmurs. The bell is used to detect low-pitched murmurs.

Students often find difficulty in identifying whether murmurs or added sounds are in systole or diastole. The traditional advice is to time the murmur by palpating the carotid artery, the impulse of which, in practice, coincides with the first heart sound. This is a difficult skill to master, but if the patient has a palpable apex beat, a systolic event will be heard when the stethoscope is seen or felt to be lifting. A diastolic event will be heard when the stethoscope bell is returning. As it happens, the most sensitive form of auscultation would be to place your ear on the patient's chest wall, but this is not recommended!

GRADING

Heart murmurs are graded clinically into five grades:

- *Grade 1* is just audible with a good stethoscope in a quiet room.
- *Grade 2* is quiet but readily audible with a stethoscope.
- *Grade 3* is easily heard with a stethoscope.
- *Grade 4* is loud and obvious.
- *Grade 5* is very loud, heard not only over the precordium but elsewhere in the body.

'Innocent' murmurs (those not associated with structural abnormalities of the heart or with abnormal blood turbulence) are always systolic (conversely, diastolic murmurs are usually significant). They are always less than Grade 3 and unassociated with cardiac abnormalities

on clinical examination, chest X-ray and electrocardiogram.

Palpable murmurs (thrills) are always pathological and are usually caused by stenosed or incompetent valves, or septal defects.

Changing or newly developed murmurs are caused by acute valvular dysfunction or by increases in blood flow and, if associated with febrile illness, should always suggest infective endocarditis in which the heart valves develop vegetations. Severe endocarditis may cause valve rupture, but 'mild' endocarditis causes prolonged fever with signs including splinter haemorrhages, clubbing and splenomegaly.

HEART SOUNDS

First and second

Heart sounds are abrupt brief sounds. The first heart sounds (Fig. 3) are caused by the closure of mitral and tricuspid valves. The second heart sounds are caused by closure of the aortic and pulmonary valves. Both are normal findings. The first and second heart sounds are predominantly created by the left-sided valves (because higher pressure gradients in the left heart cause more abrupt valve closure). The relevant heart sounds are loud if the causative valve shuts more quickly or forcibly than normal (e.g. because of hypertension). In atrial fibrillation or complete heart block the first heart sounds may vary because ventricular systole may occur when the mitral valve is in varying positions.

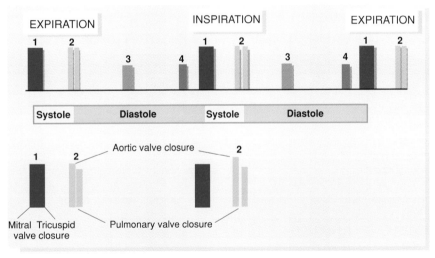

Fig. 3 **The heart sounds as recorded in shorthand notation.**

Third and fourth

The third and fourth heart sounds (Fig. 3) are usually, but not always, abnormal findings. A third heart sound is associated with rapid ventricular filling in ventricular diastole, whereas a fourth heart sound is associated with the end of atrial emptying in ventricular diastole. Both left and right ventricles can give rise to third and fourth heart sounds, but, because of the higher pressure involved, the left ventricular sounds are louder. Either a third or a fourth heart sound may give rise to a triple or a 'gallop' rhythm, and if both third and fourth heart sounds are audible, a quadruple 'summation gallop' rhythm results. Because fourth heart sounds are associated with atrial contraction, it is impossible to have a fourth heart sound in the presence of atrial fibrillation.

A (left ventricular) third heart sound may be found in severe hypertension, myocardial infarction (which usually

affects the left side of the heart), left heart failure or mitral incompetence. A third heart sound can be normal in athletes who have slow pulse rates, in febrile conditions and during pregnancy. In mitral incompetence, blood regurgitates into the left atrium during ventricular systole and, during ventricular diastole, the unusual amount of blood in the left atrium rapidly re-enters the left ventricle thereby causing a third heart sound. A right ventricular third heart sound may occur in massive pulmonary embolism, in tricuspid incompetence or in cor pulmonale.

Other heart sounds

Other added sounds include clicks (very brief sounds notably occurring in mitral valve prolapse) and snaps (notably in

mitral stenosis). These are detailed later. Prosthetic heart valves cause added clicks.

Basic principles

- Systole or diastole refers to ventricular systole or diastole.
- The pitch of heart murmurs is related to valve size and pressure gradient across the valve.
- First and second heart sounds are normal findings .
- Third and fourth sounds are usually abnormal findings.

MAJOR SYMPTOMS OF CARDIOVASCULAR DISEASE

There are four major symptoms of cardiac dysfunction:

- chest pain
- palpitations
- shortness of breath
- peripheral tissue swelling (oedema).

Cough and haemoptysis may also be symptoms of cardiovascular disease: these are discussed in the section on the respiratory system.

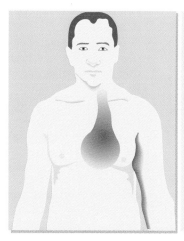

Sites of pain

○ Central chest pain:
   band-like
   constricting

○ Radiating to:
   shoulder
   arm
   neck

○ Worse on exertion
   and in the cold

○ Relieved by resting

Fig.1 **Anginal pain.**

CHEST PAIN

Chest pain of cardiac origin may be caused by angina, myocardial infarction, aortic dissection or pericarditis.

Angina

The pain of angina (Fig.1) occurs when the heart muscle is starved of oxygen (usually caused by narrowing of the coronary arteries, Fig. 2). This causes accumulation of anaerobically generated metabolites.

Angina pain is:

- tight
- bandlike
- crushing
- felt across the front of the chest
- classically brought on by exertion and relieved within 5 minutes of rest or administration of trinitrin.

Pain may radiate to the jaw, to the back, or down into one or both arms. It may be worsened by extra circulatory burdens such as a heavy meal or cold weather. Hypotension of any cause may precipitate angina by causing inadequate perfusion of the coronary arteries. If pain lasts for longer that about 20 minutes, myocardial infarction should be strongly suspected. Angina does not cause brief stabs of pain.

There are several variants of angina:

- **Decubitus angina** (angina on lying down flat) is usually only experienced when there is severe myocardial ischaemia.
- **Nocturnal angina** awakens the patient at night.
- **Acute coronary insufficiency** is a severe attack of angina suggesting myocardial infarction, but without any investigatory confirmation of infarction.
- **Unstable angina** is angina that has become significantly worse within the previous 4 weeks or so. It may have started then or progressed from

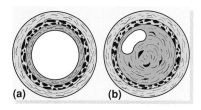

Fig.2 **Narrowing of coronary arteries.**
(a) Normal coronary artery.
(b) Arterial narrowing.

previously stable angina. Angina at rest, crescendo angina, or angina unrelieved by trinitrin usually develops.
- **Crescendo angina** comprises anginal attacks which, over a short period of time, have become progressively more frequent or severe. It is usually a pre-infarctive condition.

Myocardial infarction

Myocardial infarction pain is usually caused by inadequate oxygenation of heart muscle such that there is necrosis. There may have been a history of preceding angina. The pain of myocardial infarction is usually:

- of sudden onset
- severe
- often described as heavy and tight ('vice-like')
- associated with sweating.

Although pain may radiate in the same distribution as angina, the pain of myocardial infarction is not transient and is not relieved by rest or trinitrin. Other less specific symptoms may include shortness of breath (especially if there is left ventricular failure), faintness and collapse. On occasion, symptoms of myocardial infarction may be atypical or vague (e.g.

suggesting indigestion), and sometimes myocardial infarction may be painless.

Aortic dissection

Dissection occurs when there is a tear in the innermost layer of an arterial wall. Blood then dissects the vessel wall into two layers which interfere with the normal blood flow (unless the dissection breaks back into the main lumen).

The pain of aortic dissecting aneurysms is severe and tearing in nature. The pain is situated in the chest if there is dissection of the ascending and/or descending aorta, or in the abdomen if there is dissection of the abdominal aorta. There may be symptoms and signs in the organs supplied by the aortic branches which have been stripped off.

Pericarditis

The pain of pericarditis is typically sharp, of sudden onset and may be indistinguishable or indeed coexistent with that of myocardial infarction. The pain may be affected by breathing and may persist for several days. Recurrent bouts may occur. Pericarditis is often presumed to have a viral aetiology, and in these circumstances there may be a history of a preceding flu-like illness.

PALPITATIONS

Palpitations are whatever the patient thinks they are. Therefore, always define exactly what it is that the patient is experiencing (Table 1). It is sometimes helpful to get the patient to tap out with a finger what he notices when he/she has palpitations.

Table 1 **Possible causes of a patient's complaint of 'palpitations'**

- Abnormal awareness of a normal heart beat or rate
- Ectopic beats experienced as sudden forceful 'thumps' or the awareness of the compensatory pause after ectopic beats
- Awareness of a regular fast heart rate (atrial flutter or tachycardias of various causations)
- Awareness of an irregular fast heart rate (atrial fibrillation — usually noticed only when of recent occurrence)
- Awareness of a slow heart rate

Anxious patients may be aware of their (normal) heart beat.

Isolated forceful beats ('thumps in my chest') are usually caused by ectopic beats either of atrial or ventricular origin. The patient either notices the 'extra thump' of the next beat or the compensatory pause that follows: 'my heart missed a beat'.

A rapid and regular heart beat may occur in:

- atrial flutter
- paroxysmal supraventricular tachycardia
- ventricular tachycardia.

In **atrial flutter**, the atria are driven by an ectopic atrial pacemaker at a rate of about 330 per minute, and the atrioventricular node can only transmit a proportion of these beats (Fig. 3). Patients usually notice the change in heart rate when the proportion of beats is doubled or halved. In **paroxysmal supraventricular** tachycardia, the routine pacemaking function of the sinoatrial node is taken over by a rapidly discharging focus in the atria or atrioventricular node. The patient notices a sudden onset of a fast heart rate of about 150 per minute. It is usually a benign, although alarming, condition affecting young people. **Ventricular tachycardia** involves a rapidly discharging ectopic

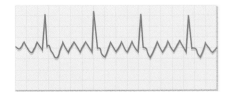

Fig. 3 **Atrial flutter with typical saw-tooth P waves and a regular ventricular response.**

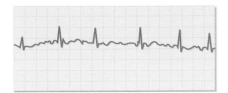

Fig. 4 **Atrial fibrillation.**

pacemaker in the ventricles which takes over as pacemaker, producing a heart rate of about 130–200 beats per minute.

A rapid *irregular* pulse may occur in **atrial fibrillation** (Fig. 4). In this condition the atria contract chaotically providing the atrioventricular node with about 600 totally irregular impulses a minute: only a proportion of these impulses survive to initiate a ventricular contraction. The patient may note a fast irregular fluttering in the chest. Unlike the fluttering due to frequent ectopic beats, there are no following compensatory pauses.

Slow pulse rates may be noticed by the patient usually because of the more forceful ventricular contractions which occur consequent to the bradycardia-induced extra ventricular filling. A slow heart rate may be found in very fit patients, in hypothyroid patients, in patients on digoxin or β blockers, or in complete heart block.

SHORTNESS OF BREATH

Cardiac shortness of breath is usually caused by excessive pressure or accumulation of blood in the lungs, caused by failure of the left heart to deal with the oxygenated blood returning from the lungs in the pulmonary veins. Because of this, patients feel they need to breath more, but there is no sensation of airways blockage unless there is gross pulmonary oedema.

Other forms of shortness of breath (dyspnoea) which are usually of cardiac origin (thus representing heart failure) include:

- **Orthopnoea.** This is dyspnoea which develops when the patient lies down flat and which is relieved by sitting up.
- **Paroxysmal nocturnal dyspnoea.** Classically, the patient is awoken with severe shortness of breath and classically has to stand or sit up with legs dependent for several minutes before relief is obtained. The mechanism is similar to that of orthopnoea, but symptoms tend to be more severe as the decompensation is more severe as the patient has to be awoken.
- **Acute pulmonary oedema.** There is usually marked shortness of breath with sweating and cyanosis. Frothy sputum may be produced, which may be pink due to rupture of congested blood vessels.

With shortness of breath (or angina), it is useful to describe an individual patient's limitations in regard to their particular life situation. Relevant questions would thus include the patient's exercise tolerance, the distance that can be walked on the level, the number of flights of stairs that can be mounted, how many flights of stairs can be managed, and whether the patient can manage routine day-to-day living tasks.

SOFT TISSUE SWELLING DUE TO OEDEMA

There are two main characteristics of cardiovascular oedema. First, it is dependent, being most apparent in the lowermost part of the body, such as in the ankles in ambulant patients and in the sacral area in those confined to bed. Second, pressure applied with a single finger for several seconds results in transient pitting (Fig. 5). The commonest cause of cardiovascular oedema is right-sided heart failure. Other causes include vascular lesions — varicose veins, inferior vena caval obstruction, or intrapelvic pressure on veins due to neoplasm or pregnancy. Prolonged immobility can cause dependent oedema.

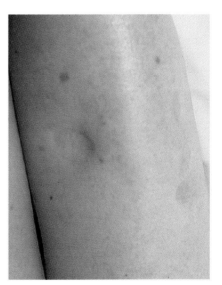

Fig. 5 **Pitting oedema.**

Major symptoms of cardiovascular disease

- Any change in angina is likely to be significant.
- Always define in medical terms what the patient means by palpitations.
- Define the pattern of shortness of breath.
- Always ascertain the limitations that the symptoms impose onto the patient.

GENERAL EXAMINATION AND THE PULSE

GENERAL EXAMINATION

A general assessment of the cardiovascular system (Table 1) should take into account the patient's age and sex. It is also essential to determine if the patient:

- is in pain
- is experiencing shortness of breath
- has a cough
- is pale or cyanosed
- has evidence of fluid retention
- has the 'mitral' facial appearance (dilated cyanotic vessels over the cheek bones)
- has chest operation scars
- has tar-stained fingers
- has signs of hyperlipidaemia (including fat deposits in the skin).

The first part of the patient that a doctor usually comes into contact with is the hands, and their temperature and colour should be noted. Peripheral cyanosis in the absence of central cyanosis might suggest inadequacy of peripheral circulation, as would coldness of the peripheries. Clubbing, in the presence of heart disease, suggests either cyanotic congenital heart disease or infective endocarditis. Splinter haemorrhages suggest infective endocarditis.

Table 1 **Review of cardiovascular examination**

- Assess the whole circumstances surrounding the patient's presentation
- Assess the patient's general condition looking specially for signs of hyperlipidaemia such as xanthelasma
- Assess the patient's hands
- Assess the characteristics of the radial pulses and symmetry of radial pulse
- Assess other pulses if appropriate
- Take the blood pressure
- Assess the jugular venous pressure
- Inspect the chest wall
- Palpate the precordium
- Auscultate, assessing the heart sounds, added sounds, and murmurs
- Look for signs of right or left-sided heart failure

THE PULSE

The pulse impulse as felt in the arteries is the pressure wave initiated by ventricular systole and usually, but not always, reflects blood flow and cardiac output. Traditionally, the pulse is assessed by gently compressing the radial artery against the lower end of the radius, using the pulps of the index and middle fingers. Palpation of the carotid pulse may give much more information about the pulse character.

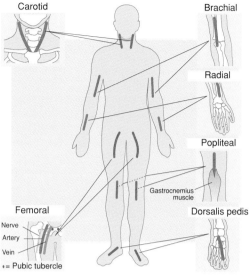

Fig. 1 **The routinely palpated pulses.**

When palpating the pulse, pay particular attention to five major characteristics:

- rate
- rhythm
- volume
- character
- state of the vessel wall.

At some stage of the examination, the rest of the peripheral pulses (Fig. 1) should be felt. When the radial pulse is being palpated it is useful to compare the two sides.

RATE

A fast pulse, about 100–150 beats per minute, may occur in:

- exercise
- heart failure
- fever
- thyrotoxicosis
- severe anaemia
- acute haemorrhage
- ectopic pacemakers(s) either in the atria or ventricles.

Ectopic pacemakers occur in such conditions as atrial flutter, paroxysmal supraventricular tachycardia, ventricular tachycardia and multiple individual ectopic beats (either atrial or ventricular). A slow pulse, about 50 beats per minute or less, may be caused by:

- extreme fitness
- hypothyroidism
- complete heart block
- digitalis overdosage
- β-blocker therapy.

RHYTHM

The pulse rhythm may be regular or irregular. If the pulse is irregular, the apex beat rate should be ascertained and compared with the pulse rate at the wrist. A slower pulse at the wrist than at the apex of the heart constitutes a pulse deficit. This means that not all ventricular contractions are forceful enough to produce a detectable peripheral impulse. It is important to detect a pulse deficit as a normal peripheral pulse rate may conceal an inefficient fast heart rate. A pulse deficit may be found in atrial fibrillation, 'extra' heart beats (extrasystoles) and in heart block. In atrial fibrillation the pulse rate is irregular and, unlike the pulse in atrial or ventricular ectopics (in which there are predictable compensatory pauses after each ectopic beat), the timing and force of the following pulse is unpredictable.

VOLUME

The term 'pulse volume' refers to movement of the palpating finger and not necessarily to the volume of blood flowing.

A small volume pulse is found in blood flow obstruction, the causes of which include:

- narrowing of the heart valves (stenosis)
- a low blood volume (as in gastrointestinal haemorrhage or dehydration)
- post-heart-attack (myocardial infarction) state
- any state in which the heart cannot contract efficiently
- generalized or localized peripheral circulatory inadequacy for any reason
- in shock states (p. 138).

VESSEL WALL

Clinical assessment of arterial wall hardening (previously thought to reflect arteriosclerosis) is liable to error.

PULSE CHARACTER (Fig. 2)

Deep inspiration normally increases the pulse rate . Inspiration increases the chest volume, thus the lungs can contain more blood than otherwise. This leads to a reduced return of blood to the left side of the heart, which then speeds up to compensate for the reduced blood volume presented to it. If marked, this will constitute sinus arrhythmia (Fig. 2), which is a cyclical variation in the pulse rate, speeding up during inspiration and slowing down during expiration. It is a common finding in young people.

The ability to appreciate a normal pulse character can only be gained from experience.

Collapsing pulse

A collapsing pulse is caused by a large difference between the systolic and diastolic blood pressure. A collapsing pulse is thus best ascertained by taking the blood pressure and finding a wide pulse pressure. However, it is traditionally appreciated by raising the arm while monitoring the pulse, and feeling a forceful jerk of brief duration with several fingers. Sometimes this wide pulse pressure imparts a distinctive jerking movement of the neck structures because of the marked carotid artery pulsation. In addition, the arterial capillaries may exhibit visible pulsation. This is best seen if the nails are gently compressed against the nailbed when the arm is elevated. The causes of a collapsing pulse include:

- aortic incompetence
- high output cardiac states such as found in thyrotoxicosis
- severe anaemia
- arteriovenous communications
- high fevers
- complete heart block.

Pulsus paradoxus

Pulsus paradoxus is a diminution in pulse volume during inspiration which may occur with pericardial effusions, constrictive pericarditis or in serious bronchoconstriction. The blood pressure also falls during inspiration.

Plateau pulse

A plateau pulse is a sustained but small volume pulse which is found in aortic stenosis.

Pulsus alternans

Pulsus alternans is an alternation of normal and small volume pulses, representing failure of the left ventricle to provide the normal impulse with each contraction. When the blood pressure is taken, the pulse rate suddenly doubles as the sphygmomanometer mercury falls (see p. 25). There are in effect two different systolic blood pressures.

Pulsus bisferiens

Pulsus bisferiens is a double impulse which is found in combined aortic stenosis and incompetence.

EXAMINATION OF THE CAROTID ARTERIES

In patients with cerebrovascular symptoms it is important to evaluate the carotid arteries, as neurosurgical intervention may be possible. A murmur or a thrill not transmitted from the heart (or absent pulsation) may be indicative of impaired or absent blood flow. Only palpate the carotid arteries one at a time, and if there is no pulsation in the first ensure you do not occlude the second on palpation.

PERIPHERAL PERFUSION

If there is poor peripheral perfusion, the hands and feet may be cyanosed (because of increased extraction of oxygen from the blood associated with the slower circulation). The temperature of extremities may be diminished as the slowly circulating blood cannot supply heat to the peripheries fast enough. Normally, blanching of the skin caused by digital pressure only lasts for a few seconds, but in the presence of peripheral circulatory failure the blanching time is prolonged. The blood pressure may be low (if it can be measured) in arteries which supply the area involved.

Acute limb ischaemia

In acute limb ischaemia there may be a history suggesting a source for an occluding embolism, a predisposing hyperviscosity state of the blood or severe peripheral vascular disease. The limb affected is typically:

- painful
- pale
- pale on elevation, with dusky pink or redness on subsequent dependency
- cold
- pulseless.

Later ulceration and gangrene may develop (Fig. 3).

Chronic limb ischaemia

In chronic limb ischaemia, the history ranges from muscle pain on exercise, relieved by rest (claudication), in the calf, thigh, or buttock to persistent pain or non-healing ulcers and gangrene. Relevant pulses will be diminished or absent.

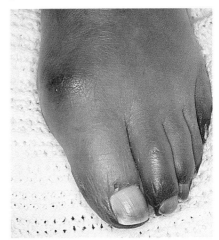

Fig. 3 **Gangrene.**

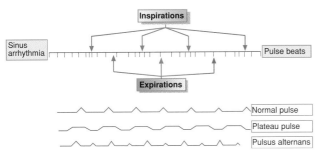

Fig. 2 **The pulse character.**

General examination and the pulse

- If a peripheral pulse is reduced, always check for bruits.
- Blood pressure measurement often assists in the assessment of pulse abnormalities of cardiac origin.
- Always palpate carotid arteries gently: if the non-palpated artery is thrombosed as cerebral blood flow could be compromised.
- Acute circulatory blockage may be reversible.

THE NECK VEINS AND BLOOD PRESSURE MEASUREMENT

THE NECK VEINS

The internal jugular veins drain directly (without valves or other obstructions) into the right atrium, and significant sustained elevations indicate that the right heart cannot cope adequately with the returning venous blood. In examination of the jugular veins the patient should be at 45° to the horizontal (Fig.1).

Venous impulses in the neck (unlike the arterial impulses):

- cannot usually be palpated (except in severe tricuspid incompetence)
- are relatively easily occluded (except in severe tricuspid incompetence)
- are made more prominent if the patient lies flat
- have two or more flickerings with each impulse.

With normal venous pressure the top of the blood column in the internal jugular vein should not be visible more than 4 cm above the manubriosternal angle (Fig. 1) and falls on inspiration as the chest capacity is expanded (as if blood is being sucked into the chest).

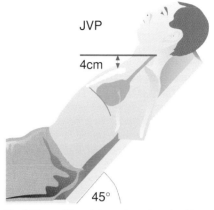

Fig. 1 **The position of the patient when checking jugular venous pressure.**

The internal jugular vein should be used to assess the jugular venous pressure, but often the external jugular is used (Fig. 2). In this case, always ensure that the external jugular pressure is not (falsely) elevated by kinking as it passes through the cervical fascia. Turning the head should relieve the kinking and cause the pressure to fall.

Jugular venous pressure waves (Fig. 3)
The **a wave** represents atrial systole if the atria are contracting in a controlled fashion (in atrial fibrillation the a waves will be absent). The a wave is followed by the x descent. The **c wave** is simultaneous with carotid pulsation and is not normally discernable. The **v wave** represents the building up of venous blood returning to the almost full right atrium which occurs in late ventricular systole.

Prominent a waves. These occur in severe pulmonary stenosis or tricuspid stenosis. There is blockage of blood flow through the right side of the heart, and contraction of the right atrium causes the extra 'held up' blood to be forced back into the jugular veins.

Cannon waves. These are very large a waves which occur in conditions when the atria contract and the atrioventricular valves are shut (in atrioventricular dissociation states) as may occur when there is complete block of transmission of electrical impulses from atria to ventricles (complete heart block). In such circumstances the first heart sound often has a varying intensity. Cannon waves occasionally occur in ventricular tachycardia. They cannot be found in uncomplicated atrial fibrillation, as the cannoning of the a waves depends on coordinated atrial contraction

Very large v waves. These occur in tricuspid incompetence because the

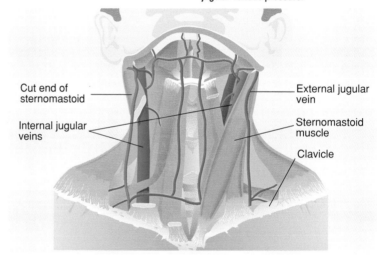

Fig. 2 **The anatomical situation of the juglar veins.**

Cut end of sternomastoid

Internal jugular veins

External jugular vein

Sternomastoid muscle

Clavicle

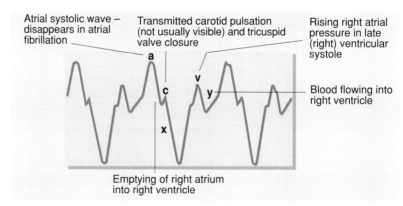

Atrial systolic wave – disappears in atrial fibrillation

Transmitted carotid pulsation (not usually visible) and tricuspid valve closure

Rising right atrial pressure in late (right) ventricular systole

Blood flowing into right ventricle

Emptying of right atrium into right ventricle

Fig. 3 **The jugular venous pressure waves.**

incompetent tricuspid valve allows ventricular blood to rush up into the right atrium and jugular veins.

Marked y descents. These indicate a diastolic collapse of jugular venous pressure and may occur when the heart is imprisoned by its enclosing structures in constrictive pericarditis or cardiac tamponade. Ventricular systole can empty the right ventricle rapidly to evacuate the small amount of blood it had been able to

accommodate and then, during ventricular diastole, the right ventricle fills rapidly, thus precipitously emptying the veins near to the heart. If the jugular venous pressure is very high (as it might well be) this collapse will not be visible.

Causes of a raised jugular venous pressure

Causes of raised jugular venous pressure include the following:

- **Superior mediastinal obstruction** by large space-occupying lesions will yield a raised but non-pulsatile jugular venous pressure.
- **Right heart failure** in which the right side of the heart cannot cope with the returning venous blood causes a backup of blood in jugular veins. A raised jugular venous pressure increases the filling pressure on the heart, which may stimulate a failing heart.
- **Slow heart rates** may delay the processing of returning venous blood, thereby raising the venous pressure.
- **Tricuspid incompetence** allows excessive ventricular blood to be regurgitated into the right atrium and thereby into the jugular veins, causing a raised jugular venous pressure.
- **Restriction of heart movement** by pericardium or pericardial fluid (constrictive pericarditis and cardiac tamponade respectively) obstructs venous return and, thus, the venous pressure may rise.
- **Hyperdynamic circulation** may result in excessive venous return and a raised venous pressure. This may be found in thyrotoxicosis, high fevers and in pregnancy.
- **General increased blood volume** may occur in excessive intravenous fluid administration or in kidney failure if fluid intake is not restricted, leading to increased jugular venous pressure.

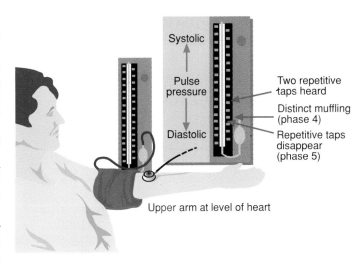

Upper arm at level of heart

Fig. 4 **Measurement of blood pressure.**

MEASUREMENT OF BLOOD PRESSURE

The blood pressure is an important indication of the 'circulatory force' that is generated by the heart. A high blood pressure (hypertension) requires extra work by the heart and puts more stress on the arteries which may become damaged. A low blood pressure (hypotension) implies either a low 'circulating force' generated by the heart, a low blood volume, excessive vasodilation (leading to relative hypovolaemia) or circulatory blockage to the relevant part of the body. Particularly if there is a low blood volume, the blood pressure as taken when the patient is lying flat may fall upon sitting upright or on standing.

A sphygmomanometer is used to measure the blood pressure. It is important that the sphygmomanometer is upright and this means *not* resting it upon the bed. The systolic pressure is the higher pressure in the arteries (during ventricular systole) and the diastolic pressure is the lower pressure (when the ventricles are in diastole).

Always explain to the patient what you are about to do. The arm used for measurement should be horizontal at the level of the midsternum (Fig. 4). Pregnant patients should lie on their side or sit (to avoid problems caused by the uterus interfering with blood flow).

Applying the cuff

Apply the uninflated cuff firmly yet comfortably to the upper arm with the tubing exiting superiorly (so that it does not interfere with the auscultating stethosope) with the bladder over the brachial artery. The bladder should surround at least 80% of arm circumference to give accurate readings. Large arms may require an extra large cuff and bladder.

Estimating the systolic pressure by palpation

Gradually inflate the cuff until it becomes impossible to palpate the radial arterial pulsation: this is the approximate systolic pressure. This step is very important because on auscultation there may be a silent gap between the higher 'true' systolic sound and a lower 'apparent' systolic sound. A falsely low systolic pressure may be recorded unless palpation has identified the true level of the systolic blood pressure. In pregnant or shocked patients, one may have to rely upon palpation alone because the systolic pressure may be difficult to measure accurately by auscultation.

Measuring the systolic and diastolic pressure using auscultation

Gently press the stethoscope over the brachial artery in the antecubital fossa and inflate the cuff to just above the palpated systolic pressure, and then reduce the cuff pressure by a 1 mm per second. The systolic pressure is the point at which at least two repetitive clear 'taps' are heard. Continue reducing the pressure slowly and a distinct muffling of the 'tapping' sounds occurs ('phase four'). Continue the pressure reduction and the diastolic pressure is the point at which repetitive 'taps' disappear ('phase five'). Occasionally 'tapping' persists until the sphygmomanometer is recording zero: in

such circumstances utilize phase four muffling. In pregnant patients, phase four is more reliable. Always record which phase was used for the diastolic recording.

Measure the systolic and diastolic pressures twice to the nearest 2 mm of mercury (although such precision is optimistic). If the two sets of readings do not agree closely, repeat the recordings after a period of resting the patient.

The blood pressures in hypertensive patients should be measured in both arms. If there is a systolic difference of 20 mm or more, or a diastolic difference of 10 mm or more, the pressures should be ascertained for both arms simultaneously. If patients are taking antihypertensive therapy, it is more relevant to measure the blood pressure before a dose to ascertain what the worst pressure is.

A normal systolic pressure is usually taken to be 100–140 mm of mercury, and a normal diastolic 60–90 mm of mercury. Increases in either the systolic or diastolic pressure are associated with increased cardiovascular morbidity and mortality. The difference between systolic and diastolic pressure is the pulse pressure.

The neck veins and blood pressure measurement

- A visible double impulse in the jugular venous pressure does not occur in atrial fibrillation.
- A raised jugular venous pressure in heart failure may be temporarily reduced shortly after diuretic administration.
- Always ascertain the systolic blood pressure by palpation.

CARDIAC EXAMINATION

The technique of cardiac examination can be divided into inspection, palpation, percussion (rarely) and auscultation.

INSPECTION AND PALPATION OF THE HEART

The position and character of the apex beat should be noted. The position of the apex beat is usually taken to be the lowermost and outermost impulse which is easily papable (Fig. 1). It is usually in the fifth intercostal space in the midclavicular line if the patient has a normal shaped chest and is sitting up at 45°. The normal apex beat should just be felt by the finger, rather than moving the finger outwards.

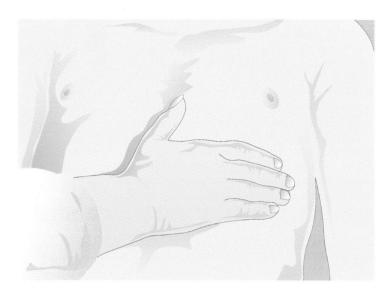

Fig. 1 **Position of the hand in heart palpation.**

PALPATION OF THE APEX BEAT

To palpate the apex beat, the fingers of the examiner's right hand should be lightly pressed onto the chest wall along the axis of the ribs, with the pad of the middle finger more lateral and inferior to the fifth intercostal space in the midaxillary line. The fingers should be gently slid, slowly and medially, towards this position. The pad of the middle finger is used to define the outermost and lowermost impulse, whilst the index finger can ensure that a more apparent impulse is not present above. The ring and little fingers can ensure that a more apparent impulse is not lateral or inferior to a putative apex beat identified by the middle finger.

It might be thought that the apex beat should be an indrawing of the apex as the heart is anchored by the great vessels of the upper mediastinum, but in fact the apex beat is an *outward* movement because the heart rotates anteriorly during ventricular systole.

A thrill (palpable murmur) felt by the palpating hand implies particularly turbulent blood flow. Systolic thrills are usually associated with left-sided pathology because the pressures are higher. Thrills felt over the heart may be caused by aortic stenosis, ventricular septal defects or mitral regurgitation. Occasionally, the diastolic murmur of mitral stenosis is palpable.

Abnormal situation of the apex beat

If the apex beat is displaced either downwards or outwards, this implies chest deformity, mediastinal displacement, pleural or pulmonary pathology, or (statistically more likely) cardiac enlargement.

Abnormal characteristics of the apex beat

Heaves are a lifting of the palpating finger(s). A heaving or thrusting apical impulse is sustained and forceful, and lifts the palpating finger. It may be found (particularly with left ventricular enlargement) either due to hypertrophy of cardiac muscle (often found in pressure overload) or dilatation of the heart (often found in volume overload).

An **impalpable apex beat** may be caused by:

- obesity
- a thick chest wall
- emphysema
- constrictive pericarditis.

Systolic retraction of the apex beat can occur in constrictive pericarditis because rotation of the heart is impaired by the imprisoning pericardium. Systolic retraction may also occur in tricuspid incompetence, as rapid overemptying of the right ventricle means that the left ventricle has a less firm foundation for rotation anteriorly.

A **tapping apex beat** may be caused by 'palpably loud' mitral valve closure, or a left ventricle pushed forward by an enlarged left atrium. It is often the first clinical clue to mitral stenosis.

Lower-sternal heaves may be caused by right ventricular hypertrophy. Sometimes right ventricular hypertrophy occurs secondary to lung disease, and an expanded chest may make it difficult to palpate the right ventricle over the heart. However, it may still be possible to feel a labouring right ventricle from the abdomen by palpating upwards from just below the xiphod process.

Left-sided midsternal heaves may occur in anterior mycardial infarction or when there is a left ventricular aneurysm.

A **forceful apex beat** occurs if the cardiac output is increased as after exercise.

A **poorly localized apex beat** may occur with heart muscle disease, either caused by cardiomyopathy or after myocardial infarction.

PERCUSSION OF THE HEART

Percussion of the heart rarely yields useful information. Sometimes it is possible to percuss a large pericardial effusion or a giant left atrium (in severe long-standing mitral stenosis).

AUSCULTATION

To auscultate the heart, both the diaphragm and the bell of the stethoscope should be used, the former to detect high-pitched murmurs and the latter to detect low-pitched murmurs. The positions of the heart valves and auscultatory areas are

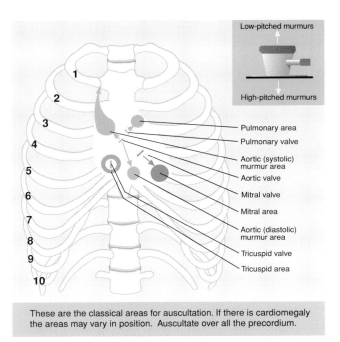

Low-pitched murmurs

High-pitched murmurs

Pulmonary area
Pulmonary valve
Aortic (systolic) murmur area
Aortic valve
Mitral valve
Mitral area
Aortic (diastolic) murmur area
Tricuspid valve
Tricuspid area

These are the classical areas for auscultation. If there is cardiomegaly the areas may vary in position. Auscultate over all the precordium.

Fig. 2 **Position of the heart valves and auscultatory areas.** Note that most murmurs are heard away from the valve that created them (because murmurs are transmitted in the direction of the abnormal blood flow).

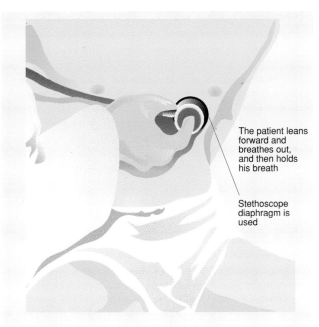

The patient leans forward and breathes out, and then holds his breath

Stethoscope diaphragm is used

Fig. 3 **Auscultation of aortic regurgitation.** Patient leans forward in expiration and the diaphragm of the stethoscope is used.

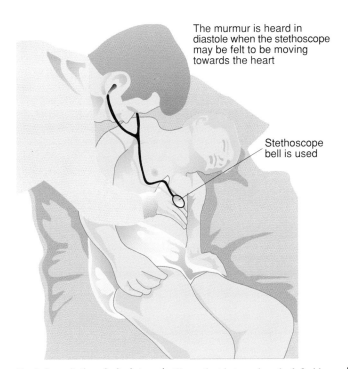

The murmur is heard in diastole when the stethoscope may be felt to be moving towards the heart

Stethoscope bell is used

Fig. 4 **Auscultation of mitral stenosis.** The patient is turned on the left side and the bell of the stethoscope is used.

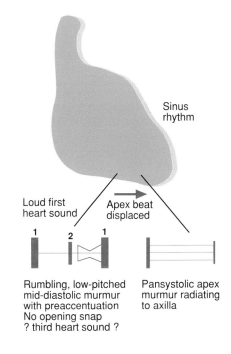

Sinus rhythm

Loud first heart sound

Apex beat displaced

Rumbling, low-pitched mid-diastolic murmur with preaccentuation No opening snap ? third heart sound ?

Pansystolic apex murmur radiating to axilla

Fig. 5 **The recording of heart abnormalities on clinical examination.**

illustrated in Figures 2, 3 and 4. Until clinical recognition of various valve lesions becomes second nature, it is recommended that the first and second sounds are identified and characterized, the third and fourth heart sounds specifically sought, and murmurs (if any) characterized. If there are any abnormalities, the aim should be to describe them accurately in writing (which may be tedious) or preferably by means of a diagram (Fig. 5).

Cardiac examination

- A displaced apex beat may be found in ventricular hypertrophy or dilatation.
- Use the stethoscope diaphragm to listen for high-pitched sounds; the bell for low-pitched sounds.
- The first heart sound occurs at the beginning of ventricular systole which is when the apex beat starts to be palpable.

AUSCULTATORY FINDINGS IN COMMON HEART LESIONS (I)

Rather than concentrate exclusively on general auscultatory findings, it is useful to deal with the findings in various common heart lesions. In most cases it is possible to anticipate auscultatory findings by interpreting findings on inspection and palpation.

The advent of echocardiography has revealed that some clinical diagnoses as described below are occasionally flawed. In particular, signs of aortic sclerosis may be associated with significant stenosis and obstruction of blood flow.

AORTIC STENOSIS

In aortic stenosis (Fig. 1) there should be a plateau pulse and possibly a palpable thrill in the neck. The apex beat in long-standing stenosis will be forceful and possibly displaced, as the left ventricular muscle will have hypertrophied because of the increased work required to force blood through the stenosed valve. As the aortic valve is small and has a high pressure gradient, the murmur will be high pitched and loud, and will be maximal during midsystole when the maximum rate of blood ejection from the left ventricle occurs. The murmur may be transmitted into the neck, occasionally along the clavicles, or sometimes over most of the anterior chest wall.

The aortic second sound is usually soft, as the stenosed valve has only a small distance to travel before it closes: it cannot snap shut. Associated hypertension is uncommon because of impaired ejection of blood.

The differential diagnosis of aortic stenosis includes aortic aneurysms and aortic sclerosis. In aortic sclerosis there is thickening of the aortic valve without stenosis and, thus, there is usually little obstruction to blood flow. Consequently, the pulse volume and character are normal, and there will be no left ventricular hypertrophy. The aortic second sound will be normal because the valve shuts more or less normally.

AORTIC INCOMPETENCE

In aortic incompetence (Fig. 2), the pulse may be collapsing with a wide pulse pressure. With long-standing aortic incompetence the left ventricle will have had a volume overload and the apex beat will be displaced. The murmur is diastolic, high-pitched and best heard using the stethoscope diaphragm whilst listening along the lower left border of the sternum. Leaning the patient forward whilst temporarily holding his breath in full expiration renders the murmur more easily audible by bringing the relevant structures closer to the chest wall. Rarely, regurgitant blood from aortic incompetence will cause a murmur by impinging upon the mitral valve, thus simulating the murmur of mitral stenosis. This is the Austin Flint murmur of aortic incompetence.

MITRAL STENOSIS

Because of the circulatory blockage in severe mitral stenosis (Fig. 3), the pulse may be of low volume and hypertension is unusual. A diastolic thrill may be detected at the apex, and loud mitral first heart sound may also be palpable as the thickened valve claps shut. The murmur of mitral stenosis is best heard between the apex beat and the left sternal border. The stethoscope bell should be used for auscultation with the patient turned to the left side.

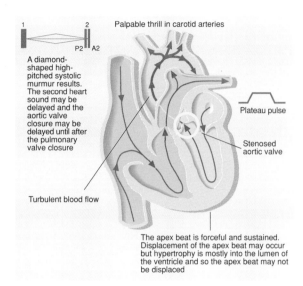

A diamond-shaped high-pitched systolic murmur results. The second heart sound may be delayed and the aortic valve closure may be delayed until after the pulmonary valve closure

Palpable thrill in carotid arteries

Plateau pulse

Stenosed aortic valve

Turbulent blood flow

The apex beat is forceful and sustained. Displacement of the apex beat may occur but hypertrophy is mostly into the lumen of the ventricle and so the apex beat may not be displaced

Fig. 1 **Aortic stenosis.**

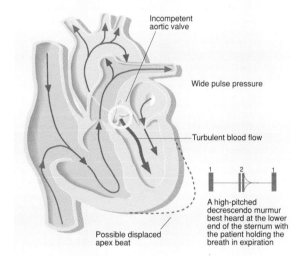

Incompetent aortic valve

Wide pulse pressure

Turbulent blood flow

Possible displaced apex beat

A high-pitched decrescendo murmur best heard at the lower end of the sternum with the patient holding the breath in expiration

Fig. 2 **Aortic incompetence.**

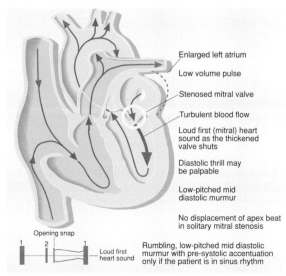

Enlarged left atrium

Low volume pulse

Stenosed mitral valve

Turbulent blood flow

Loud first (mitral) heart sound as the thickened valve shuts

Diastolic thrill may be palpable

Low-pitched mid diastolic murmur

No displacement of apex beat in solitary mitral stenosis

Opening snap

Loud first heart sound

Rumbling, low-pitched mid diastolic murmur with pre-systolic accentuation only if the patient is in sinus rhythm

Fig. 3 **Mitral stenosis.**

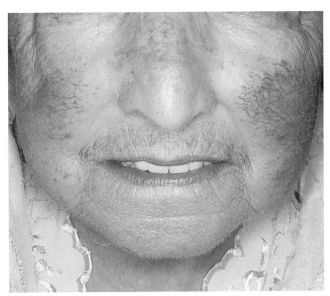

Fig. 4 **Malar flush in mitral stenosis.**

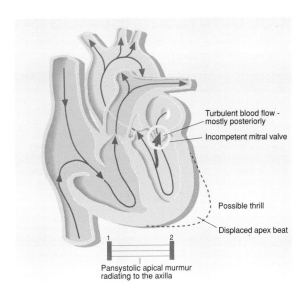

Turbulent blood flow -
mostly posteriorly

Incompetent mitral valve

Possible thrill

Displaced apex beat

Pansystolic apical murmur
radiating to the axilla

Fig.5 **Mitral incompetence.**

There may be an opening snap as the mitral valve opens in ventricular diastole. The opening snap is associated with the abrupt cessation of descent of the stenosed mitral valve leaflets into the left ventricle.

If there is combined mitral stenosis and incompetence, the presence of an opening snap suggests dominance of the stenosis, whereas a third heart sound suggests dominance of the incompetence.

The murmur of mitral stenosis is low pitched and rumbling, and is loudest in mid-diastole. If the patient is in sinus rhythm there will be a presystolic crescendo of the murmur as the contracting left atria pushes blood through the stenosed mitral valve in late ventricular diastole (this crescendo will be lost in atrial fibrillation). In severe mitral stenosis the murmur may be clinically undetectable due to minimal blood flow through the stenosed mitral valve.

The classical mitral facies (Fig. 4) comprises a reddish blue appearance over the cheek bones caused by dilated capillaries with slow blood flow. This leads to redness with cyanosis once oxygen has been extracted.

MITRAL INCOMPETENCE

Mitral incompetence (Fig. 5) may be caused by valvular disease (usually of rheumatic aetiology) or by left ventricular enlargement which interferes with mitral valve closure. If the mitral incompetence is long standing, the apex beat will be displaced because of volume overload of the left ventricle in which venous blood returning to the left atrium from the lungs

is augmented by the extra volume of regurgitated blood from the left ventricle. This augmented volume, when it returns to the left ventricle, overloads the left ventricle and is possibly associated with a third heart sound.

The first heart sound may be soft, as left ventricular pressure cannot rise rapidly (because of the valve leakage) and the mitral valve cannot be closed as fast as usual.

The murmur of mitral incompetence is systolic, loud, long (pansystolic, reaching both heart sounds) and is maximal in the region of the apex beat. It may radiate towards the axilla because the abnormal blood flow is directed posteriorly (the murmur cannot be heard at the back because of the intervening lung). The murmur thus appears to fade out as the listening stethoscope progresses laterally around the chest wall into the axilla.

There are three common causes for pansystolic murmurs, mitral incompetence, tricuspid incompetence and ventricular septal defect.

PROLAPSING MITRAL VALVE SYNDROME

Prolapsing (floppy) mitral valve syndrome is caused by:
- unusually large mitral valve
- unusually large mitral valve ring
- unusually long chordae (which normally prevent the mitral valve leaflets from ascending)
- dysfunction of the papillary muscles from which the chordae derive.

Between 2–17% of the population have this condition, and thus mild forms can be regarded as normal. However, there is a risk of infective endocarditis.

During ventricular systole one of the mitral leaflets prolapses into the left atrium and this may be associated with abnormal ventricular contraction or mitral incompetence. Symptoms include atypical left-sided chest pain (often described as 'sharp'), syncope especially on exertion, or palpitations. Signs include a mid-systolic click, possibly followed by a late systolic murmur. Occasionally classical signs of mitral incompetence are found.

Auscultatory findings in common heart lesions (I)

- Examination of the pulse, blood pressure and palpation of the precordium often enable anticipation of the findings on auscultation.
- Systolic hypotension, although it can occur, is uncommon if the left heart is failing because of valvular stenosis.
- Mitral valve prolapse is often of no haemodynamic significance.

AUSCULTATORY FINDINGS IN COMMON HEART LESIONS (II)

PULMONARY STENOSIS

In pulmonary stenosis (Fig. 1), the murmur is of the crescendo-diminuendo type and is best heard in the second left interspace. If severe, a thrill may be palpable.

With severe stenosis, blood will be held up in the right ventricle (which may therefore become enlarged and palpable). In consequence, blood may also be held up in the right atrium, causing prominent jugular venous pressure *a waves* to be seen.

PULMONARY INCOMPETENCE

In pulmonary incompetence (Fig. 2), there is a blowing diastolic murmur best heard along the left side of the sternum.

TRICUSPID STENOSIS

Tricuspid stenosis (Fig. 3) causes blood returning to the heart in the veins to be held up in the right atrium, thus producing very large 'flicking' *a* waves with diminution of the *y* descent.

There is a low-pitched mid-diastolic murmur best heard over the xiphisternum or to the right of the lower end of the sternum, with pre-systolic accentuation if the patient is in sinus rhythm. Rheumatic tricuspid stenosis is very rare as a solitary lesion and often only occurs in the presence of left-sided valvular involvement.

TRICUSPID INCOMPETENCE

Tricuspid incompetence (Fig. 4) may occur if the valve is damaged, or if the valve ring becomes distended because of enlargement of the right ventricle (as may occur in right ventricular failure). Functional obstruction to the outflow of blood from the right ventricle (as may occur in pulmonary stenosis or in cor pulmonale) can also be a cause.

Regurgitated ventricular blood flows into the venous system and may cause marked *v* waves in the jugular veins, and an enlarged pulsating liver.

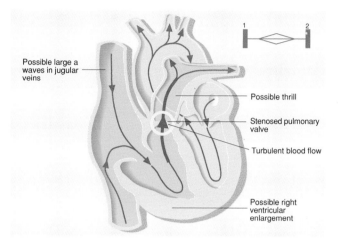

Fig. 1 **Pulmonary stenosis.**

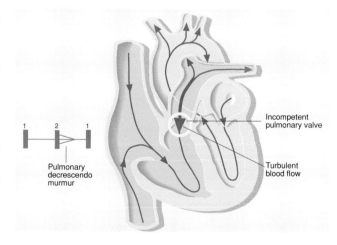

Fig. 2 **Pulmonary incompetence.**

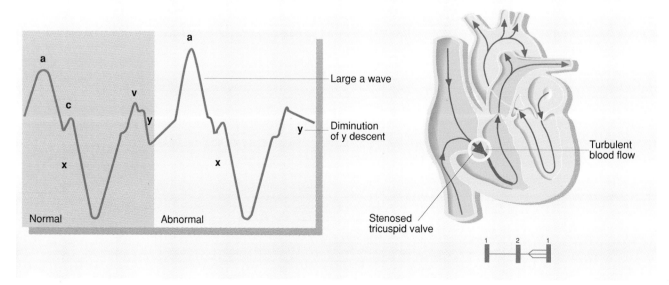

Fig. 3 **Tricuspid stenosis.**

The murmur is pansystolic and best heard over the lower end of the sternum, and may be louder during inspiration. Tricuspid murmurs, unlike mitral murmurs, are increased when inspiration expands the lungs which can then accommodate extra blood from the right ventricle. This allows extra blood to pass through the right side of the heart, thereby accentuating murmurs. To demonstrate these increased murmurs, the patient should ideally take a slow deep inspiration and hold the breath briefly in full inspiration.

It is often difficult to correlate the patient's state of respiration and the sound of the murmur. If the murmur does vary in intensity, it is easier to close one's eyes to enable exclusive concentration upon auscultation and, when the murmur is maximal, open one's eyes and observe whether the patient is breathing in or out.

SCHEMATIC ATRIAL SEPTAL DEFECT

In atrial septal defect (Fig. 5), oxygenated blood returns from the lungs into the left atrium and then passes through the defect into the (lower pressure) right atrium and thence (again) to the lungs. Thus, cyanosis does not occur in uncomplicated atrial septal defects. In theory, an atrial septal murmur should be heard in ventricular diastole (i.e. atrial systole), being caused by passage of blood through the defect between the left and right atrium. However, because of the low pressures involved and the largeness of most atrial septal defects, a murmur generated by the defect itself is rarely audible. In practice, the murmur of atrial septal defect is in ventricular systole and is caused by the augmented right ventricular blood volume passing through the pulmonary valve (thus simulating a pulmonary stenosis murmur). The augmented blood flow through the right heart may also cause a mid-diastolic tricuspid flow murmur.

With atrial septal defects there may be a fixed splitting of the second heart sound. Normally, the second heart sound is split in inspiration with the aortic valve closing before the pulmonary valve (because of the higher aortic pressures). During inspiration more blood can be accommodated in the lungs, which in turn passes into the right ventricle during diastole which then causes prolonged right ventricular systole (it takes longer to eject the increased amount of blood). The prolonged systole delays pulmonary valve closure. Thus the normal second heart sound may be split, and the split is accentuated during inspiration.

With an atrial septal defect, the two atria can be regarded as one chamber and blood flow into both ventricles is similar. Both ventricular systolic times are therefore identical, and both valve closures are delayed equally. Thus, there is a split second sound which does not vary with respiration.

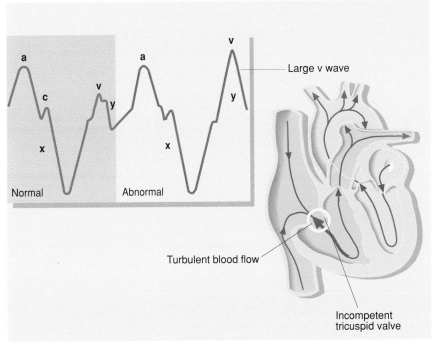

Normal   Abnormal

Large v wave

Turbulent blood flow

Incompetent tricuspid valve

Fig. 4 **Tricuspid incompetence.**

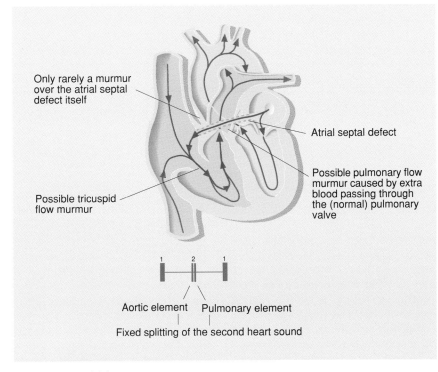

Only rarely a murmur over the atrial septal defect itself

Atrial septal defect

Possible pulmonary flow murmur caused by extra blood passing through the (normal) pulmonary valve

Possible tricuspid flow murmur

Aortic element   Pulmonary element

Fixed splitting of the second heart sound

Fig. 5 **Atrial septal defect.**

> ### Auscultatory findings in common heart lesions (II)
>
> - Right-side rheumatic valve disease is almost invariably associated with left-sided disease.
> - With atrial septal defects there is splitting of the second heart sound which does not vary with respiration.
> - The murmur of atrial septal defect is caused by extra blood flow through the pulmonary valve–a systolic murmur.

AUSCULTATORY FINDINGS IN COMMON HEART LESIONS (III)

VENTRICULAR SEPTAL DEFECT

With a ventricular septal defect (Fig. 1), left ventricular pressure is higher than right ventricular pressure, and thus blood is forced through the defect from left to right. The murmur is loud, long and is best heard down the left border of the sternum. There may be a thrill. As expected, the smaller the defect, the louder and the higher the pitch of the murmur produced.

The murmur of ventricular septal defects can be differentiated from the murmur of aortic stenosis (which may produce a murmur audible all over the front of the heart), as the former is rarely audible in the neck. If there is right-to-left blood flow through a ventricular septal defect (as may occur in severe pulmonary hypertension), there may be cyanosis as the deoxygenated 'cyanosed' right ventricular blood enters the left ventricle and, thus, into the general circulation. This constitutes a reversed shunt.

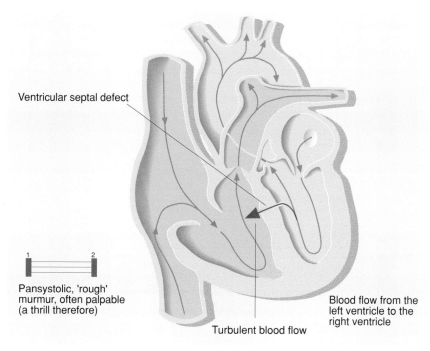

Fig. 1 **Ventricular septal defect.**

PATENT DUCTUS ARTERIOSUS

In patent ductus arteriosus (Fig. 2), both the systolic and diastolic pressures in the aorta normally exceed the maximum pressure in the pulmonary artery. There is a continuous rumbling murmur occupying both systole and diastole caused by aortic blood continuously entering the pulmonary artery. Because oxygenated blood from the high pressure aorta passes into the pulmonary artery, cyanosis is not usually a feature of uncomplicated patent ductus arteriosus.

The murmur may be heard (and a thrill palpated) to the left of the sternum in the region of the second rib interspace. There will be a collapsing pulse and a wide pulse pressure because the aortic diastolic pressure is lower than normal due to the continued drainage of blood from the aorta into the pulmonary artery.

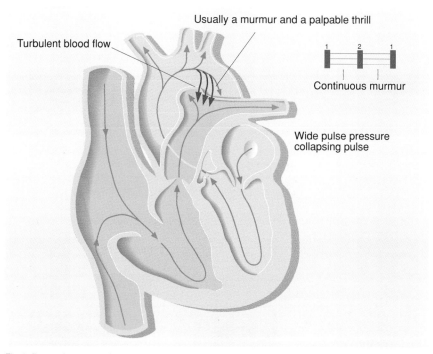

Fig. 2 **Patent ductus arteriosus.**

CONSTRICTIVE PERICARDITIS

With simple pericarditis there is usually a rub which may be transient and vary with posture. With constrictive pericarditis (Fig. 3), the heart is imprisoned by a tight pericardium. The neck veins are engorged with prominent y descents, and pulsus paradoxus may be detectable. If the constricting pericardium is also adherent to the pleura, there may be rib retraction during systole (the heart is anchored by

the great vessels and the constriction prevents the rotation of the heart during ventricular systole). A pericardial knock may be heard in association with rapid ventricular filling, as if the rapidly expanding ventricles knock against their constricting pericardium. Ascites, usually without much peripheral oedema but possibly with liver or splenic enlargement, may be found in constrictive pericarditis.

CARDIOMYOPATHY

With **dilated cardiomyopathy** the left and/or right ventricle becomes dilated and functions abnormally. Ventricular dilatation leads to stretching of the valve rings, and mitral or tricuspid incompetence may result. The symptoms and signs are those of heart failure or of the possible associated dysrhythmias or emboli.

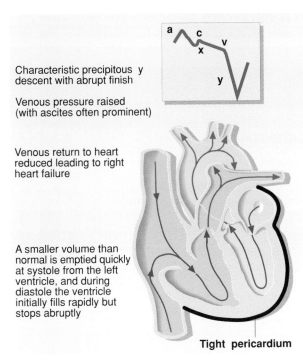

Characteristic precipitous y descent with abrupt finish

Venous pressure raised (with ascites often prominent)

Venous return to heart reduced leading to right heart failure

A smaller volume than normal is emptied quickly at systole from the left ventricle, and during diastole the ventricle initially fills rapidly but stops abruptly

Tight pericardium

Fig. 3 **Constrictive pericarditis.**

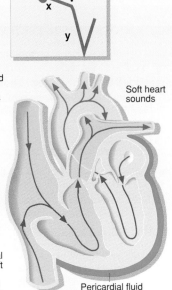

Sharp early diastolic y descent

Reduced cardiac output

Venous pressure raised and increases on inspiration

Venous return to heart reduced leading to right heart failure with (often massive) oedema

Paradoxical pulse – accentuation of normal drop in arterial blood pressure on inspiration (more than 10-15mmHg in absence of bronchospasm)

Tamponade is produced by rapid accumulation of small amounts of fluid or slow accumulation of larger amounts

A smaller volume than normal is emptied quickly from the left ventricle at systole, and at diastole the left ventricle fills rapidly but stops filling abruptly

Soft heart sounds

Pericardial fluid

Apex beat not usually palpable

Fig. 4 **Cardiac tamponade.**

With **hypertrophic cardiomyopathy** there is hypertrophy of the ventricular septum or the ventricles themselves. Ventricular contraction is distorted and ventricular filling during diastole may be impaired. Signs include a double apical impulse (the forceful atrial contraction required to fill the ventricular cavity causes a palpable and audible fourth heart sound), an abrupt carotid pulse (caused by abrupt obstruction to left ventricular emptying), a systolic murmur if there is left ventricular outflow obstruction, and a mitral incompetence murmur.

In **restrictive cardiomyopathy**, ventricular filling is restricted because of ventricular muscle abnormality, and the symptoms and signs are thus similar to those of constrictive pericarditis (a raised jugular venous pressure with abrupt fall in ventricular diastole and elevation of the jugular venous pressure on inspiration). Thrombus formation is common.

CARDIAC TAMPONADE

Cardiac tamponade (Fig. 4) is caused by compression of the heart by accumulation of fluid between the pericardium and heart. This presses on, and prevents adequate filling of, the right atrium and ventricle. Diastolic filling of the heart with blood is impaired and, in consequence, the neck veins become distended. Unlike the normal occurrence, this distension increases during inspiration (venous pulsus paradoxus).

The jugular venous pressure may be hard to see if grossly elevated, and in this

situation the collapsing hand vein sign is useful. If the dependent hand is raised slowly the veins on the back of the hand collapse at the approximate jugular venous pressure level.

The pulse will be rapid and of low volume. Pulsus paradoxus may be detectable, and the heart sounds may be muffled. Despite the obvious haemodynamic manifestations, there may be little central evidence of heart disease (no cardiac enlargement and no abnormal sounds or murmurs) and, thus, the diagnosis of tamponade (a rare disorder) may easily be missed.

The blood pressure will be low and the heart rate will be fast as the heart attempts to maintain cardiac output by increasing the number of fixed volume contractions.

COARCTATION OF THE AORTA

Coarctation (focal narrowing of the aorta) may be associated with aortic valve abnormalities and weakness of the aortic wall. Aortic dissection (blood forcing its way between the layers of the arterial wall)

may occur as a complication.

With uncomplicated coarctation there will be a raised blood pressure in the arms but a lower pressure in the legs. This is because most coarctations occur distal to the point of origin of the arm arteries from the aorta. Femoral pulsation may be delayed when compared with the radial pulse (normally the femoral pulse slightly precedes the radial pulse as the pressure wave travels faster along the wider aortic route to the femoral arteries).

There may be a systolic murmur distal to the coarctation if sufficient blood passes directly through the obstruction. Occasionally, dilated arteries over the scapula may be seen or felt as the blood in the aorta proximal to the coarctation finds routes to bypass the obstruction.

CONGENITAL HEART DISEASE

Only Fallot's tetralogy will be mentioned. This is a tetrad of pulmonary stenosis, ventricular septal defect, an overriding aorta which accepts blood from both ventricles, and right ventricular hypertrophy.

Auscultatory findings in common heart lesions (III)

- The flow of blood in ventricular septal defects is from left to right unless there is substantial impairment of right ventricular outflow.
- Small ventricular septal defects often produce louder murmurs than larger ventricular septal defects.
- With constructive pericarditis and cardiac tamponade there are often no cardiac murmurs.

COMMON CARDIOVASCULAR CONDITIONS

ACUTE MYOCARDIAL INFARCTION

Patients with myocardial infarction are usually anxious and pale (Fig. 1). The blood pressure may be abnormal, and there may be signs of left ventricular failure (vide infra) if the left ventricle is involved and, more rarely, signs of right ventricular failure if the right ventricle is involved. A fourth heart sound is more common than a third heart sound. If there has been a large anterior infarction there may be a thrusting systolic impulse over the heart as the infarcted segment of muscle 'balloons out' (a cardiac aneurysm). If papillary muscle function is impaired there may be mitral incompetence with an apical systolic murmur. Circulatory failure with shock may supervene.

DEEP VENOUS THROMBOSIS

Deep venous thromboses (DVT) usually affect the calf, thigh or pelvic veins. About half of DVTs are locally asymptomatic but may present with pulmonary embolism in which a blood clot breaks off and impacts in the lungs. It is particularly those DVTs in which clots float free in the veins without surrounding inflammation that often present with pulmonary embolism. The clinical symptoms of clinical DVT range from an aching pain in the calf or thigh or, if venous obstruction is complete, a severe bursting pain.

On examination there may be local tenderness in the calf or thigh, and oedematous swelling distal to the DVT. Homan's sign (an increased resistance to dorsiflexion of the foot associated with pain) is a time honoured yet unhelpful (indeed possibly dangerous) sign of a calf DVT, as it is positive in almost all cases of a painful calf. Other signs of DVT include cyanotic discoloration with dilated superficial calf veins. The limb affected by DVT is often warmer than its fellow (caused by cutaneous

re-routing of blood), and the peripheral pulses are likely to be intact (unless total venous obstruction causes venous gangrene in which arterial blood cannot pass through the limb).

HYPERTENSION

To assess the clinical effects of raised blood pressure look for:

- a heaving and/or displaced apex beat
- evidence of peripheral vascular disease
- hypertensive changes in the retinal vessels
- a loud aortic second sound (possibly).

Exclude coarctation by comparing the radial and femoral pulses (p. 33), and auscultate the abdomen for renal artery bruits (p. 53).

Hypertension is unusual if heart valve lesions (particularly aortic stenosis or mitral stenosis) restrict the volume of blood that can be abruptly delivered to the aorta.

LEFT HEART FAILURE

In left heart failure the patient may be short of breath, and pulsus alternans or a triple rhythm may be detectable (Fig. 2). Pulmonary oedema results when the left heart fails to cope with the blood returning from the lungs, and the lungs therefore become waterlogged. Inspiratory crepitations may be audible. The crepitations are inspiratory because small respiratory passages are occluded by their oedematous walls and are opened up during inspiration (the crepitations thus produce a similar sound to that of pulling apart two opposed plates of glass). Free fluid within the air passages with production of frothy mucoid sputum only occurs in severe pulmonary oedema.

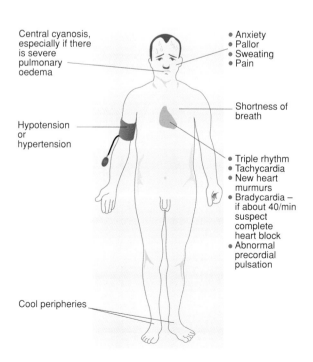

Fig. 1 **Symptoms and signs of myocardial infarction.**

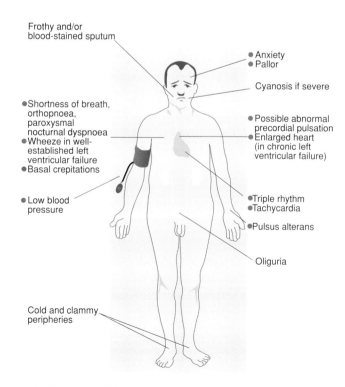

Fig. 2 **Symptoms and signs of left heart failure.**

In severe left heart failure, circulatory failure supervenes with hypotension, shock, confusion and oliguria. The peripheries may be cold and cyanosed.

Pure right ventricular failure may occur in severe pulmonary disease (cor pulmonale), and pure left ventricular failure may occur in severe hypertension, aortic valve disease or, acutely, in myocardial infarction (which usually involves the left ventricle).

Frequently both sides of the heart fail simultaneously, and if heart failure is of long duration, cardiac enlargement is an almost invariable finding.

PULMONARY EMBOLISM

An embolism is an impaction of a blood clot in a blood vessel which *may* cause infarction of the tissue supplied unless there is another route of blood supply. A pulmonary embolism (PE) may present with sudden collapse and hypotension if the embolism is large enough to cause acute circulatory blockage. Smaller PEs may present with faintness, tachycardia, fevers, or unexplained shortness of breath. If there is pulmonary infarction there may be pleuritic-type chest pain and haemoptysis.

RHEUMATIC FEVER

Acute rheumatic fever is very uncommon in the United Kingdom, but is still common in developing countries. Streptococcal-induced immune responses affect the heart and heart valves, and also cause fever, migratory joint pains, heart murmurs, subcutaneous nodules, chorea and erythema marginatum. Rheumatic heart valve damage tends to be slowly progressive, and because it has been relatively rare in recent years, most affected patients are middle aged or older. Right heart involvement is rare in the absence of left-sided involvement. Mitral stenosis is commoner than mitral incompetence, and pure mitral stenosis is about twice as common as combined mitral stenosis and incompetence.

RIGHT HEART FAILURE

In right heart failure (Fig. 3), the right side of the heart fails to cope with the returning blood and thus the neck veins are distended. The raised venous pressure may cause congestion and enlargement of the liver (which may be tender). The extra hydrostatic pressure in the veins causes passage of fluid into tissues, leading to peripheral oedema or ascites. The abnormal amount of tissue fluid gives rise to swelling which can be indented by a finger (Fig. 5, p. 21) and remains indented for a short while after the finger is removed. The oedema of right heart failure is dependent (accumulating in the feet of those who are ambulant or in the sacral area of those confined to bed). Severe right heart failure may cause oedema which may extend upwards onto the chest.

SUPERFICIAL THROMBOPHLEBITIS

An acute superficial thrombophlebitis is characterized by pain over the superficial vein involved. On examination there is a tender cord-like vein, perhaps with surrounding inflammation.

VARICOSE VEINS

Varicose veins are abnormally dilated superficial leg veins, usually associated with incompetent valves (which normally only allow superficial venous blood to drain into the deep veins) and/or incompetence affecting the area where the saphenous veins drain upwards into the femoral vein. Varicose veins become more apparent when the patient stands, and empty when the patient lies down or the legs are elevated. Chronic venous insufficiency may cause chronic oedema or varicose ulcers (Fig. 4) which typically occur just above the malleoli.

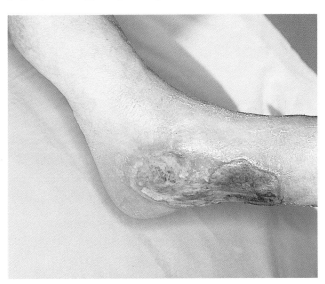

Fig. 4 **Varicose ulcer around medial malleolus.**

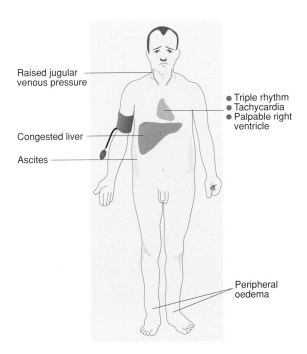

Raised jugular venous pressure

Congested liver

Ascites

Triple rhythm
Tachycardia
Palpable right ventricle

Peripheral oedema

Fig. 3 **Symptoms and signs of right heart failure.**

Common cardiovascular conditions

- Most myocardial infarctions affect the left ventricle.
- A displaced apex beat in myocardial infarction suggests previous hypertension or heart valve disease.
- Rheumatic heart valve disease tends to be slowly progressive.
- Severe lung disease may cause right ventricular failure.

BASIC PRINCIPLES

STRUCTURE AND FUNCTION

Before examining the chest, it is obviously necessary to know the surface markings of the lungs and the reference points from which these can be clinically identified. The inferior limits of the lungs are indistinct because the surfaces are dome shaped and, the diaphragms move on respiration (Fig. 1). The sternal angle is opposite the second anterior rib end, and thus each anterior rib can be numbered. Posteriorly, the spinous process of the seventh cervical vetebra (vertebra prominens) usually protrudes, enabling other spinous processes to be numbered.

The lower border of the lungs usually passes from the sixth costochondral junction to the spinous process of the tenth thoracic vertebra (the pleura extend lower than this). The oblique fissure (which separates the left upper from the lower lobe, and the right lower from the upper and middle lobe) passes obliquely from the sixth costochondral junction anteriorly to the fourth thoracic spinous process posteriorly. The horizontal fissure (on the right) passes laterally from the fourth costochondral junction to meet the oblique fissure in the midaxillary line.

Inspiration occurs through expansion of the chest cavity by elevation of the ribs into a more horizontal position, and by contraction of the diaphragm. Expiration is largely a passive process assisted by elastic recoil of lung tissue. Women tend to breath more with their intercostal muscles (thoracic respiratory pattern), whereas men tend to use their diaphragms (abdominal respiratory pattern).

RESPIRATORY HISTORY

The respiratory history should include questions about:

- smoking
- history of tuberculosis in the patient or contacts
- chest injuries
- chest operations
- previous episodes of pneumonia (recurrent pneumonias in the same part of the lung suggest bronchiectasis or obstructing lesions)
- occurrence of severe measles or whooping cough in childhood (both of which can leave residual lung damage).

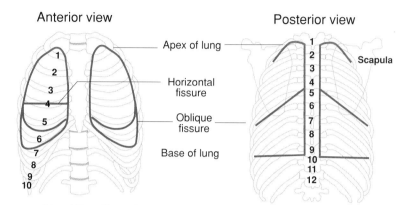

Anterior view   Posterior view

Apex of lung — Scapula

Horizontal fissure

Oblique fissure

Base of lung

The oblique fissure is approximately parallel to the medial border of the scapula when the arm is raised above the horizontal

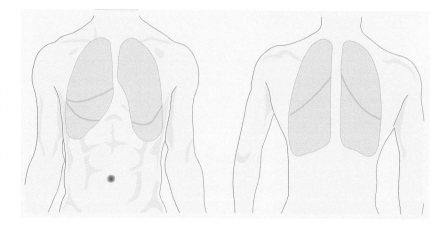

Fig. 1 The surface markings of the lungs. The position of the lung bases and the horizontal and oblique fissures vary with inspiration.

Certain occupations predispose to respiratory tract problems. For example, dust-related diseases occur in:

- coal miners
- foundry workers
- masons
- asbestos workers.

Exposure to birds may be associated with an allergic alveolitis (inflammation of the air sacs) or psittacosis.

Patients who smoke should be made aware at an appropriate stage of the risks (Fig. 2). A useful guide is that each cigarette smoked statistically takes 5 minutes off a lifetime.

There are six main respiratory symptoms:

- cough
- sputum production
- haemoptysis
- breathlessness
- chest pain
- wheezing.

COUGH

The duration, productiveness and characteristics of cough should be ascertained. It is easy to identify the laryngeal cough which is, in the absence of tuberculosis or diphtheria, almost always of viral aetiology. Hoarseness invariably accompanies significant laryngitis. A deep, often productive, 'chesty' cough often occurs in bronchopneumonias. A deep, unproductive cough suggests primary involvement of lung parenchyma (an interstitial process) rather than involvement of the airways. 'Interstitial' coughs may occur in lobar pneumonias, atypical pneumonias, viral pneumonias and in lung infiltrated by pathological tissue. A muffled bronchitic cough occurs in measles.

The repetitive, paroxysmal, expiratory and stacatto cough of pertussis (whooping cough) is easy to identify even if the whoop (an inspiratory high-pitched noise made as air is sucked into the 'empty' lungs) does not follow the cough. Vomiting characteristically follows coughing paroxysms. Children usually swallow

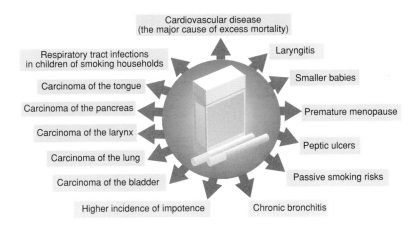

Fig. 2 **The risks associated with smoking.**

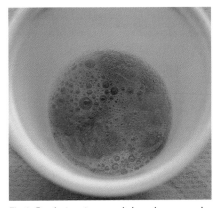

Fig. 3 **Purulent sputum seen in bronchopneumonia.**

sputum, but pertussis is one condition in which (thick tenacious) sputum is produced. Adults with pertussis rarely whoop, but the other cough characteristics alone often provide the clue.

Prolonged episodes of coughing may be caused by asthma, and severe coughing bouts may cause cough syncope because the raised intrathoracic pressure reduces venous return to the chest and, thus, cardiac output. Bronchial carcinoma may damage a recurrent laryngeal nerve and cause vocal cord paralysis, leading to a 'bovine' cough.

Coughs are often worse at night, possibly provoked by a change in temperature or humidity in the bedroom.

> Every smoker with a cough ought to be told that coughing is abnormal, and production of sputum is an unequivocal sign of pulmonary problems.

SPUTUM PRODUCTION

Sputum production is usually absent or minimal in interstitial pneumonias (inflammation of lung parenchyma rather than the airways). Patients with bronchopneumonias usually produce discoloured sputum (Fig. 3). Patients with bronchiectasis (abnormal dilatation of the bronchi) or freely draining lung abcesses or cavities usually produce large amounts of sputum which may be malodorous. Sparse, rusty coloured sputum is a common feature of pneumococcal lobar pneumonia.

HAEMOPTYSIS

Haemoptysis is coughing up of blood from the lungs (more proximal sources of bleed-

ing should be excluded). If infection in the chest is the cause, the blood is often mixed with purulent sputum. Blood alone may be coughed up in pulmonary infarction. Copious haemoptysis is usually secondary to tuberculosis, lung abscesses or cavitating carcinomas. The main causes of haemoptysis include carcinoma of the bronchus, bronchiectasis, tuberculosis or severe pulmonary oedema, but *not* uncomplicated chronic bronchitis or emphysema. Haemoptysis always demands an aetiological explanation.

BREATHLESSNESS (DYSPNOEA)

Both of these terms are somewhat ambiguous and require further definition. Does the patient report difficulty in breathing in or out (favouring a respiratory aetiology, usually obstructive), or is it a feeling that the patient needs to breathe more without any feeling of respiratory obstruction or restriction (favouring early pulmonary oedema or, rarely, acute onset severe anaemia)? In other words, patients with acute onset shortness of breath of cardiac origin can pant (at least in the early stages) whereas those with acute onset of obstructive airways disease cannot. Some patients complain of chest tightness and it is important to define whether this is a feeling of restriction (respiratory) or pain (most likely cardiac). Acute onset severe breathlessness is a medical emergency, as it suggests tension pneumothorax, asthma or acute left heart failure.

CHEST PAIN

Respiratory chest pain may be pleuritic (a sharp, stabbing, well-localized pain made worse on deep inspiration) which is caused by irritation of the outer pleura by inflammatory processes, infarction (death of tissue caused by anoxia), malignancies or occasionally by a pneumothorax.

Fractured ribs (which may be caused by a coughing bout) also give rise to pain on chest movement, but this pain is superficial and the ribs tender. Pain may be referred to the relevant shouldertip or to the upper abdomen if the diaphragmatic pleura is involved.

Superficial chest pain is caused by chest wall lesions, including rib fractures (which may occur in a coughing bout), inflammation of the costochondral junctions (Tietze's syndrome), nerve root pain including shingles and intercostal muscle cramps or Bornholm syndrome (intercostal myalgia of viral aetiology). Tracheitis produces a raw upper sternal pain, possibly in association with laryngitis. Large intrapulmonary malignancies may cause vague, dull and continuous central chest pain.

Tracheal pain is felt behind the sternum, and mediastinal pain may be similar to cardiac pain but will not be exacerbated by exercise.

WHEEZING

Wheezing may be episodic as in asthma. Some patients have obvious wheezes on auscultation with the stethoscope, but do not give a history of audible wheeze.

> **Basic principles**
> - Symptoms associated with disease caused by smoking usually occur late when the disease has established itself.
> - There are definite risks to others from passive smoking.
> - Pregnant women who smoke may harm their fetus.
> - Tar – not nicotine – stains the fingers.

RESPIRATORY SOUNDS

TYPES OF RESPIRATORY SOUNDS

Respiratory sounds comprise breath sounds (vesicular or bronchial) and added sounds (crackles, wheezes, rubs, and amphoric sounds) (Fig. 1). Normal breath sounds are vesicular, having a rustling quality, and are predominantly heard during inspiration (Fig. 2).

ABNORMAL BREATH SOUNDS

Breath sounds are produced by airflow through the larynx during breathing. Abnormal breath sounds are produced by abnormal creation, or by abnormal conduction of normally created breath sounds to the chest wall. Conduction of breath sounds to the stethoscope is reduced or absent if there is airways obstruction (either generalized as in asthma or focal as in obstructing carcinoma), pleural fluid, pleural thickening or pneumothorax. The breath and voice sounds will also be reduced.

BRONCHIAL BREATH SOUNDS

Turbulent airflow in the upper airways causes high-pitched bronchial sounds which, in normal individuals, can only be heard over the trachea and upper chest. Although bronchial sounds are transmitted to the rest of the lung, the higher frequencies are filtered out leaving the softer, lower-pitched sounds which are normally heard at the lung bases. The smaller airways distal to the trachea and bronchi usually do not create breath sounds, as they have a slower, laminar-type airflow. Bronchial breathing can be simulated by softly saying 'her...er' with the 'her' in expiration and the 'er' in inspiration after a brief pause. Bronchial breathing represents more effective unchanged transmission of upper airways sounds through the lung and is almost always associated with increased voice sounds (Fig. 2). Bronchial breathing is found with consolidation (if the airways remain open).

CRACKLES (CREPITATIONS)

Inspiratory crackles are produced in the smaller lower airways when the walls of previously collapsed airways snap open. Occasionally, coarse crackles are initiated

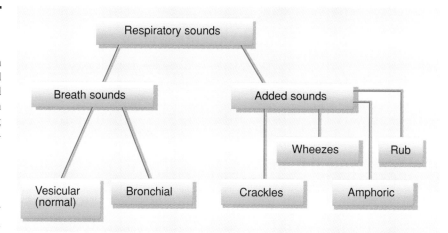

Fig. 1 **The breath sounds and added sounds.**

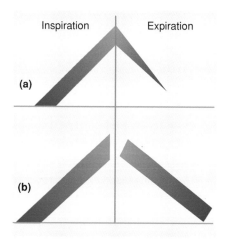

Fig. 2 **Normal vesicular breath sounds (a) compared with bronchial breath sounds (b).**

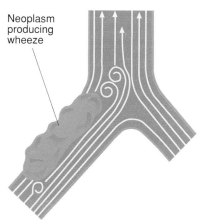

Fig. 3 **A fixed wheeze can be a sign of a bronchial neoplasm.**

by fluid bubbling in the airways as may occur in severe pulmonary oedema, bronchiectasis or severe bronchopneumonia. As might be expected, these crackles may be moved by coughing or postural drainage. Late inspiratory crackles are produced by conditions which predominantly affect the alveoli (the terminal air sacs of the lung) and are heard in pneumonia and pulmonary fibrosis.

WHEEZES (RHONCHI)

Wheezes are produced when there is turbulent airflow in diffusely or focally narrowed airways. This produces a musical increase in sound intensity by vibrating the airway walls. Because the airways are usually narrower during expiration, rhonchi are more prominent during expiration. A fixed wheeze (one which is

constant in position) is caused by a focal partial stenosis of an airway, such as may occur with a bronchial neoplasm or an inhaled foreign body (Fig. 3).

PLEURAL RUB

A pleural rub is a scratchy, creaking sound produced when one layer of irritated pleura has to slide over another layer (Fig. 4). Often the rub is well localized and audible in both inspiration and expiration. Increased pressure exerted by a stethoscope may increase the rub. Occasionally a pleural rub may be confused with coarse crackles. However coughing may move crackles but not a pleural rub.

A pleural rub may be associated with pleuritic-type chest pain. If a patient has localized chest pain, always listen carefully over the painful area for a pleural rub.

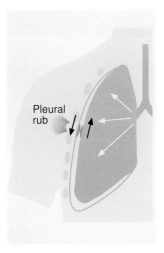

Fig. 4 **A pleural rub is produced when one layer of irritated pleura slides over another.**

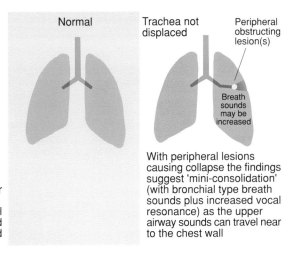

Trachea pulled over to side of lesion

Breath sounds reduced

Proximal obstructing lesion

With proximal lesions with peripheral collapse the upper airway sounds are not well transmitted to the chest wall and so the breath sounds and vocal resonance are reduced

Normal

Trachea not displaced

Peripheral obstructing lesion(s)

Breath sounds may be increased

With peripheral lesions causing collapse the findings suggest 'mini-consolidation' (with bronchial type breath sounds plus increased vocal resonance) as the upper airway sounds can travel near to the chest wall

Fig. 5 **Differing signs in collapse caused by proximal and peripheral obstructing lesions.**

Apologize to the patient in advance and then ask him to take a breath sufficient to cause the pain and listen carefully over the site of the pain for the rub. Pleural rubs may be transient because the irritated pleura often initiates a lubricating pleural exudate. A pleural rub implies inflammation of the pleura (pleurisy) or pulmonary infarction.

AMPHORIC BREATH SOUNDS

Amphoric breath sounds are similar to the sound produced by blowing across a glass jar, and are created by airflow associated with a comunicating lung cavity.

ABNORMAL CONDUCTION OF BREATH SOUNDS

There are seven major anatomical causes for abnormal conduction of breath sounds:

- consolidated lung
- emphysematous lung
- fibrosis
- pleural thickening
- pleural fluid
- pneumothorax
- collapsed lung.

Note that reduced breath sounds are not necessarily associated with 'poor air entry' and thus this later term should not be used.

CONSOLIDATED LUNG

Consolidated lung (as classically occurs in streptococcal lobar pneumonia) conducts upper airway sounds more efficiently than a normal lung, and consequently the consolidated lung transmits bronchial breath sounds (often high pitched) to more distant sites than usual. If the bronchus is blocked, bronchial breath sounds will not be heard unless the consolidation is in the upper lobes and close to the trachea. Voice sounds, which are created in the larynx, are also transmitted more efficiently resulting in:

- increased vocal resonance in which the patient's voice sounds are much louder than normal when heard through the stethoscope
- whispering pectoriloquy in which a whisper by the patient becomes abnormally loud and transmitted to unusual sites
- aegophony in which the voice sounds have a high-pitched bleating quality.

EMPHYSEMATOUS LUNGS

Emphysematous lungs are less efficient conductors of upper airway sounds and, thus, the sounds should be reduced in emphysema. In practice the assessment of breath sounds reduced by emphysema is subjective and unreliable.

FIBROSIS

Localized areas of fibrotic lung tissue conduct upper airway sounds more effectively and thus breath sounds may be bronchial in nature (often of low pitch) and voice sounds are increased.

PLEURAL FLUID AND THICKENING

Pleural thickening reduces transmission of breath sounds. Pleural fluid (fluid between the two layers of pleura and thus between the lungs and the chest wall) almost totally blocks sound transmission. The major differentiation between con-

solidation and pleural fluid is the increased breath sounds with underlying consolidation and the reduced or totally absent breath sounds associated with pleural fluid.

It is a common mistake to regard the above signs as those of pleural *effusion* (implying an exudate or transudate) because a haemorrhage between the pleura or an empyema will have the same signs but will usually require very different treatment.

PNEUMOTHORAX

Pneumothorax (air between the lungs and the chest wall) causes breath sounds to be reduced because air is a poorer conductor of breath sounds than normal lung.

COLLAPSED LUNG

Large portions of collapsed lung conduct breath sounds less well than a normal lung and breath sounds are therefore reduced (Fig. 5). This is a major differentiating point from consolidation which produces increased (bronchial) breath sounds.

Respiratory sounds

- Assessment of breath sounds can be assisted by asking the patient to breath audibly ('heavy breathing') as this produces more laryngeal sound.
- Listen carefully over localized areas of pleuritic type chest pain. A pleural rub may be audible or, less commonly, the crunching of a fractured rib.

COMMON LUNG ABNORMALITIES

There are nine possible anatomical diagnoses of lung abnormality:

- bronchial narrowing
- cavitation
- collapse
- consolidation
- fibrosis
- pleural fluid
- pleural rub
- pleural thickening
- pneumothorax.

The differentiating points are summarized in Table 1, and the differentiation between the four important common anatomical lesions is illustrated in Figure 1.

BRONCHIAL NARROWING

If bronchial narrowing is generalized, the patient is often short of breath and will be using accessory muscles of respiration to elevate the upper chest in order to help suck in more air. There will usually be wheezing on auscultation, providing that sufficient air is passing through the air passages. Wheezes may not be heard in very severe bronchial narrowing. If obstruction is severe, patients sit upright with their arms resting forward and horizontally to enable the back muscles (notably latissimus dorsi) to pull the ribs upwards to increase chest capacity (Fig. 2). Breathing out with pursed lips keeps the airway pressure high even in expiration, thus minimizing small airway collapse.

CAVITATION

Chest movements will be diminished over a large cavity, and if a large cavity communicates with a bronchus, post-tussive suction may be heard (a sucking, hissing sound heard after the patient coughs). Amphoric breathing and crackles may also be heard. Bronchial breathing and whispering pectriloquy may be heard if the cavity is surrounded by consolidation. A patient with a communicating cavity usually produces large amounts of sputum.

COLLAPSE

Chest movements on the side affected by lung collapse will be diminished (Fig. 3). The trachea may be pulled over to one side if an upper lobe is involved or, if a lower lobe is involved, the heart may be pulled over towards the affected side. The percussion note is dull, breath sounds are variable and voice sounds are reduced. Upper lobe collapse may cause an increase in bronchial breathing and increased breath sounds, probably because the trachea is pulled nearer to the chest wall of the side involved.

Table 1　**Possible clinical signs of lung pathologies detectable on clinical examination**

Pathology	Chest wall movement	Mediastinal position	Percussion note	Breath sounds	Vocal resonance	Accompaniments
Consolidation	Reduced on side affected	Normal	Dull	High-pitched bronchial	Increased and whispering pectriloquy	Crackles
Major collapse	Reduced on side affected	Shift towards side of lesion	Dull	Reduced or absent	Usually reduced	
Cavitation (large)	Reduced on side affected	Variable	Increased but decreased if surrounded by consolidation	Variable	Variable	Coarse crackles ? amphoric breathing
Pneumothorax	Reduced on side affected	Shift away from side of lesion	Increased if large	Usually reduced or absent	Usually reduced or absent	"Tinkling" crackles
Pleural thickening	Usually normal, reduced if extensive	Normal	Usually normal. reduced if extensive	Usually normal. reduced if extensive	Usually normal. reduced if extensive	? Rub
Pleural rub	Possibly reduced	Normal	Normal	Normal	Normal	Rub
Pleural fluid	Reduced on side affected	If large shift away from lesion	Stony dull	Absent	Reduced or absent	
Emphysema	Reduced symmetrically	Normal	Normal	Reduced or prolonged expiration	Normal	Often coarse crepitations
Localized fibrosis	Reduced on side affected	Normal or shift towards lesion	Normal or reduced	Low pitched bronchial	Increased	Often coarse crackles
Bronchial narrowing (diffuse)	Reduced symmetrically	Normal	Normal	Prolonged expiration, high pitched	Normal	Wheeze

The findings in many lung pathologies depend on their extent and on whether there is surrounding consolidation.

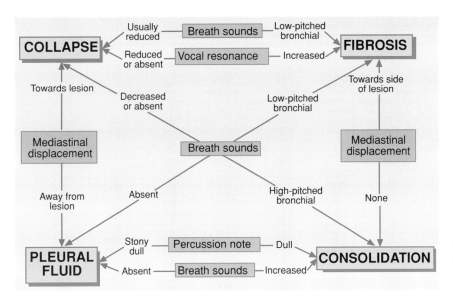

Fig. 1 **The clinical differentiation between four important lung pathologies.**

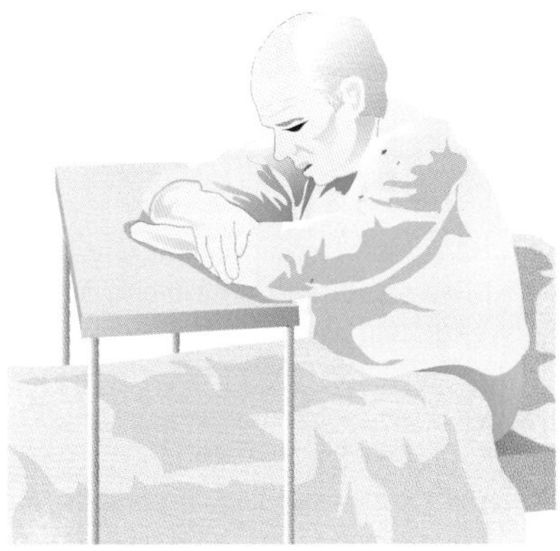

Fig. 2 **Patient using accessory muscles of breathing, and pursed lips to maintain airway pressure.**

CONSOLIDATION

Chest movements over the area affected may be diminished and the percussion note will be dull: the mediastinum remains central. Bronchial breathing should be audible with increased vocal resonance and whispering pectriloquy, and crackles may be heard. There may be a pleural rub if the pleura is also involved by inflammatory conditions that have caused the consolidation.

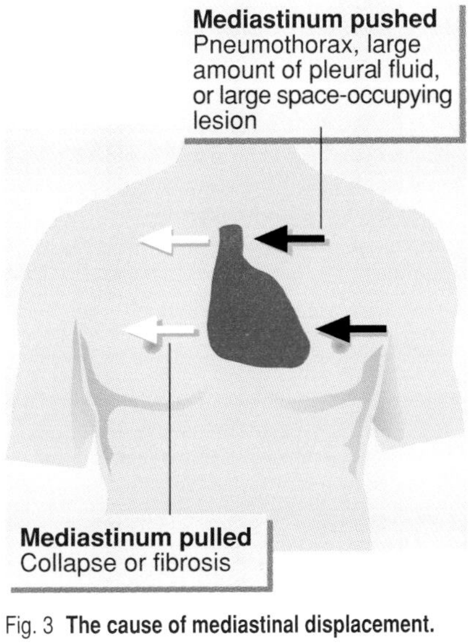

FIBROSIS

Fibrosis produces vesicular or bronchial breath sounds and increased voice sounds. Mediastinal displacement may be evident if fibrosis is predominantly unilateral and, if extensive, there may be flattening of the overlying chest wall and the percussion note may be dull. Crackles may be heard. Bilateral symmetrical fibrosis may be difficult to detect clinically.

PLEURAL FLUID

The heart may be pushed to the opposite side if there is a large quantity of pleural fluid. On the affected side, chest movements are diminished and the percussion note will be markedly dull (stony dullness). The breath sounds are grossly reduced or absent and vocal resonance is reduced. Over the top of pleural fluid the clinical signs may suggest consolidation with bronchial breathing and a curious bleating of transmitted voice sound (aegophony). Paradoxically, the percussion note above pleural fluid may be excessively resonant (skodiac resonance). Pleural fluid has to be at least 300 ml in volume before clinical signs are apparent (Fig. 4).

PNEUMOTHORAX

Movements of the affected side may be reduced and the mediastinum may be pushed away from the affected side. The percussion note may be hyperresonant or tympanitic (drum-like). Vocal resonance and breath sounds are reduced and sometimes bronchial or amphoric breathing may be heard if there is a communication between the pneumothorax and the airways. A tension pneumothorax will result (with marked breathlessness and mediastinal displacement) if there is a one-way flutter valve effect (rather than a free communication) between the lung and the air in the pneumothorax. Occasionally a crunching noise is audible with each heart beat, probably representing the heart crunching against the surrounding tissue without the intervening cushion of expanded lung. The coin sign may be positive: a coin placed on the affected chest wall tapped with another coin produces a ringing sound.

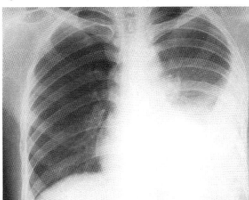

Mediastinum pushed
Pneumothorax, large amount of pleural fluid, or large space-occupying lesion

Mediastinum pulled
Collapse or fibrosis

Fig. 3 **The cause of mediastinal displacement.**

Fig. 4 **Left pleural fluid seen on chest X-ray.** Note that the fluid appears to 'lip up' into the axilla.

Common lung abnormalities

- Patients suffering from bronchial narrowing often use accessory muscles of breathing.
- Chest movements will be diminished over a large cavity.
- Lung collapse will lead to diminished chest movements over the affected side.
- Fibrosis produces bronchial breath sounds and increased voice sounds.

RESPIRATORY EXAMINATION (I)

INTRODUCTION

It is often easier to examine the chest with the patient standing if possible. Certainly percussion and assessment of respiratory movements of the lung bases at the back is difficult if the patient is sitting in bed. The possible signs of acute respiratory disease are shown in Figure 1 and chronic respiratory disease in Figure 2. Before utilizing the conventional sequence of inspection, palpation, percussion and auscultation, three observations should be made.

Observe the breathing pattern

Prolonged expiration occurs in bronchial narrowing or in inflammation of the bronchi and smaller airways (as in bronchitis). Restrictive lung disease, as may be found in diffuse fibrosing processes, may be suspected (but not actually diagnosed) if the diminuendo of expiratory wheeze ceases abruptly (as the restricted lungs suddenly reach the end of their elastic recoil potential). In contrast, the wheeze of bronchial narrowing often progressively diminuendoes away to nothing without a cutoff point.

Stridor is a wheezing noise generated at the larynx or above. Unlike lower respiratory tract wheezing, the wheezing of stridor is audible well away from the patient and is of approximately equal intensity and duration in both inspiration and expiration.

Examine the sputum pot

Yellow or green sputum usually signifies infection (numerous eosinophils in allergic lung disease can also discolour the sputum). Copious amounts of sputum suggest bronchiectasis or lung cavities that are draining into the air passages. Mucoid (watery) sputum may be found in severe pulmonary oedema, asthma, or in uncomplicated viral pneumonias. Foul-smelling sputum suggests infection with anaerobic bacteria.

Voluntary cough

Ask the patient to cough and note the characteristics as outlined previously (p. 36).

INSPECTION

Observe the pattern of shortness of breath and the respiratory rate. Observe the patient's colour.

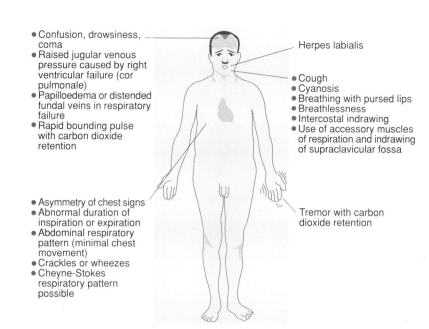

Fig. 1 **The possible clinical findings in acute respiratory disease.**

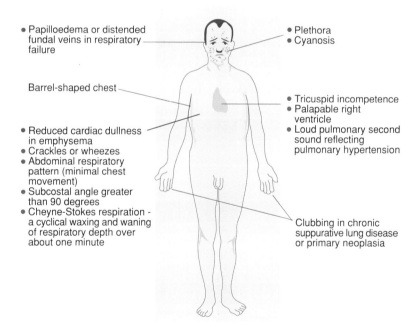

Fig. 2 **The possible findings of chronic respiratory disease. Signs of acute disease may be superimposed.**

Cyanosis

Cyanosis is a bluish discoloration which may be central or peripheral in distribution. Central cyanosis is best identified by observing the tongue which, being central and warm, cannot develop a cyanosis of peripheral causation.

Cyanosis may occur if the oxygen saturation of blood leaving the lungs is about 75% or less. Cyanosis requires about 5g or more of desaturated haemoglobin: thus patients with a severe anaemia of less than 5g cannot become cyanosed. Patients with polycythaemia (who have excessive

haemoglobin) are often cyanosed. Some patients fight cyanosis by hyperventilation ('pink puffers') whereas others surrender and become 'blue bloaters' (Fig. 3).

In contrast, peripheral cyanosis (in the absence of central cyanosis) signifies an impaired peripheral circulation such that the haemoglobin in the sluggishly circulating red blood cells becomes significantly more deoxygenated than normal, thus causing cyanosis. The causes of peripheral cyanosis are thus those of an impaired circulation rather than respiratory disease.

Causes of central cyanosis (caused by desaturated blood being distributed by the arterial system) include asphyxia, hypoventilation, impaired oxygen transfer across the lungs or venous to arterial shunting of blood. Chronic central cyanosis caused by respiratory disease is most often caused by chronic obstructive airways disease or fibrosing alveolitis. Because cyanosis induces vasodilation, the peripheries are often blue, warm, and with full bounding pulses.

The depth, frequency and character of breathing

The depth, frequency (normally between 15 and 20 per minute) and character of breathing should be noted. Not whether the patient uses unusual accessory muscles of respiration (e.g. the sternomastoids) to attempt adequate ventilation of the lungs, or whether there is an abnormally expanded chest wall such that abdominal muscles have to be used for respiration. Note also whether there are scars from previous chest surgery and if the chest wall is asymmetric or flattened. Obvious skeletal deformities of the spine include a kyphosis (an excessively curved thoracic spine in the anterior posterior dimension) and scoliosis (a laterally curved spine), either of which may interfere with chest ventilation. Assess whether respiratory excursion is limited, although in the absence of previous measurements this must be rather subjective.

If there is chest asymmetry or reduced movement on one side then the side of pathology is almost invariably the side of *reduced* movement. Never say that there is increased movement on one side of the chest but rather say that there is reduced movement of the other side.

Suspect chronic obstructive airways disease if the chest is barrel shaped. This appearance is caused by an increase in the antero-posterior diameter of the chest, horizontal ribs and clavicles, and a subcostal angle greater than 90° because the chest wall muscles have been attempting to ensure maximum ventilation by maximum elevation of the ribs.

Other signs

Other signs which may be seen include clubbing (p. 8) or enlarged lymph nodes and Horner's syndrome (a unilateral ptosis, a small pupil, a slightly sunken eyeball and loss of sweating; p. 99). Horner's syndrome may be a sign that malignant tissue has invaded and interrupted the sympathetic nerve supply to the eye.

In hospital practice the nursing observation chart should be noted. If the patient is febrile from any cause, the respiratory rate is usually increased by about five for each degree centigrade rise in temperature, but if respiratory infection is the cause the respiratory rate rise is often greater than this.

PALPATION

Position of the mediastinum

The position of the mediastinum should be determined by ascertaining that the trachea and the apex beat are in their normal position (very slightly to the right of the midline and the fifth intercostal space in the midclavicular line respectively). Palpation of the trachea is best performed (with the patient's neck in the normal upright position) by placing the index finger in the suprasternal notch and ascertaining that it is slightly easier to push to the left of the trachea than to the right (Fig. 4). If there is airways obstruction, the trachea is moved ('tugged') downwards on inspiration. This can be best appreciated by feeling movements of the thyroid cartilege. Displacement of the mediastinum occurs when it is pushed from one side (by a pneumothorax, a large accumulation of pleural fluid or by other space-occupying lesions), or pulled to the other side (by pulmonary collapse or fibrosis).

Respiratory excursion

Respiratory excursion of all areas of the chest should be assessed, comparing the right side with the left side. To determine whether there is asymmetry of chest movement, place your relaxed hands symmetrically on either side of the patient's chest with your fingers over the two areas to be compared. Then concentrate on feeling chest movements. Simultaneous inspection often detracts from this assessment. The technique of looking to see whether the thumbs (used in a caliper-like fashion) are asymmetrically displaced by chest movement is reserved for those who are only interested in the gross lung pathology which should have been evident on inspection.

Assessing the voice

Tactile vocal fremitus is appreciation of voice sounds by a palpating hand: vocal resonance, which used the stethoscope to pick up the same voice sounds, yields the same results. Most physicians rarely use tactile vocal fremitus, preferring the more easily assessable vocal resonance.

Other signs

Air may enter the subcutaneous tissue (usually with a tension pneumothorax or in association with therapeutic chest needling) causing swelling and a curious crackling sensation on palpation of the skin.

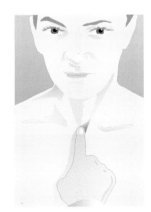

Fig. 4 **Palpation to ascertain the position of the trachea.**

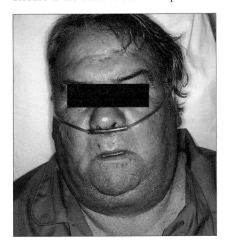

Fig. 3 **A typical 'blue bloater'.**

Respiratory examination (I)

- A full sputum pot suggests bronchiectasis.
- An empty sputum pot in a patient with chronic respiratory symptoms suggests a non-respiratory aetiology, an interstitial pulmonary process or asthma.
- Chronic chest conditions may cause secondary right ventricular failure – cor pulmonale.
- Crackles or wheezes may occur in patients with a normal chest X-ray: believe your stethoscope.

RESPIRATORY EXAMINATION (II)

PERCUSSION

Percussion is a method of assessing the state of underlying tissue by the quality of the elicited sound. The most effective way to produce a satisfactory sound is to percuss the midpoint of the middle finger of the left hand (just distal to the proximal interphalangeal joint) with the tip of the middle finger of the right hand. The right hand should remain firm, but not rigid and the percussing action is fulfilled by letting gravity flex the right wrist (Fig. 1). The percussing finger should only be in contact with the percussed finger for a brief time to avoid obscuring the note produced. Percussion produces:

- a resonant note over normal lungs
- a hyperresonant note over air (in a pneumothorax)
- a lower frequency 'dull' note over consolidated lung
- a very low frequency ('stony dullness') over fluid.

The chest should be percussed systematically and symmetrically, with particular attention to the comparison between notes obtained at symmetrical points either side of the chest. Percusssion is best performed with the percussing finger lying along the rib interspace because there is an easily audible difference between a percussion note obtained over a rib and percussion in the space between the ribs. Direct percussion of the chest without the examiner's finger interposed is useful but it may cause the patient discomfort and it may not be easy to tell whether you are percussing between or over ribs. Percuss in two bands down the front of the chest, then percuss each axilla, and finish by percussing the back of the chest (Fig. 2).

Never forget to percuss in the supraclavicular fossae and the clavicles, beneath which is the classical site for secondary complex tuberculosis. When percussing the back of the chest it helps if the patient's arms are folded across the front of the chest, as this moves the scapulae laterally.

In thin individuals it is possible to assess movement of the diaphragms. With the patient taking normal breaths, percussion is performed down the patient's back until the percussion note becomes dull. The patient then takes a slow deep breath. If the diaphragm is moving normally, the initially dull note will become more resonant as the lungs descend. A paralysed diaphragm will be sucked upwards as the

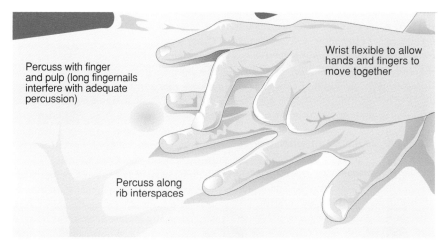

Percuss with finger and pulp (long fingernails interfere with adequate percussion)

Wrist flexible to allow hands and fingers to move together

Percuss along rib interspaces

Fig. 1 **The technique of percussion.**

Compare right and left at each level

Do not forget to percuss the clavicles

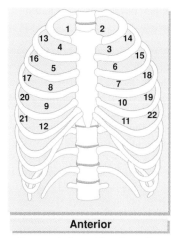

Anterior

Percuss in two strips down the anterior chest (the numbered order is the most logical)

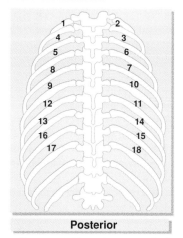

Posterior

Percuss in the order suggested, then percuss each side from above downwards

Fig. 2 **Pattern of percussion of the chest.**

chest wall expands, and thus the percussion note will remain dull, and may indeed be duller higher than previously (Fig. 3).

AUSCULTATION

Some physicians listen for lung sounds using only the bell of the stethoscope whereas others prefer the diaphragm. Sense dictates using the diaphragm to listen for high-pitched sounds and the bell for lower- pitched sounds. The sites for auscultation should be those of percussion, again not omitting the supraclavicular fossae. Vocal resonance is elicited by asking the patient to say '99'. With consolidation, the '99' is increased in volume compared with normal, but with pleural fluid, pneumothorax or pleural thickening it is reduced. Whispering pectriloquy is also found. Ask the patient to breath with an open mouth. Do not ask a patient to take a deep breath if there is obviously a chest infection (this is guaranteed to evoke a coughing bout), but rather ask the patient to take a moderate breath and ideally demonstrate how you want him/her to breathe.

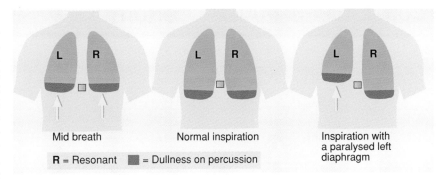

Mid breath   Normal inspiration   Inspiration with a paralysed left diaphragm

R = Resonant   ■ = Dullness on percussion

Fig. 3 **Explanation of the findings when a diaphragm is paralysed.**

EXAMINATION OF THE BREASTS

Examination of the breasts has been included in the respiratory section because routine breast examination almost invariably is performed along with examination of the respiratory system.

The patient should be undressed to the waist and examined in a good light (to avoid embarrassment a preliminary explanation is mandatory). On inspection note any asymmetry or local abnormality of nipple or skin.

Various positions assist palpation (Fig. 4):

- the patient hands resting on her hips (underlying pectoralis major muscle relaxed)

- the patient's pressing on her hips with elbows pointing outwards, or the arms raised above the head (pectoralis major muscle contracted in both positions)

- the patient leaning forward such that the breasts are pendulous

- the patient lying flat on her back.

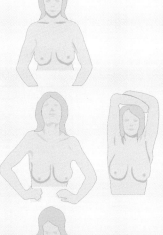

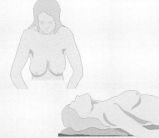

Fig. 4 **Various positionings of the patient which may assist breast palpation.**

Each of the breast quadrants and the axillary tail should be examined with the four fingers of the examining hand providing a single palpating surface which should be moved with a slight rotatory action (enabling edges of any swelling to be detected).

Swellings

Any focal palpable swellings should be further characterized according to the scheme for examination of swellings detailed on page 6, particularly noting mobility, fixation or tethering of the skin. The axillae and supraclavicular fossae should also be examined to detect associated lymph node enlargement.

The multiple small nodules of fibrocystic disease 'chronic cystic mastitis' usually cannot be palpated with the flat of the hand. Fibrocystic disease tends to be bilateral and comprises numerous small nodular areas which are firm, rubbery, well-circumscribed, possibly tender and easily moved short distances in the breast. Do not forget that fibrocystic disease and carcinoma may both be present.

Breast abscesses are usually associated with nipple changes and usually occur during lactation, especially if there are cracked nipples. The breast becomes engorged and tender, and a very tender focal area of swelling results.

Suspect carcinoma if there is a palpable firm or hard swelling which is non-tender. Tethering of the skin, skin retraction, infiltration of the skin (giving an orange-skin-like stippled appearance), a bloodstained nipple discharge or impaired mobility demand further investigation. Later skin nodules or ulceration may develop. Paget's disease (a chronic eczematous appearance) of the nipple is caused by intraductal carcinoma.

Discharge

A minimal discharge from the nipple may be normal in pregnancy or lactation. Breast infections may cause a purulent discharge from the nipple. Carcinoma, particularly intraductal carcinoma, may cause a bloodstained discharge. Any discharge in the absence of lactation should be treated with suspicion.

Respiratory examinations (II)

- Do not forget to percuss and auscultate in the supraclavicular fossae.
- One woman in 13 will develope breast carcinoma.

- Patients who obviously have a chest infection should be asked to take moderate breaths – deep breaths usually precipitate a coughing bout.

COMMON RESPIRATORY CONDITIONS

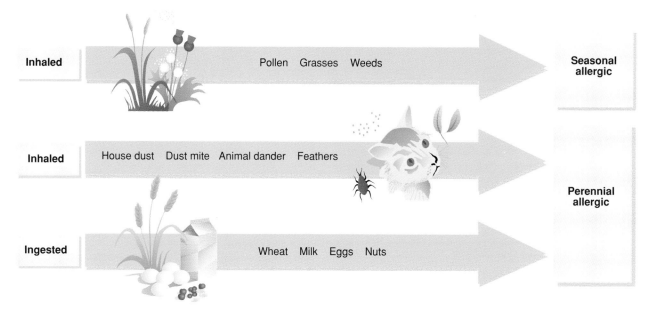

Fig. 1 **Common allergens that can trigger attacks.**

ASTHMA

Asthma is difficult to define: 'a reversible airways obstruction not caused by other disease'. Extrinsic asthma is precipitated by exposure to allergens such as pollens or external irritants (Fig. 1). Intrinsic asthma is triggered by known or unknown internal factors. Symptoms of asthma include wheezing, difficulty in breathing, chest tightness, shortness of breath or cough.

On examination, patients may be only slightly inconvenienced or may be fighting for breath with an increased respiratory rate and wheezing. Patients may prefer to sit up or lean forward to enable effective use of accessory muscles of respiration. Pulsus paradoxus (p. 23) may be evident. On auscultation the breath sounds are prolonged in expiration and wheezes are audible. Clinical signs should be symmetrical unless there is a complicating pneumothorax, pulmonary collapse, or pneumonia.

In a severe attack patients may:

- be unable to speak
- be cyanosed
- be confused or lethargic.

In such circumstances breath sounds may be much diminished because of poor air entry and mucous plugging of airways. Thus, the absence of wheezing in a patient with asthma is an ominous sign. With chronic asthma there may be chest deformity (Fig. 2) and, not uncommonly, signs of hypercortisolism caused by corticosteroid therapy.

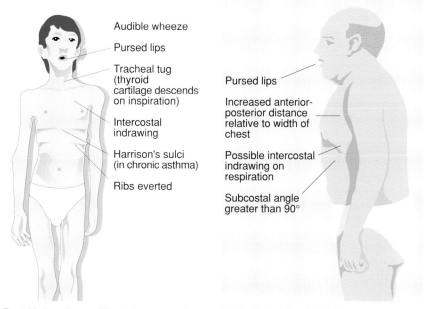

Fig. 2 **Various abnormalities that may occur in a child with chronic asthma.**

Fig. 3 **Clinical signs in COAD.**

ACUTE BRONCHITIS

Acute bronchitis is acute inflammation of the bronchial tree. There may be a history of previous attacks, exposure to air pollutants or smoking. Initially there may be upper respiratory tract symptoms (coryza, sore throat), and an initially unproductive cough. Later sputum is produced but if secondary bacterial infection supervenes the sputum becomes purulent.

On examination there may be fever and prolonged expiratory breath sounds with bilateral symmetrical wheezes on auscultation. Crackles may be heard but these usually imply additional inflammation of non-bronchial tissue and thus may indicate pneumonia, pulmonary oedema or bronchiectasis.

CHRONIC OBSTRUCTIVE AIRWAYS DISEASE (COAD)

COAD is a descriptive term indicating a generalized airways obstruction which is only partially reversible. The major causes are chronic bronchitis and/or emphysema.

The history is variable, often with a smokers' cough with occasional wheezing, followed by progressive exertional dyspnoea and associated right-heart strain possibly culminating in symptoms and signs of right-sided heart failure (cor pulmonale).

The findings on examination (Fig. 3) are variable but respiratory outflow obstruction is characteristic (clinically manifest as an inability to exhale totally within 4 seconds). Later a barrel-shaped chest develops. Such patients often learn to breathe with pursed lips to keep end-expiratory pressure high. Cyanosis may develop with plethora if there is secondary overproduction of the oxygen carrying red blood cells (polycythaemia) in response to hypoxaemia.

CHRONIC BRONCHITIS

Chronic bronchitis is said to exist when there is a chronic recurrent cough with expectoration, persisting for more than 3 months each year for a minimum of 2 years. As respiratory function declines some patients eschew cyanosis and hyperventilate ('pink puffers') but others surrender to cyanosis and do not hyperventilate ('blue bloaters'). If there is carbon dioxide retention there may be a flapping tremor of the outstretched hands. The peripheries may be warm with a full bounding pulse caused by carbon dioxide induced vasodilatation.

EMPHYSEMA

Emphysema is a permanent abnormal enlargement of part or all of the alveoli (the gas exchange part of the lung) with destruction of lung tissue. The history is of shortness of breath, and on examination there may be reduced chest expansion and diminution of the normal areas of heart and liver dullness to percussion (caused by the interposed hyperinflated lung). It is not possible to make an unequivocal diagnosis of emphysema purely on clinical grounds.

INFLUENZA

In influenza the history is distinctive with:

- abrupt onset fever
- malaise
- shivering
- a hacking cough
- musculoskeletal aches and pains
- an irritated throat
- slight nasal discharge.

Most 'flu-like' illnesses are not influenza-like (a streaming head cold is not a

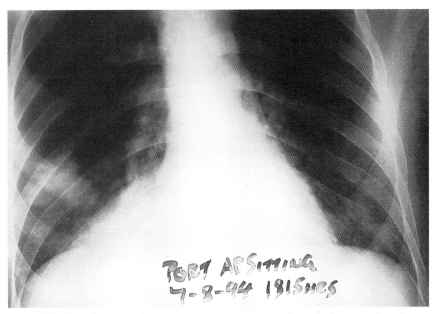

Fig. 4 **CXR of bronchopneumonia.** There is patchy shadowing and the patient had a cough productive of purulent sputum.

feature of influenza). On examination there may be signs of acute bronchitis or pneumonia.

LARYNGITIS

Usually there is a barking cough, hoarseness and possible laryngeal tenderness.

PNEUMONIA

Pneumonia is inflammation of the lung with alveolar involvement, usually caused by microorganisms. Classical streptococcal lobar pneumonia presents with a few hours history of fever, a dryish cough (occasionally with rusty coloured sputum), shortness of breath, and pleuritic-type chest pain. On examination there are signs of consolidation, and later signs of complicating pleural fluid may develop. Classical bronchopneumonia (Fig. 4) often starts as an acute bronchitis but fever and discoloured sputum develop.

Coarse crackles, usually bilateral, may be heard.

Atypical pneumonia is a term which refers to interstitial pneumonias usually with minimal (clear) sputum production. Clinical signs are less than a chest X-ray would suggest and extrapulmonary manifestations (such as headache, diarrhoea, vomiting and cerebral dysfunction) are often found. Symptoms specific to the respiratory tract may occur late in the course of the illness. Causes of atypical pneumonia include mycoplasma infection, Q fever, psittacosis, Legionnaire's disease and viral pneumonias.

Pneumocystis pneumonia in HIV infection usually presents as progressive shortness of breath developing over weeks rather than days, as there is interference with oxygen transfer to the pulmonary capillaries. Usually cough is not prominent and sputum production is minimal. Progressive decrease in exercise tolerance is typical.

Common respiratory conditions

- Absence of wheezes on auscultation is an ominous sign in asthma.
- Influenza should not be diagnosed in a patient returning from a malarial area until blood films are negative.
- Pneumocystis pneumonia does not present like a typical or atypical pneumonia. It usually presents with progressive shortness of breath and decreasing exercise tolerance.
- Carbon dioxide retention causes vasodilation with full bounding pulses and warm peripheries.
- With atypical pneumonias the chest X-ray is often more dramatic than clinical examination would suggest.
- Causes of atypical pneumonias include mycoplasma infection, Q fever, psittacosis, Legionnaire's disease and viral pneumonias.

ABDOMINAL SYMPTOMS (I)

INTRODUCTION

The alimentary system is a multifunctional tube comprising the lips, mouth, oropharynx, oesophagus, stomach, duodenum, jejunum, ileum, caecum, appendix, colon, rectum and anus. The liver, gallbladder and pancreas are included in this account. Urological and genital causes for abdominal symptoms or signs are detailed on pages 66 and 60–63 respectively. The intra-abdominal contents are shown in Figure 1.

The questions that could be asked routinely are shown in Table 1. In the following account history and examination are occasionally dealt with together to avoid separation of related features.

ABDOMINAL PAIN (Fig. 2)

Aortic pain

Aortic pain is usually severe and may have a tearing component especially if associated with an expanding, leaking, or dissecting aneurysm. Abdominal pain is usually most marked in the back and, especially with dissecting aneurysms, may originate in the chest and spread downwards to the legs.

Anal pain

Anal pain is usually well localized and most often caused by fissures or piles. It is exacerbated by defaecation. Anal fissures are narrow splits in the perianal skin, usually in the midline posteriorly, which extend towards the anal edge where a 'sentinel' pile may be found. Fissures are characteristically very painful.

Appendix pain

Classically a persistent pain starts in the central abdomen and then localizes to the right lower quadrant.

Biliary tract pain

Biliary tract pain is predominantly felt in the right upper quadrant, possibly radiating towards the midline; it may also be referred to the region of the right scapula. Often the pain is a minor discomfort but, especially if a gallstone is passing down the biliary tract, biliary colic may result. The main characteristic of biliary colic is that it is *not* colicky, but rather a rapid onset pain which crescendos over about 15 minutes, remains constant for a variable period of time, and diminuendos.

Bladder pain

Bladder pain is a midline suprapubic pain often associated with frequency, dysuria, or other symptoms of urinary tract infec-

Table 1 **Major questions that could be asked concerning gastrointestinal pathology**

Question	Detail
Appetite	Good/bad. Recent alteration? Specific food intolerance?
Weight	Loss/gain/steady? How much over how long?
Dysphagia	Any difficulty swallowing? Caused by pain or by sticking? What type of food? Perceived situation of blockage? When does it happen? Does regurgitation occur?
Diet	Include questions about drugs (especially purgatives, gastric irritant drugs, antibiotics and steroids)
Alcohol consumption	See page 5
Abdominal pain/dyspepsia/indigestion	Situation? Radiation? Associations? Effect of food? Effect of antacids? Effect of bowel movements?
Vomiting	How much? How often? Content? Any blood or coffee ground material?
Abdominal distension	Pain? Vomiting? Bowel movements reduced/absent? Passage of flatus?
Diarrhoea	How often? Small or large amounts often? Blood? Mucous? Pus? Associated symptoms? Recent travel abroad?
Jaundice	Previous episodes? Associated pain? Duration? Urine colour change? Stool colour change? Feverishness?
Stool	Diarrhoea? Constipation? Melaena?

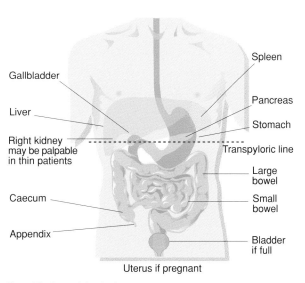

Fig. 1 **The intra-abdominal contents.** The position of most of the viscera is variable.

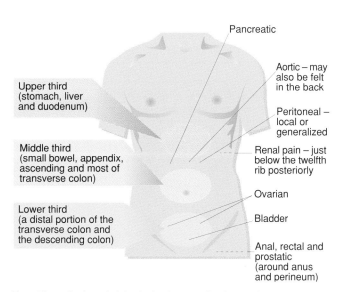

Fig. 2 **The main sites of abdominal pain emanating from various organs.** Pain derived from each third of the gut is localized appropriately.

tion. Uncomplicated bladder inflammation (cystitis), unlike renal tissue inflammation (pyelonephritis) does not usually cause fever or renal pain. Acute retention of urine is usually very painful and palpation is resisted by the patient.

Colic

A colicky pain is a squeezing pain which varies in intensity. Patients often indicate the squeezing nature by clenching their fist. Colic almost invariably denotes abnormality in hollow organs including gut, ureters or Fallopian tubes.

Gastric and duodenal pain

Gastric and duodenal pains are often ill-defined upper abdominal pains which may be felt in the back and which tend to occur at regular times in relationship to meals. The pain is often described as gnawing and may be relieved (or exacerbated) by meals and relieved by antacids.

Duodenal pain is occasionally localized by the patient pointing precisely to the xiphisternal area. Pain when the stomach is empty, especially pain that wakens the patient at night, is suggestive of duodenal lesions. Traditionally pain exacerbated by food is gastric and relieved by food is duodenal. With the advent of endoscopy, it has become apparent that most of the above are fallible generalizations.

Pain radiating to the back suggests posterior penetration of a gastric or duodenal ulcer.

If an ulcer perforates there is an abrupt change in the nature of the pain with pain becoming generalized unless the perforation is small and localized.

'Dyspepsia' means whatever the patient thinks it means. Always define what the patient means by complaints such as 'indigestion, tummy ache, gastritis' etc.

Hepatic pain

Damage to the liver tissue does not give rise to pain: it is the stretching of various other tissues, notably the hepatic capsule, which causes pain. Hepatic pain is usually a mild diffuse right upper quadrant discomfort, but if the capsule is stretched rapidly (by acute hepatitis or heart failure for example) pain may be severe.

Large intestinal pain

Large intestinal (colonic) pain tends to be felt predominantly in the central abdomen if the ascending or transverse colon is the source whereas descending colonic pain may be felt in the lower abdomen in the midline below the umbilicus.

Oesophageal pain

Oesophageal pain is midline and retrosternal, occasionally simulating cardiac pain. It may radiate to the back or down the arms in a similar fashion to myocardial pain (the autonomic sensory supplies are at the same spinal cord level).

Oesophageal pain is made worse when hot or bulky foods are swallowed.

Heartburn is a warm burning sensation in the chest caused by regurgitation of gastric acid into the oesophagus when the cardia (the lower end of the oesophagus) is incompetent (possibly in association with a hiatus hernia). Predictably heartburn is made worse by lying down, relieved by standing, or by alkali.

Achalasia is spasm of the lower end of the oesophagus with loss of peristalsis and failure of the cardia to relax. Pain is retrosternal, may be severe, and occurs in bouts. It may be sufficiently severe to simulate angina or myocardial infarction, and, confusingly, may be relieved by trinitrin.

Ovarian pain

The characteristics of ovarian pain are detailed on page 63.

Pancreatic pain

Pancreatic pain is felt in the upper quadrants and usually also in the back. Pain may be worse when the patient is lying down (as the pancreas is 'indented' by the spine) and relieved by bending forwards. The pain of acute pancreatitis (usually secondary to alcohol abuse or biliary tract disease) is a severe constant pain which may simulate perforation or other intra-abdominal emergency.

Peritoneal pain

Peritoneal pain is caused by irritation of the peritoneum. Focal irritation produces localized pain but generalized peritonitis with generalized irritation produces generalized pain. There is rebound tenderness.

Prostatic pain

Prostatic pain is predominantly perineal and possibly associated with other prostatic symptoms. A loaded rectum or a digital rectal examination may exacerbate discomfort. The findings on rectal examination are detailed on page 55.

Rectal pain

Rectal pain is usually well localized. Proctalgia fugax is a dramatic, abrupt onset, severe pain which is attributed to cramp of pelvic floor muscles.

Renal pain

Renal pain is mostly associated with stretching or irritation of the renal capsule. Classically there is a constant pain and tenderness to percussion in the back just below the 12th rib. Pain may occasionally radiate downwards in 'ureteric' fashion.

Small intestinal pain

Small intestinal pain is colicky and periumbilical when due to inflammatory or infective causes.

Small intestinal colic tends to have more frequent variations in intensity than does large intestinal colic. If there is an impaired blood supply there may be mesenteric angina with pain after eating which lasts until the demand for extra blood for the gut is over (usually for an hour or two after eating). Terminal ileal pain tends to be localized to the right lower quadrant.

Complete arterial blockage with intestinal infarction causes sudden onset central abdominal pain with circulatory collapse.

Splenic pain

Splenic pain is a left upper quadrant pain which may vary as the spleen moves with respiration. Splenic infarction, which occurs particularly in sickle cell disease (an inherited blood disease) gives rise to pain if it involves the splenic capsule.

Ureteric pain (renal colic)

Ureteric pain is a sudden onset, almost invariably unilateral, severe pain possibly with periodic exacerbations, felt in the lateral abdomen. It radiates downwards towards the external genitalia and makes the patient writhe with agony.

Uterine pain

The characteristics of uterine pain are detailed on page 63.

Abdominal symptoms (I)

- The aetiology of pain is often initially revealed by associated symptoms, not by the signs on examination.
- Biliary colic is not colicky.
- Fever and lateralized loin pain suggest pyelonephritis rather than simple cystitis.
- Achalasia may be relieved by trinitrin.

ABDOMINAL SYMPTOMS (II)

OTHER GASTROINTESTINAL TRACT SYMPTOMS

Abnormal stools

Always consider the possibility of underlying neoplasia. Progressive narrowing of the stool occurring over weeks suggests a stenosing lesion of the lower intestine. Hard pellet-like stools, possible alternating with vague looseness of the stool, may be a feature of the irritable bowel syndrome. Tarry black stools suggest melaena—stools which consist of altered partially digested blood (which, if from a brisk upper gastrointestinal tract bleed, has a characteristic smell). Treatment with iron also causes dark stools.

Stools associated with malabsorption are foul smelling, pale, bulky and contain excessive fat. They may therefore float in the lavatory pan.

Ask about changes in the character of the stool:

- changes in calibre
- changes in colour
- changes in odour
- changes in bulk
- stools which are greasy
- stools which are difficult to flush away.

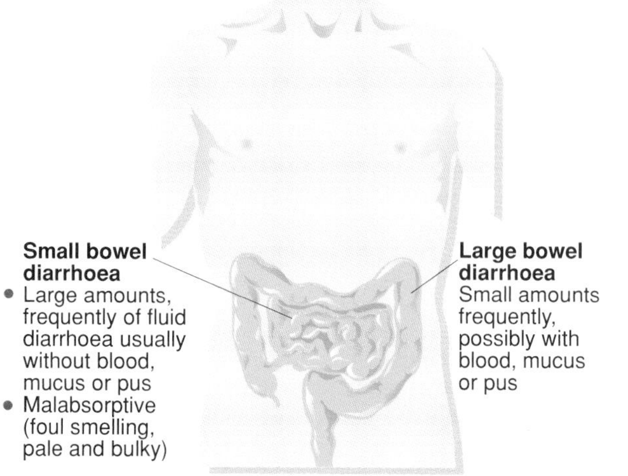

Small bowel diarrhoea
- Large amounts, frequently of fluid diarrhoea usually without blood, mucus or pus
- Malabsorptive (foul smelling, pale and bulky)

Large bowel diarrhoea
Small amounts frequently, possibly with blood, mucus or pus

Fig. 1 **Differentiation between large and small bowel diarrhoea.** Fever is usually associated if either type of diarrhoea is caused by an inflammatory process (including invasive infections). There is usually no fever if the diarrhoea is caused by a toxin-mediated process because there is usually no associated tissue inflammation.

Appetite change

Gastrointestinal causes of poor appetite include pain, gastritis, gastrointestinal malignancy, and prodromal hepatitis. A poor appetite may also occur in many other conditions including social or psychiatric disorders (alcoholism, depression, anorexia nervosa).

Constipation

Constipation is difficult or infrequent passage of stools. This may be a lifelong affliction but, if bowel habit changes are recent, an explanation is required. Causes of constipation include anatomical intestinal obstruction, paralytic ileus, stenosing lesions of the gut, dehydration, or painful anal conditions. Constipation may be a response to changes in appetite, diet, drugs or general health.

Diarrhoea

Diarrhoea is the excessive passage of fluid stools (Fig. 1). The small intestine is (second only to the kidneys) responsible for bodily fluid balance: small intestinal diarrhoea is thus watery and rarely contains blood, mucus, or pus. Large intestinal diarrhoea is often caused by processes which irritate the large intestinal wall so that the large intestine cannot fulfil its major function as a reservoir. Thus large intestinal diarrhoea usually comprises frequent passage of small amounts of stool which may contain blood, mucus, or pus.

Dysphagia

Dysphagia is painful or difficult swallowing. Complaints of food sticking in the gullet in the presence of normal mastication is a symptom that demands a definitive diagnosis.

Dysphagia caused by inflammatory conditions (which are often easily treated) is often painful (Fig. 2) whereas non-painful dysphagia may be caused by non-inflammatory conditions, notably neoplasms.

If the oesophagus is narrowed, difficulty will initially be in swallowing large boluses of inflexible foods such as meat: a rapid progression to difficulty with fluids suggests progressive malignant obstruction. Other causes of dysphagia (usually of slower onset) include peptic ulceration with fibrotic stenosis, or the (Plummer–Vinson) triad of iron deficiency anaemia, glossitis, and an oesophageal web. An oesophageal diverticulum (an outpouching of the oesophagus) may fill with food and

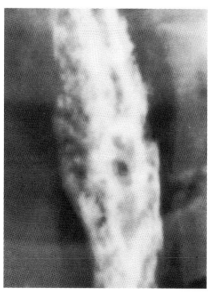

Fig. 2 **X-ray of severe oesophageal candida in an AIDS patient.** Dysphagia is typically very painful.

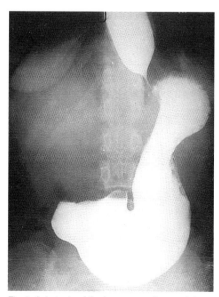

Fig. 3 **Achalasia of the lower oesophagus giving rise to the classical 'rat's tail appearance'.** Malignancies tend to have abrupt 'shouldering'.

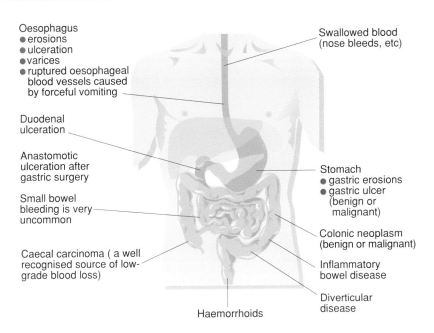

Oesophagus
● erosions
● ulceration
● varices
● ruptured oesophageal
  blood vessels caused
  by forceful vomiting

Duodenal
ulceration

Anastomotic
ulceration after
gastric surgery

Small bowel
bleeding is very
uncommon

Caecal carcinoma (a well
recognised source of low-
grade blood loss)

Swallowed blood
(nose bleeds, etc)

Stomach
● gastric erosions
● gastric ulcer
  (benign or
   malignant)

Colonic neoplasm
(benign or malignant)

Inflammatory
bowel disease

Diverticular
disease

Haemorrhoids

Fig. 4 **Common sources of gastrointestinal bleeding.**

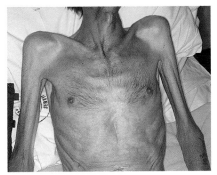

Fig. 5 **Severe weight loss in a patient with two infections—AIDS and tuberculosis.**

compress the oesophagus causing dysphagia in which gurgling and a visible swelling in the neck may provide clues.

Achalasia (Fig. 3) is a disease of unknown aetiology with slowly progressive diminution of lower oesophageal peristalsis which usually presents with a long history of progressive, initially intermittent, dysphagia. Retrosternal pain may be associated with oesophageal contractions.

Gastrointestinal bleeding

Although a brisk upper gastrointestinal bleed may cause gastrointestinal hurry and passage of relatively fresh blood from the rectum, the presence of blood in or on the stool usually implies large intestinal problems. Often the brighter the blood the lower is its source. Blood mixed in with the stool implies a relatively proximal site of bleeding.

Gastrointestinal bleeding may be caused by a number of conditions (Fig. 4) including ulcers (benign or malignant), oesophagitis, gastric erosions, duodenitis, neoplasia or oesophageal tears after bouts of vomiting (the Mallory-Weiss syndrome).

Irritable bowel syndrome

Patients (who are usually young and usually female) have colonic type pain, typically in the region of the sigmoid colon, in association with episodic constipation or diarrhoea. The diarrhoea of irritable bowel syndrome is not a high volume fluid diarrhoea; it is rather a sense of urgency to pass frequent small stools (which may be formed, pellety, or slightly loose).

Patients complain of pain, constipation, or a sensation of incomplete defaecation. Some patients may pass mucus but bleeding is *not* a feature of the irritable bowel syndrome. Patients may have an enhanced gastrocolic reflex in which distension of the stomach by food precipitates colicky type bowel pain.

On examination patients may have a tender descending colon. One variant of irritable bowel syndrome is painless diarrhoea usually occurring after rising in the morning or after taking food.

Vomiting

Vomiting may be caused by upper gastrointestinal pathology including

Table 1 Conditions that can cause vomiting and clues from the history or examination

Condition	Clues
Gastroenteritis	Fever, others affected
Food poisoning (toxins)	No fever, short incubation period
Obstruction	Abdominal distension
Faulty infant feeding	Dietary history
Infantile pyloric stenosis	Projectile vomiting, Age of patient, Pyloric swelling palpable
Hypotension	Measure the blood pressure
Peptic ulcer	Previous history
Pyloric stenosis (adult)	At each occasion vomiting of several previous meals
Gastritis	History of alcohol abuse?
Pregnancy	Think of diagnosis!

peptic ulceration, gastritis, malignancies, or stenosing lesions affecting the stomach or duodenum, or intestinal obstruction. Vomiting can be a non-specific response to pain or severe illness. Some conditions that can cause vomiting and various clues from the history are detailed in Table 1.

Waterbrash

Waterbrash is sudden regurgitation of fluid from the oesophagus into the mouth which may occur in gastroeosophageal reflux and other upper gastrointestinal problems.

Weight loss

The patient's weight is a non-specific indicator of health. Before investigating weight loss always ascertain that weight loss has occurred (refer to old notes if necessary).

Weight loss may result from:

● inadequate diet
● malabsorption
● excessive excretion of energy sources
  (e.g. diabetic glycosuria)
● excessive metabolism (e.g. in prolonged fever or thyrotoxicosis)
● occult malignancy or infection (Fig. 5).

Rapid weight loss (over hours) is usually caused by fluid loss and conversely rapid weight gain implies fluid retention.

Abdominal symptoms (II)

● Stool characteristics are an important but often neglected topic.
● Dysphagia may be caused by pain or difficulty in swallowing; painful dysphagia is likely to be inflammatory in aetiology.
● Bleeding is not a feature of irritable bowel syndrome.
● Weight loss should be confirmed (by previous notes) if possible.

PRINCIPLES OF EXAMINATION (I)

Abominal examination is best performed with the patient lying comfortably and relaxed on the back, arms by the sides and preferably breathing through the mouth. It may be helpful to have the patient flex the knees and hips which allows the abdominal muscles to relax (Fig. 1). The examining doctor should be comfortable and relaxed, and this may mean that either the bed should be raised or that the examiner should kneel by the bedside. The examiner should have warm hands to avoid reflex muscle tensing by the patient.

INSPECTION

After general inspection of the patient and his/her immediate environment, inspect the abdomen to check the following:

- Does it move freely when the patient breathes?
- Does the patient obviously have abdominal pain?
- Does the patient have peritoneal irritation in which abdominal movements are minimized?
- Are there scars from previous surgery?
- Is there obvious abdominal distension?
- Are there dilated veins?
- Is there visible peristalsis?
- Is there any other visible abnormality?

Generalized distension is classically caused by fat, fluid, fetus, or flatus, whereas the causes of localized swellings include hernia, or specific organ enlargement. With generalized abdominal distension, particularly if caused by ascites, the umbilicus may be filled in or protruberant.

Other abnormalities on inspection may include small red maculopapular spots of no significance (Campbell de Morgan spots), and signs of pancreatitis such as periumbilical bruising (Cullen's sign) or bruising of the back of the abdomen (Gray Turner's sign).

Visible peristalsis (waves of intestinal contractions) may be seen in normal thin individuals, but otherwise is only seen proximal to obstructing lesions of the gut.

Dilated veins may be seen if blood returning from the gut to the liver cannot pass through the liver because of raised pressure or thrombosis in the portal vein (which drains blood from the gut

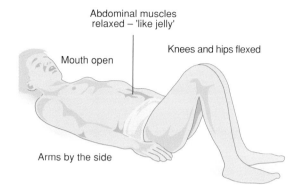

Fig. 1 **Flexion of the knees and hips to assist abdominal examination.**

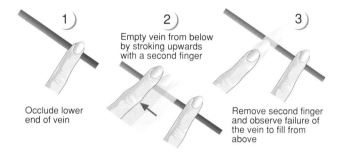

Fig. 2 **Procedure to demonstrate blood flow in dilated abdominal veins.** Repeat the procedure but stroke downwards from the first finger with the second finger, then lift the second finger and observe filling of the vein from below.

into the liver). The blood flow in the dilated veins will be away from the umbilicus, either upwards towards the superior vena caval system or downwards towards the inferior vena caval system.

If there is inferior vena caval obstruction the blood flow will be uniformly from below upwards to pass over the costal margin. Identify the upward direction of blood flow by obstructing the lower part of a vein with a finger, empty the vein by stroking the blood upwards with another finger, then observe failure of filling from above. To confirm upward blood flow reverse the procedure and lift the lower finger to observe filling of the empty vein from below (Fig. 2).

PALPATION

It is important to examine the abdomen systematically, especially if the patient has abdominal pain. Always ask the patient where the pain is maximal and examine this region last. Abdominal contents may be mobile, semi-solid, hidden behind other organs, on the posterior abdominal wall, have to be felt through abdominal muscles, or all five. As a result palpation is difficult to do well (even experienced doctors often hide their uncertainty by using terms such as 'equivocal' organomegaly).

Relaxation of the palpating hand is essential: this can be assisted by resting the palpating hand on the abdomen and providing the palpating pressure with the other hand (Fig. 3).

Palpate each quadrant in turn, initially without exerting much pressure but later palpate deeply (provided that no painful regions have been volunteered or identified). Then palpate specifically for certain organs (see p. 54).

When feeling for intra-abdominal organomegaly it is often sensible to feel for the edges rather than the 'body' of the organ in question—the contrast in consistency between the organ and the contiguous organs often being apparent only at the edges. Organ edges can be identified more easily if they can be made to move by having the patient take moderately deep breaths. When palpating for intra-abdominal organs that move on respiration do not plunge in the palpating hand when the

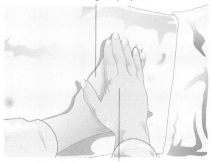

Fig. 3 **Palpation with the hand underneath concentrating on palpation whilst the overlying hand provides the palpating pressure.**

patient breathes in: rather allow the organ in question to move to touch your fingers.

Paradoxically when attempting palpation of organs that move on respiration it helps to ask patients to breathe out when you really want them to breathe in. Patients, especially male patients, often tense up their abdominal muscles when asked to take deep breaths in but hardly ever tense their abdominal muscles whilst taking in the necessary deep breath after a deep expiration.

If an organ or abnormal swelling does *not* move on respiration a gentle rotatory movement of the examiner's hand may be required to provide the relative movement.

When an abnormal swelling is detected, and providing palpation does not provoke pain, define its situation and character-istics (p. 6). If a swelling is pulsatile (suggesting an aneurysm) do not test for indentability.

Guarding is a reflex localized tense-ness of the abdominal muscles which cannot be abolished by a patient's conscious efforts. Guarding is a sign of peripheral peritoneal irritation or marked tenderness of an underlying organ. Confirm guarding by light percussion over the affected area.

PERCUSSION

Percussion may be valuable (especially in obese patients) to confirm suspected enlargement of certain organs, in particular the liver, spleen or bladder. Always percuss from areas of resonance to areas of dullness, with the examiner's percussed finger being parallel to the anticipated organ edge.

Shifting dullness is a stony dullness percussable below the horizontal surface of intraperitoneal fluid (ascites). It is best to elicit the shifting element on the opposite side to an enlarged liver or spleen in order to avoid their interfering with findings on percussion: for similar reasons the bladder should have been emptied before testing for ascites. Starting in the midline, position the percussed finger parallel to the expected fluid level and percuss laterally until the note becomes markedly dull, then return the percussed finger to the less dull area. Keeping the percussed finger in position, ask the patient to roll over gently towards the finger. Wait about

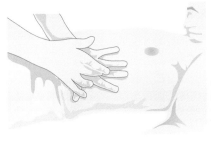 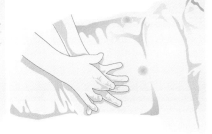

Percussed finger which stays on abdominal wall at position at which percussion becomes more resonant (above fluid level)

Position of percussed finger unchanged, now less resonant

Fig. 4 **Demonstration of ascites by detecting shifting dullness.**

20–30 seconds for any ascitic fluid to percolate downwards then percuss the finger again. If there is ascites the note should be markedly duller than that induced by the previous percussion (Fig. 4).

To elicit the fluid thrill of ascites the examiner rests a hand on one side of the abdomen and then taps the other side of the abdomen whereupon a fluid-transmitted shock wave is appreciated. In order to avoid detecting misleading impulses transmitted through the abdominal wall the edge of an assistant's (or the patient's) hand should be pressed gently along the midline. Occasionally in gross ascites the liver 'floats' within the abdomen and it may be possible for palpating fingers to 'tap' onto the liver.

AUSCULTATION

Only clinical experience can teach what are normal bowel sounds. An examiner may have to listen for several minutes before he can say confidently that bowel sounds are absent.
Increased bowel sounds may be found in:

- any cause of increased peristalsis
- bowel obstruction
- diarrhoeal illness
- if there is blood in the gut from an upper gastrointestinal haemorrhage (which causes intestinal hurry).

Reduced or absent bowel sounds are found in:

- intestinal paralysis (ileus)
- perforation
- generalized peritonitis.

Patients with severe abdominal pain due to gastroenteritis may simulate peritonitis but their overactive bowel sounds speak against generalized peritonitis (in which bowel sounds should be absent).

Aortic or femoral systolic bruits may be heard over aneurysmal or stenosed arteries. Always ascertain that such murmurs are not transmitted from the heart. Renal artery bruits may be heard in the lateral abdomen or in the back. Systolic bruits over the liver may be almost inaudible but may indicate vascular neoplasm, angioma, primary liver cancer or alcoholic hepatitis.

A continuous venous hum may indicate inferior vena caval obstruction or portal vein obstruction.

Hepatic or splenic rubs are uncommon but are important because they locate abnormal tissue.

A useful confirmatory sign of ascites is to request the patient to remain in the rolled over position, and to place a stethoscope in the midline of the abdomen. Then percuss the abdomen directly with a finger tip at points symmetrically equidistant from the midline. A marked difference in the sounds produced suggests a marked difference in sound propagating ability of the intra-abdominal contents, and thus implies the presence of ascites.

Principles of examination (I)

- Examine painful areas last.
- Organ edges are often easier to palpate than the organ 'body'.
- Allow organs that move on respiration to palpate your waiting fingers.
- Percuss for shifting dullness well away from enlarged intra-abdominal organs if possible.

PRINCIPLES OF EXAMINATION (II)

EXAMINATION FOR SPECIFIC ORGANS

Bladder swellings

A full bladder is usually palpable and percussable in the midline midway between the symphisis pubis and the umbilicus. One cannot get below a bladder and, unlike the uterus and other possible pelvic swellings, the bladder gets smaller after micturition. In bladder outflow obstruction the bladder may remain palpable after micturition. The size at which a palpable bladder becomes pathologically enlarged is variable but it would be unusual for a normal bladder to be palpable at or above the umbilicus.

Chronic overdistension of the bladder is usually painless and easily missed unless palpated for specifically. Palpate for the bladder by starting well above the umbilicus and move the palpating hand downwards with the index finger parallel to the expected bladder edge, and with the middle, ring and little finger being successively deeper (Fig. 1).

Colonic swellings

The palpability of the normal colon depends upon its contents and this depends upon the interrelationship between diet (input) and defaecation (output). The normal colon thus has a variable palpability and the persistence of any mass should be confirmed by palpation several hours later.

Colonic swellings may be caused by colonic distension (either focal or generalized) or by masses within the colonic lumen or wall.

Colonic masses may be fixed or mobile depending on their situation (caecal masses tend to be fixed but transverse colonic masses may be mobile). Multiple swellings along the line of the descending colon are likely to be faecal in nature. If intra-abdominal mass lesions are identifiable and 'squelshy' then they are usually either in the stomach or colon.

The kidneys

Normal kidneys are impalpable, except in thin patients in whom the lower pole of the right kidney may be felt.

Kidney swellings are usually felt lateral to the spine in the upper abdomen. Swellings usually have well-defined lower borders, and usually move slightly on respiration unless there is fixation to extrarenal tissue. Dullness on percussion rarely occurs (because of the interposition of more resonant tissues).

To palpate for kidney enlargement the examiner's left hand should support and push forward the back of the patient's abdomen and lower ribs on each side. The examiner's palpating hand should gradually ascend from the relevant lower quadrant whilst the patient takes moderate breaths; the examiner's palpating hand should be dipped inwards towards the end of each inspiration (Fig. 2).

The liver and gallbladder

An enlarged liver usually:

- is detected in the right upper quadrant
- may extend across to the left upper quadrant
- has a definable lower border
- is impossible to get above
- moves downwards on inspiration
- is dull to percussion.

Palpate for the liver (and gallbladder) with the patient lying on his back, relaxed, and taking moderate breaths through an open mouth. It is very helpful to have the patient flex his hips and knees. Start palpation in the right lower abdomen just lateral to the rectus sheath and move the palpating hand upwards 1 or 2 cm successively after each time the patient takes a breath in. Keep the index finger parallel to the expected liver edge with the middle, ring and little fingers successively deeper (you then get four chances of feeling the liver edge) (Fig. 3). Some physicians prefer to use their palpating hand 'finger tips first'.

If a swelling is felt below the rib cage then palpate laterally and medially to confirm that it is liver enlargement and not a palpable gallbladder. If the liver is enlarged a gentle circular motion with the fingers above the liver edge may reveal the presence of focal swellings within the liver or on its surface.

The gallbladder is usually found at the junction of the rectus sheath and the rib cage: a normal gallbladder cannot be felt. An enlarged gallbladder will have a rounded lower edge and, if the liver is also enlarged, there may be a shallow groove between the two. Gallbladder enlargement caused by bile duct blockage is usually painless whereas with any inflammatory cause (cholecystitis or empyema of the gallbladder, for example) the gallbladder

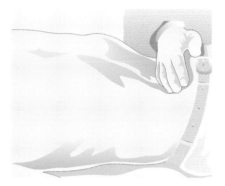
Fig. 1 **Palpation of the bladder.**

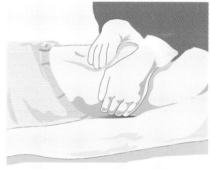
Fig. 2 **Palpation for an enlarged kidney.**

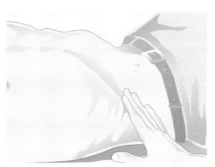
Fig. 3 **Palpating for a liver edge.** When the rib cage is approached by the palpating hand it is helpful to rest the index finger along the rib cage and to palpate with the middle, ring and little fingers.

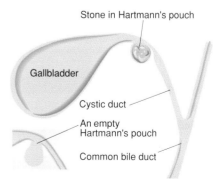

Stone in Hartmann's pouch

Gallbladder

Cystic duct

An empty Hartmann's pouch

Common bile duct

Fig. 4 **The mechanism of jaundice caused by a stone in Hartmann's pouch.**

is usually tender. Gallbladder tenderness will be worsened if a patient takes a deep breath against the examiner's palpating fingers (Murphy's sign).

Gallstones cause fibrosis of the gallbladder wall which prevents the gallbladder from enlarging if there is biliary tract obstruction. Thus an enlarged gallbladder in the presence of jaundice is unlikely to be caused by gallstone obstruction of the biliary tract—the only exception being a stone formed in Hartmann's pouch (Fig. 4).

Percussion may be used to identify the upper border of the liver. Percussion to delineate the upper and lower borders may be the only clinical way to identify a small (usually cirrhotic) liver.

The position of the lower edge of the liver may be confirmed by listening with a stethoscope over the right upper quadrant and stroking a fingernail from above downwards over the suspected liver edge. As the fingernail passes over the liver edge the note changes in quality.

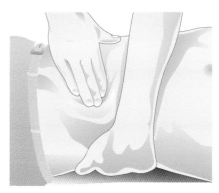

Fig. 5 **Use of the left hand to support the patient's ribs to assist splenic palpation.**

The pancreas and suprarenal glands

These organs, because of their position on the posterior abdominal wall, only become palpable when enlarged. As they are deep seated they tend to be less dull on percussion, unlike other solid intra-abdominal organs which are situated more anteriorly. Pancreatic masses tend to be fixed.

Splenic enlargement

An enlarged spleen moves from beneath the left costal margin towards the right lower abdomen. It is possible to feel below but not above a splenic swelling. The spleen is dull on percussion and a normally sized spleen should not be percussable anterior to the anterior axillary line. The spleen, unlike the kidney, moves easily on inspiration.

Commence palpation for the spleen in the right lower abdomen with the right hand index finger parallel to the possible spleen edge and with the middle, ring and little fingers successively deeper. Ask the patient to take moderate breaths and advance the palpating hand a centimetre or two towards the left costal margin each time the patient breathes out: traditionally the left ribs are simultaneously supported with the left hand (Fig. 5). Sometimes it is helpful to have a patient on the right side with the knees drawn up towards the chest. An enlarged spleen will touch your finger on inspiration and if there is a very enlarged spleen a notch may be felt in the medial border. As the left rib cage is approached it is useful to rest your right index finger along the rib cage and to palpate with the middle, ring, and little fingers (this avoids confusing the ribs with the spleen).

It should be stressed that palpation-induced rupture of an enlarged spleen is a possibility. Therefore restrict both the number and vigour of your attempts to feel the spleen.

The stomach

An empty stomach is impalpable. After a meal or drinking the stomach may be palpable in the left upper quadrant. Its edges will be smooth and a splash or gurgle may be heard if a palpating hand is suddenly withdrawn or the patient (gently) rolled from side to side. Alternatively the stethoscope can be used to listen over the stomach. The longer after a meal such a splash is heard, the more likely there is to be delayed gastric emptying.

Rectal examination

Rectal examination is an essential part of a comprehensive examination.

The procedure should be explained to the patient including the information that the examination should normally be no worse than the passage of a normal but constipated stool. The patient is traditionally examined in the left lateral position with the buttocks on the edge of the bed, and the knees tucked into the chest.

The anus is examined for evidence of skin lesions including the purplish coloration suggestive of Crohn's disease, fissures,

fistulae, skin tags, or haemorrhoids. A well-lubricated gloved index finger is then gently inserted with the finger pulp entering first. If there is reason to anticipate a painful examination a prior local analgesic lubricant or suppository would be indicated (pain may be caused by haemorrhoids, fissure, or anxiety).

If the anal sphincter is tight (often reflecting a tense personality) it can be useful to ask the patient to smile as this usually causes a temporary relaxation of the anal sphincter.

The walls of the normal anus and rectum should be tubular, smooth, non-tender, and soft. The major possible findings are shown in Figure 6. The findings related to the female genital tract and prostate are detailed on pages 64 and 61 respectively.

The examiner's finger should methodically feel laterally and then posteriorly, sweeping down the curve of the sacrum. In the female the cervix is felt anteriorly in the midline whereas in the male the prostate is felt anteriorly in the midline.

The faecal content of the rectum should be assessed. Diarrhoea or hard impacted stools are easily identified and the examiner's finger should be inspected for the presence of blood or mucus. If indicated the stool on the glove can be tested for occult blood.

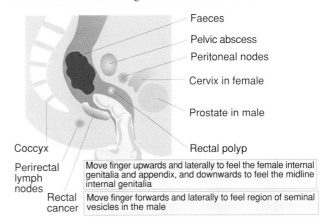

Faeces
Pelvic abscess
Peritoneal nodes
Cervix in female
Prostate in male
Rectal polyp

Coccyx
Perirectal lymph nodes
Rectal cancer

| Move finger upwards and laterally to feel the female internal genitalia and appendix, and downwards to feel the midline internal genitalia |
| Move finger forwards and laterally to feel region of seminal vesicles in the male |

Fig. 6 **Rectal examination.**

Principles of examination (II)

- Acute retention of urine is painful while chronic retention is often painless.
- Do not assume a mass in the right upper quadrant is the liver as it might be the gall bladder.
- The spleen should not be percussable anterior to the anterior axillary line.
- It is possible to rupture an enlarged spleen: palpate gently.

ABDOMINAL CONDITIONS

AORTIC ANEURYSM

Aneurysms in general are immobile, fixed and usually have smooth borders. The characteristic feature of an aneurysm is the expansile pulsation of a swelling which is larger in extent than expected of the normal blood vessel. Palpation using fingers of both hands is necessary to appreciate this expansion (Fig. 1). Once a pulsatile swelling has been identified examination should thereafter be exceptionally gentle as over-vigorous palpation may induce rupture. Swellings anterior to the aneurysm may exhibit transmitted pulsation, but such pulsation is never expansile.

Aortic aneurysms are more common in the elderly and may be felt in the midline or in any of the quadrants. The abdominal aorta may be tortuous without being aneurysmal and in this case the pulsatile swelling will not be expansile and will have a diameter in keeping with a normal-sized aorta. Systolic bruits may be heard over an aneurysm or over a tortuous aorta.

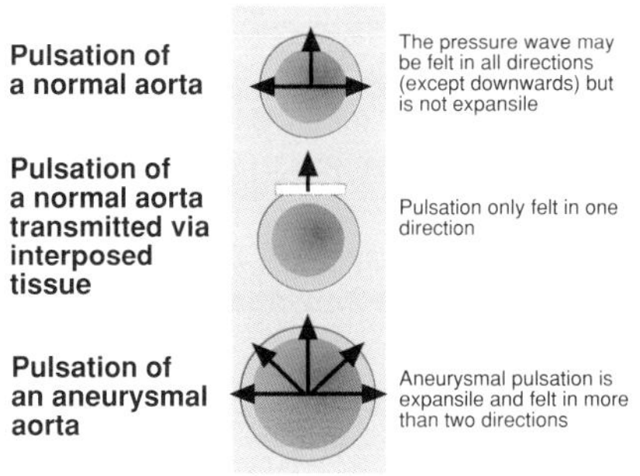

APPENDICITIS

Pain is classically persistent and commences in the central abdomen, thereafter localizing to the right lower quadrant. Constipation, rather than diarrhoea, is typical.

On examination there may be fever, signs of localized peritonitis with tenderness, rebound tenderness and guarding in the right lower quadrant maximal at McBurney's point (one third of the way along a line from the anterior superior iliac spine to the umbilicus). Extension of the right hip (the psoas sign) commonly causes pain by stretching the appendix. Symptoms and signs of appendicitis depend on the localization of the appendix – long appendices may lie almost anywhere in the abdomen.

ASCITES

Ascites is the presence of free fluid in the peritoneal cavity. The signs of ascites are:

- generalized abdominal distension
- shifting dullness (p. 53)
- a fluid thrill (p. 53)
- filling in or eversion of the umbilicus.

BOWEL OBSTRUCTION

Bowel obstruction may be partial or complete, mechanical or physiological (paralytic ileus), or secondary to bowel strangu-

Fig. 1 **Palpation of a pulsatile swelling to ascertain whether an aneurysm is present.**

lation and/or infarction. There will usually be vomiting, colicky abdominal pain and distension, perhaps with visible peristalsis proximal to the obstruction. Bowel sounds are increased, high pitched and 'tinkling'.

Proximal obstruction causes marked rapid onset vomiting which rapidly becomes malodourous and faeculent in nature. Abdominal distension tends to be mild whereas distal obstructions cause marked abdominal distension and less marked vomiting. Proximal obstruction causes a precipitous clinical decline because of rapid dehydration and electrolyte problems.

Large bowel obstruction is usually of slower onset, with abdominal distension more marked in the lateral abdomen (occasionally massively so as in twisting of the large bowel: a volvulus). Vomiting occurs later than in small bowel obstruction and pain is often less severe. With partial lower large bowel obstruction the stools may become smaller in quantity and calibre. In complete obstruction constipation is absolute and flatus is not passed.

Paralytic ileus is a physiological failure of gut peristalsis (not of mechanical aetiology) which produces abdominal distension and absent bowel sounds; visible peristalsis is never seen. A small amount of diarrhoea may 'run out' as fluid accumulates within the bowel lumen.

DIVERTICULOSIS

Diverticulae are small mucosal herniations through bowel wall muscle. Patients with diverticulosis are asymptomatic unless complications occur.

Diverticulitis is inflammation of diverticulae (usually of the sigmoid and descending colon), initially forming small abscesses which may discharge into the colon or may adhere to adjacent organs perhaps with fistula formation. On exami-

nation the patient with diverticulitis will usually be febrile, and have cramping pain and tenderness in the left lower quadrant. Symptoms may be caused in nearby organs by contiguous inflammation. Depending on the progression there may be signs of frank peritonitis or abscess formation. Diverticulitis is thus often likened to 'left-sided appendicitis'. Complications include obstruction, perforation with peritonitis, rectal bleeding and pelvic or subphrenic abscess formation.

FISTULA IN ANO

A fistula is a track opening onto two epithelial surfaces (sinuses only have one such opening). A fistula in ano is usually initiated by anorectal abscess formation. There is perianal purulent discharge and recurring abscess formation. Pain may be severe.

HAEMORRHOIDS (PILES)

Haemorrhoids are varicosities of the anal vascular cushions. Any cause of vascular congestion may precipitate symptoms. Bleeding from haemorrhoids is bright red, often present on toilet paper or, if bleeding is brisk, the lavatory pan may be dripped upon. Haemorrhoids which thrombose may present as perianal lumps. Pain may be severe.

Internal haemorrhoids are covered by mucous membrane, not skin. External haemorrhoids are small, purplish, skin-covered swellings which become more prominent when the patient strains. They may be asymptomatic unless thrombosed, when they become painful, bleed, and cause painful defaecation.

HERNIAS

Hernias are protrusions (usually of the bowel) out of the abdominal cavity at points of anatomical weakness (Fig. 2). Hernias which contain intestine are not resonant to percussion and do not transilluminate. They are made worse by raised intra-abdominal pressure and are (quite literally) brought out when the patient stands up or coughs. Non-incarcerated hernias may be returned to the abdominal cavity by gentle pressure whereas incarcerated hernias cannot be reduced. Common hernias include:

- *Femoral hernias* lie in the femoral canal below and lateral to the pubic tubercle.
- *Direct inguinal hernias* are found above

the inguinal ligament and do not extend into the scrotum.

- *Indirect inguinal hernias* push downwards through the internal inguinal ring and may travel down through the inguinal canal into the scrotum (or labium major in the female). Pressure over the mid-inguinal point will contain an indirect hernia but not a direct hernia.
- *Self-correcting umbilical hernias* are not uncommon in babies and occasionally persist.
- *Epigastric hernia* contain either intra-abdominal fat or bowel and may occur through a small defect in the midline linea alba tendon connecting the rectus abdominis muscles. In multiparous women the recti may divaricate (split apart) and abdominal contents herniate outwards.

LYMPH NODE ENLARGEMENT

Any abdominal swelling may be an enlarged lymph node and the clue to the nature of the swelling may be the finding of either lymph node enlargement elsewhere or associated splenomegaly. Always palpate for the inguinal and femoral lymph nodes. The inguinal nodes are found just below the inguinal ligament and the femoral (saphenous) nodes in the femoral triangle below.

PELVIC ABSCESS

There may have been clinical symptoms suggestive of an initiating gastrointestinal or gynaecological septic focus. Usually there is a soft, tender, occasionally appreciably warm, pelvic swelling that may bulge into the rectum. A mass may be palpable on rectal or vaginal examination.

PERFORATION OF THE GUT

Perforations may be localized and produce effects local to the perforation but 'free' perforations affect the whole of the peritoneal cavity and produce generalized peritonitis. The patient experiences a sudden, intense, non-colicky pain in the part of the abdomen relevant to the perforation, and the pain may spread rapidly to involve the whole abdomen, such that the patient has to lie still taking shallow breaths to avoid moving the abdominal contents.

On examination the abdominal muscles are rigid with tenderness and rebound tenderness and bowel sounds are much diminished or absent. Referred pain from irritated diaphragms may be felt in the shoulder tips.

Perforation into the lesser sack, intermittent small perforations, or prior steroid treatment may not result in classical signs of perforation.

PERIANAL ABSCESS

Perianal abscesses usually arise from infection of rectal and anal glands. They are painful and usually clinically obvious with perianal pain and swelling. Ischiorectal abscesses are more deeply situated with tenderness deep in the buttocks and on rectal examination. The patient is often fevered and unwell.

PERITONITIS

Localized peritonitis may occur secondary to inflammatory lesions such as diverticulitis or appendicitis.

Generalized peritonitis may occur spontaneously or secondary to abdominal organ sepsis or perforation of a viscus. Usually there is severe localized or diffuse abdominal pain. Spasmodic gut contractions (peristalsis) cease and abdominal distension develops possibly with nausea, vomiting, and sometimes diarrhoea.

On examination there is guarding, tenderness and rebound tenderness. Once generalized peritonitis is established systematic features emerge with fever, rigors, tachypnoea and tachycardia. Patients thereafter become dehydrated, acidotic and collapsed.

STRANGULATION OF A VISCUS

Strangulation is impairment of blood supply by a mechanical obstruction of supplying blood vessels. Classically the onset is rapid with severe pain. Symptoms are initially those of obstruction but later becomes those of ileus and/or peritonitis. Bowel sounds disappear, the abdomen become rigid with either focal or generalized tenderness, and the patient's general condition deteriorates rapidly. Bleeding from strangulated and therefore ischaemic bowel may present as rectal bleeding.

SUBPHRENIC ABSCESS

There may have been symptoms suggestive of previous perforation or an intra-abdominal septic focus such as diverticulitis or appendicitis. General symptoms such as feverishness may predominate with few clues to suggest subphrenic pus but usually upper abdominal pain is evident. Diaphragmatic irritation may cause referred shoulder tip pain, and pulmonary crepitations or 'sympathetic' pleural effusions may occur. The diaphragms may be immobile on respiration, either clinically or on X-ray screening.

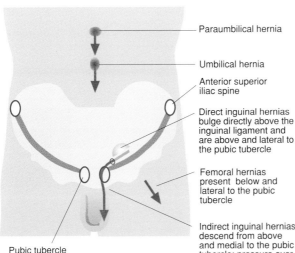

Paraumbilical hernia

Umbilical hernia

Anterior superior iliac spine

Direct inguinal hernias bulge directly above the inguinal ligament and are above and lateral to the pubic tubercle

Femoral hernias present below and lateral to the pubic tubercle

Indirect inguinal hernias descend from above and medial to the pubic tubercle: pressure over the internal inguinal ring (at the mid-inguinal point) will prevent an indirect, but not a direct, hernia from descending via the inguinal canal

Pubic tubercle

The pubic tubercle is the crucial landmark
- A hernia medial to the pubic tubercle should be an indirect inguinal hernia
- A hernia above and lateral to the pubic tubercle should be a direct inguinal hernia
- A hernia below and lateral to the pubic tubercle should be a femoral hernia

Fig. 2 **Anatomy of lower abdominal hernias.**

Abdominal conditions
- Palpation must be very gentle if an aneurysm is suspected.
- In upper bowel obstruction, vomiting is present and distension is mild.
- In lower bowel obstruction, vomiting is less common and distension more marked.
- Focal perforations start with focal symptoms and signs which may then become generalized.

LIVER DISEASE

SIGNS

The main signs of liver disease are summarized in Figure 1. If patients present acutely yet have any of the signs of chronic liver disease then both diagnosis and management are affected.

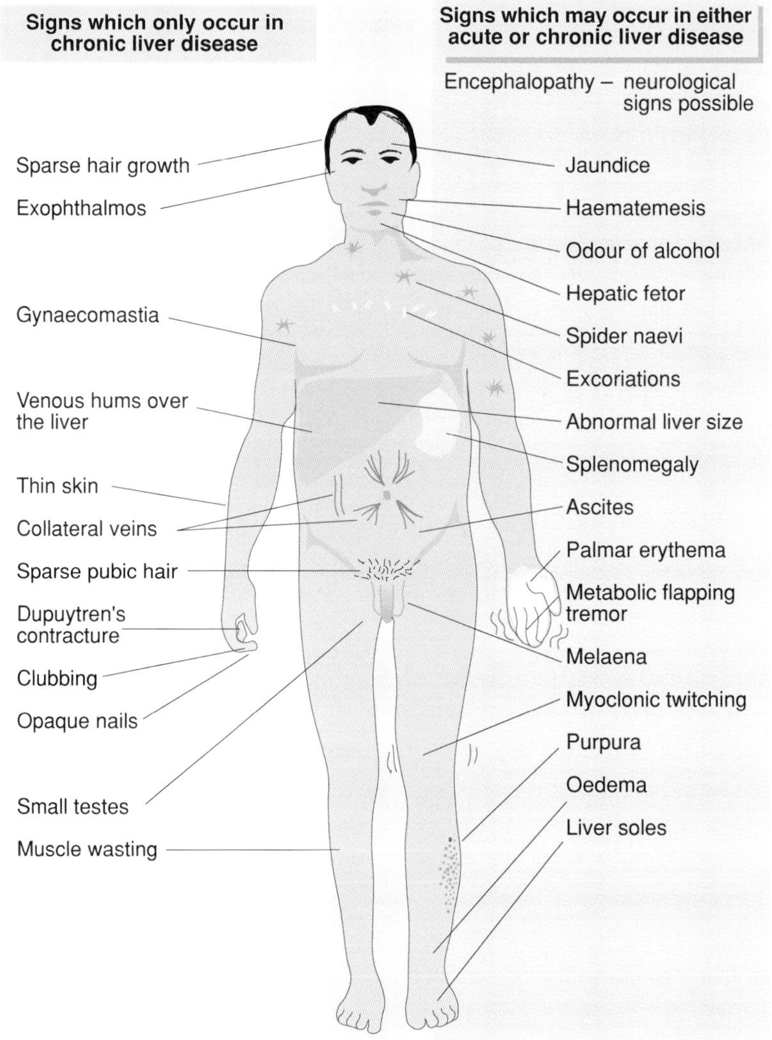

JAUNDICE

Jaundice (Fig. 2) may be caused by four mechanisms (Fig. 3):

- haemolysis
- decreased uptake or conjugation of unconjugated bilirubin by the liver
- diffuse cholestasis
- mechanical obstruction to bile flow.

Haemolysis

Breakdown of haemoglobin and other similar pigments produces unconjugated bilirubin and jaundice results if the ability of the liver to conjugate this is exceeded. Because unconjugated bilirubin is insoluble in water the excess bilirubin is not excreted into the urine (causing an acholuric jaundice). There may be a family history of haemolytic disease or a history of ingestion of haemolysis-inducing drugs. The jaundice is usually mild and yellowish, the liver is not usually tender and splenomegaly may be found in certain haemolytic anaemias.

Decreased uptake or conjugation of unconjugated bilirubin

This causes an *unconjugated* hyperbilirubinaemia. There may be a history of mild jaundice with previous non-hepatitic illness. Apart from mild jaundice examination is normal.

Diffuse cholestasis (medical jaundice)

This is associated with decreased secretion of conjugated bilirubin into the biliary tract without a causative focal space-occupying lesion. *Conjugated* hyperbilirubinaemia results and, as this is water soluble, the excess bilirubin spills over into the urine. The jaundice is of greenish hue and the stools are pale because of lack of secretion of bile pigments into the gut.

With acute viral hepatitis the liver is often diffusely enlarged and diffusely tender.

Causes of diffuse cholestasis include hepatitis A, B, C and non-A, non-B hepatitis, glandular fever, certain other infections, and drug reactions.

Mechanical obstruction to bile flow (surgical jaundice)

This is caused by lesions such as impacted gallstones or neoplasia obstructing the common bile duct.

A history of previous biliary tract surgery would provide circumstantial evidence for biliary stricture or gallstone impaction.

Signs which only occur in chronic liver disease

- Sparse hair growth
- Exophthalmos
- Gynaecomastia
- Venous hums over the liver
- Thin skin
- Collateral veins
- Sparse pubic hair
- Dupuytren's contracture
- Clubbing
- Opaque nails
- Small testes
- Muscle wasting

Signs which may occur in either acute or chronic liver disease

Encephalopathy – neurological signs possible

- Jaundice
- Haematemesis
- Odour of alcohol
- Hepatic fetor
- Spider naevi
- Excoriations
- Abnormal liver size
- Splenomegaly
- Ascites
- Palmar erythema
- Metabolic flapping tremor
- Melaena
- Myoclonic twitching
- Purpura
- Oedema
- Liver soles

Fig. 1 **Signs of liver disease.**

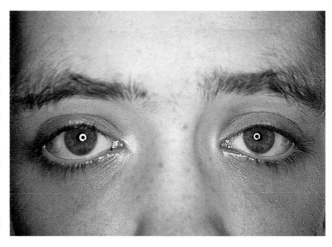

Fig. 2 **Jaundice.** The discoloration here is too profound and greenish to have been caused by a haemolytic mechanism.

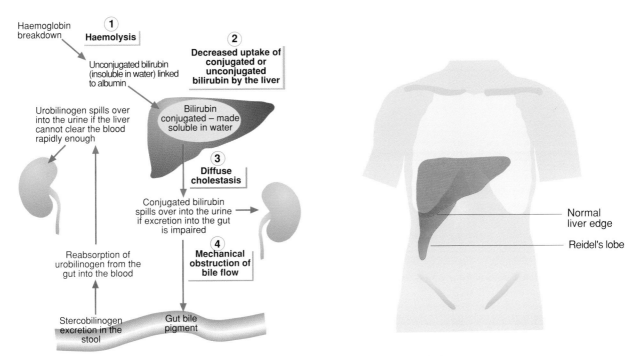

Fig. 3 **The four mechanisms of jaundice production.**

Fig. 4 **Riedel's lobe of the liver.**

With gallstone impaction there may be a history of biliary colic preceding the passage of dark urine.

Focal, rather than diffuse, liver tenderness suggests mechanical jaundice. An irregular liver surface or edge suggests malignancy or cirrhotic nodule formation. As in diffuse cholestasis there is bile in the urine and the stools are pale.

SIGNS OF HEPATOCELLULAR DYSFUNCTION

Signs of chronic or acute-on-chronic hepatocellular dysfunction are shown in Figure 1. A metabolic flap of the outstretched hands (p. 96) or altered mental state is often the first sign of encephalopathy. Later hyperventilation, dilated pupils and decerebrate or decorticate rigidity may develop.

ABNORMALITIES IN LIVER SIZE

In normal individuals the liver is impalpable but in thin patients the liver may just be palpable. Occasionally a Riedel's lobe is evident—a tongue-like extension of the liver downwards from the right lower lobe which may be mistaken for a localized liver swelling (Fig. 4).

The liver may be *diffusely* enlarged in acute hepatitis, right heart failure, multiple metastases or in early cirrhosis whereas *focal* enlargement may be caused by primary or secondary malignancy, abscess formation, or cirrhotic nodules.

Liver abscesses may occur in relation to intra-abdominal septic foci, after infec-tive gastroenteritis, or after amoebic infection of the large bowel but, not infrequently, the initiating focus is clinically occult or asymptomatic. Patients with liver abscess are febrile and the liver becomes enlarged and tender. Later there is pain on percussion of the right ribs laterally (most abscesses are in the right lobe of the liver). If untreated, abscesses may rupture into the peritoneum or lungs.

A small liver may be caused by cirrhosis or acute hepatic necrosis.

LIVER TENDERNESS

Liver tenderness may be found in the following:

- hepatitis
- right heart failure
- abscesses
- cholangitis
- multiple metastases.

LIVER FAILURE

Liver failure may present with:

- jaundice
- neurological disorders
- psychiatric disorders
- bleeding
- fluid retention (oedema or ascites).

Hepatic encephalopathy leads to coma and is often a preterminal event.

Grade 1

Grade 1 liver failure may include:

- euphoria
- occasionally depression

- fluctuating mild confusion
- slowness of mentation
- blunting of affect
- slurred speech
- disordered sleep rhythm.

Grade 2

Grade 2 liver failure may include:

- drowsiness
- inadequate response to simple commands
- inappropriate behaviour.

Grade 3

Grade 3 liver failure may include:

- sleeping for most of the time
- marked confusion
- incoherent speech.

Grade 4

Grade 4 liver patients are:

- unrousable
- may or may not respond to noxious stimuli.

Liver disease

- Haemolysis does not cause bile in the urine or a deep greenish jaundice.
- Percussion is the only way to identify a small liver.
- Splenomegaly is unusual in jaundice caused by mechanical bile duct obstruction.

MALE GENITAL TRACT

The male genitalia comprise the penis, scrotum, testes, epididymis, vas deferens (spermatic cord), seminal vesicles and the prostate gland (Fig. 1).

SYMPTOMS (Fig. 2)

Pain relevant to the male genital tract is usually well localized.

Testicular pain

With testicular pain the site is usually all too obvious although radiation into the lower abdomen is occasionally prominent. Acute injury produces excruciating pain which improves rapidly, unlike the pain associated with torsion which tends to persist. Although testicular pain and swelling can be the only manifestation of mumps infection, it is very dangerous to assume the absence of torsion. Any painful swollen testicle should be surgically explored in a male:

* under 30 years of age
* no history of injury
* with no urethral discharge
* with no frequency of micturition
* no infected urine
* an absence of clinically certain mumps
* with no prostatic tenderness.

Prostatic pain

The characteristics of prostatic pain are detailed on page 49. Infection of the prostate constitutes prostatitis. Prostatic pain is often associated with dysuria, frequency, and symptoms of urinary obstruction.

Patients with acute prostatitis are unwell with fever and acute prostatic type pain. On examination the prostate in acute prostatitis is tender (sometimes exquisitely so) swollen, indurated and warm.

Patients with chronic prostatitis may be asymptomatic but they may have perineal and low back pain and may develop urinary tract infection (UTI) or septicaemia. The prostate in chronic prostatitis may be normal or moderately tender, boggy, or indurated.

Epididymal pain

Epididymal pain is usually well localized. Examination reveals marked tenderness or mild tenderness with focal bead-like thickenings.

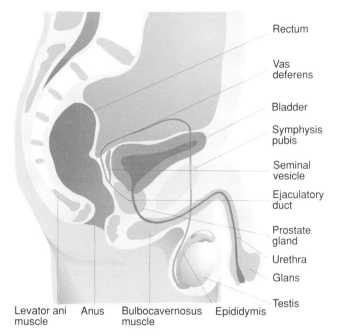

Fig. 1 **The male genitalia.**

Rectum

Vas deferens

Bladder

Symphysis pubis

Seminal vesicle

Ejaculatory duct

Prostate gland

Urethra

Glans

Testis

Levator ani muscle   Anus   Bulbocavernosus muscle   Epididymis

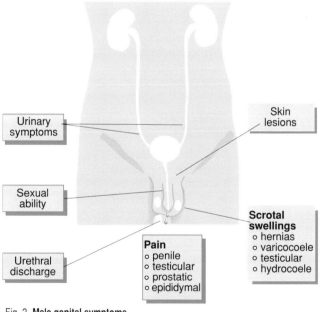

Fig. 2 **Male genital symptoms.**

Urinary symptoms

Skin lesions

Sexual ability

Urethral discharge

Pain
o penile
o testicular
o prostatic
o epididymal

Scrotal swellings
o hernias
o varicocoele
o testicular
o hydrocoele

Urethral discharge

Urethral discharge and/or urethral irritation obviously raises the possibility of sexually transmitted disease and the patient should be told that certain appropriate questions have to be asked about sexual activity and the possibility of sexually transmitted infections (p. 5) and he should be assured that confidentiality will be absolute.

Clinical diagnoses of the cause of urethral discharge are fallible and microbiological investigations are always required.

In general practice a referral to a sexually transmitted disease (STD) clinic is advisable especially as other, perhaps asymptomatic, infections must be excluded.

Sexual ability

The penis is a spongy organ surrounding the urethra which terminates in an expanded portion, the glans penis, which is surrounded (in the uncircumcised) by the foreskin. Erection depends on psychogenic or tactile stimuli and lack of psychological inhibition. Intact autonomic inner-

vation is required to produce an erection and to allow ejaculation.

'Sexual ability' questions may be relevant. Have there been any problems with fertility, erectile ability or ejaculatory ability? If so, when and how did they start? Have there been any symptoms suggestive of endocrine or neurological dysfunction? Have there been any other relevant medical problems? Is the patient receiving drugs that may interfere with sexual ability? Is stress a primary cause or a secondary phenomenon?

EXAMINATION

Always explain why it is necessary to examine the genitalia. Female examiners should have a chaperone present.

Inspect the penis

If necessary retract the foreskin (which should be easy and painless) to inspect the urethral orifice, particularly for discharge. Phimosis is a tightness of the prepuce which prevents retraction over the glans. The urethral opening is slit-like and, if the slit is opened by gentle squeezing along the long axis of the slit, then pinkish urethral mucosa without discharge should be evident. Hypospadias is a malpositioning of the urethra on the undersurface of the penis. A urethral discharge suggests infection and, although gonorrhoea is a common cause, an informed screening for other STDs should occur.

Gentle squeezing from the base to the tip of the penis may 'milk' discharge to the urethral opening. Inflammation of the glans penis is termed balantitis and if the foreskin is also involved is termed balano-posthitis.

Palpate the scrotum and its contents

The scrotum is a thin muscular bag which contains the testes and associated structures. The testes should be examined with the patient lying down and then standing up when swellings caused by dilated veins or hernias (p. 57) should become larger. The left testis is usually lower than the right. The epididymis is attached to the upper surface and upper posterior surface of the testis. The epididymis conveys spermatozoa to the vas deferens which passes upwards via the inguinal canal to join the seminal vesicles just lateral to the prostate.

Check for the following abnormalities:

- *Undescended or ectopic testicle.* If either side of the scrotum does not contain a testis (even when the patient is standing) search for an undescended or ectopic testicle which may be found in the inguinal, femoral or perineal areas. Some testes are intra-abdominal, and thus impalpable, and have a tendency to malignant change.
- *Swollen testes.* Gently palpate each testis in turn to elicit all the characteristics of swellings as detailed on page 6. Testes are usually of a rubbery consistency and are tender to gentle pressure.
- *Hydrocoele.* Fluid around the testis is a hydrocoele. As a hydrocoele surrounds most of the testis, the testis cannot be isolated for palpation. Hydrocoeles, unlike solid swellings, will transilluminate when a light is applied to the scrotum.
- *Epididymal cysts.* Unlike hydrocoeles, these are felt separate from the testis.
- *Varicocoele.* This is a varicosity (excessive tortuosity or swelling) of the veins surrounding the vas deferens in the scrotum. On palpation with the patient standing varicocoeles are separate from the testis, feel like a 'bag of worms' and briefly swell if the patient coughs.
- *Scrotal swellings.* These may be caused by indirect hernias (p. 57). It is possible to get above testicular swellings but not above hernias.

- *The epididymis and spermatic cord.* Palpate the epididymis which is usually smooth and does not feel 'knotted'. The vas deferens, which should be smooth and non-tender, can be best felt by rolling it gently between the pad of the thumb and index finger. A tender epididymis is usually caused by infection. Tuberculosis may cause an irregular thickening of the vas deferens.
- *Undersized testes.* If both testes are small then there is a non-lateralized condition such as failure of pituitary drive or primary testicular dysfunction as may occur in Klinefelter's syndrome or eunuchoidism.
- *Enlarged testis.* Suspect malignancy if it is non-tender or irregular in outline.
- *Urinary tract infection.* Symptoms of UTI may suggest bacterial epididymitis or orchitis.

Genital aspects of rectal examination

The technique of rectal examination is detailed on page 55. On rectal examination the prostate is palpable anteriorly (Fig. 3). A normal prostate is about 3.5 cm in diameter, indents the anterior rectal wall slightly, and has a midline groove. Both lobes of the prostate (each side of the median groove) should be symmetrical and should have the consistency of a firm rubber ball. Prostatic enlargement, which is common in the elderly, is often a subjective assessment. Benign prostatic enlargement may be smooth and symmetrical whereas malignant prostatic enlargement may be asymmetrical and have hard areas therein.

If the examiner has a long finger the seminal vesicles or vas deferens may be palpated on both sides (Fig. 3).

Acute pain on palpating the prostate suggests prostatitis, prostatic abscess, or, less commonly, inflammatory lesions affecting the seminal vesicles.

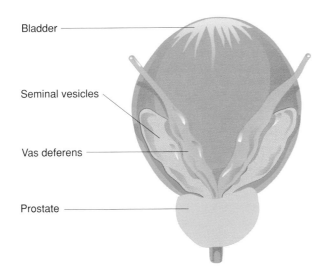

Bladder

Seminal vesicles

Vas deferens

Prostate

Fig. 3 **The anterior structures on rectal examination in the male.**

Male genital tract

- Obtain an urgent surgical opinion in all patients with a painful swollen testicle, unless mumps is certain.
- Always explain why you have to examine the genitalia.
- Presence of a chaperone avoids legal problems.
- Hydrocoeles transilluminate; solid swellings do not.

FEMALE GENITAL TRACT

The female genital tract (Fig. 1) comprises the ovaries, Fallopian tubes, uterus (including the cervix), vagina, the external genitalia (two labia minora, two labia majora) and the clitoris. Batholin's gland is present posterolaterally on each side and is a secretory gland which is not normally palpable. The hymen is a crenated fold at the entrance to the vagina which is usually partially closed in women who have not experienced intercourse or inserted tampons.

SYMPTOMS

Normally the uterus is supported by various ligaments but may prolapse and, in severe cases, appear at the entrance to the vagina. The bladder may prolapse, thereby pushing into the upper anterior vaginal wall (a cystocoele) but if the lower vaginal wall is predominantly affected the urethral area may prolapse (a urethrocoele). The rectum may also push into the posterior vaginal wall (a rectocoele) (Fig. 2).

With low oestrogen levels (e.g. after the menopause) the labia may decrease in size and the vagina may become atrophic, losing its elasticity and its self-lubricating properties. A male pattern of pubic hair (with an upward pointing triangle of hair) may suggest endocrine problems (virilization).

When dealing with such personal symptoms it is best to ask the potentially less upsetting questions first. There are a large number of questions that could be asked, but obviously not all should be asked unless relevant (Fig. 3).

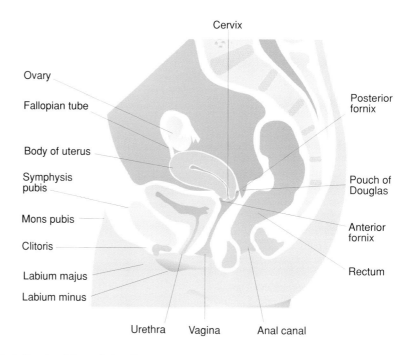

Fig. 1 **Female pelvis: sagittal section.**

DYSMENORRHOEA

Dysmenorrhoea is pain associated with menstruation. Dysmenorrhoea tends to be worse at the start of menstruation and may be continuous or spasmodic (colicky) in nature. Pain is felt in the pelvis and lower back, and if occurring several days before menstruation may be caused by endo-metriosis (ectopic uterine tissue which secretes blood).

DYSPAREUNIA

Dyspareunia is pain or difficulty with intercourse. Causes include:
- a rigid hymen
- prolapse of the ovaries into the perivaginal area
- narrowing of the vagina due to scars of previous operations
- poor coital technique
- genital tract infections.

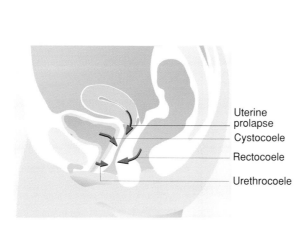

Fig. 2 **Common types of prolapse.**

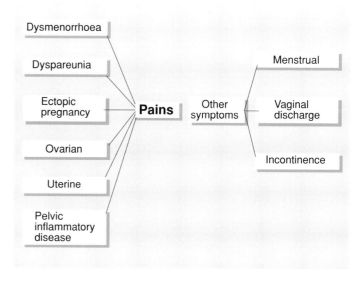

Fig. 3 **Female genital tract symptoms.**

Deep dyspareunia may be caused by:

- cervicitis
- endometriosis
- salpingitis
- malignancies (rarely).

Dyspareunia may also have psychological causes and effects.

MENSTRUATION

The normal menstruation cycle (Fig. 4) varies from 21–35 (usually 28) days from the first day of one cycle to the next. When appropriate ask about:

- age of menarche (age of onset of periods)
- duration of the menstrual flow
- length of the menstrual cycle (the first day of one cycle to the first day of the next)
- date of the first day of the last menstrual period
- amount of blood loss in terms of tampons or pads used
- menorrhagia (excessive loss of blood with regular menstruation)
- intermenstrual bleeding
- premenstrual tension
- postcoital bleeding (bleeding after intercourse) in the sexually active
- recent changes in periods
- amenorrhoea (absence of periods)
- if pregnancy is a possibility
- age of menopause (age at which periods ceased)
- occurrence of post-menopausal bleeding
- type of contraception used (if any)
- episodes of infertility
- vulval pruritus (which may be secondary to vaginal discharge or to 'general' skin conditions, particularly scabies or pediculosis, or perhaps to allergic reactions to topical preparations).

OTHER CAUSES OF PAIN

Pelvic inflammatory disease is caused by infection and can be acute or chronic. The sequence of symptoms of active infection often reflects the progression of inflammation:

- *Cervicitis* is characterized by mucopurulent vaginal discharge, possibly with 'sympathetic' urinary tract symptoms or rectal symptoms caused by spread of infection.
- *Endometritis* is inflammation of the lining of the uterus causing midline abdominal pain possibly with abnormal vaginal bleeding.

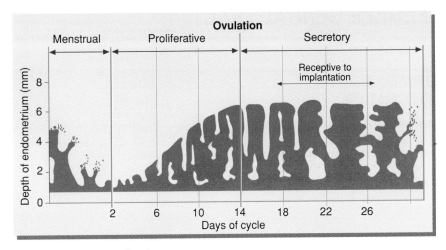

Fig. 4 **The normal menstrual cycle.**

- *Salpingitis* is inflammation of one or both Fallopian tubes with unilateral or bilateral lower abdominal pain. Swelling may be detected in the region of a Fallopian tube, and vaginal examination may cause pain on movement of the cervix.

Causes of acute pelvic inflammatory disease include gonorrhoea, chlamydia and *Gardnerella vaginalis* infection. Causes of chronic pelvic inflammatory disease include tuberculosis and chlamydia infection.

Ovarian and uterine pain

Ovarian pain is unilateral. Ovulation pain (Mittelschmerz) may occur in the middle of the menstrual cycle. Torsion of an ovarian cyst produces a unilateral lower abdominal pain and, if infarction occurs, the pain becomes very severe. Haemorrhage into an ovary or ovarian cyst produces a similar but less severe pain. Rupture of an ovary or part of an ovary (usually of small cysts or of a corpus luteum) produces unilateral pain with signs of peritoneal irritation which may simulate appendicitis.

Uterine pain is an anterior lower abdominal pain which is not lateralized, and which may be felt in the lower back. Occasionally women present with abdominal pain when in labour without consciously knowing that they are pregnant.

Ectopic pregnancy

An ectopic pregnancy is usually situated in a Fallopian tube. Other possible sites included the cervix, ovary, abdominal cavity or pelvic cavity. Unilateral colicky pain usually begins shortly after a missed period with some vaginal bleeding. The pain become severe and haemorrhage may be profuse. On examination the cervix, when moved, will cause pain and a tender swelling may be palpated laterally. Ectopic pregnancies at about 6-8 weeks may present with pain and fainting caused by profuse bleeding.

Vaginal discharge

A small amount of mucoid discharge is normal. A yellowish, irritant, pungent discharge suggests *Trichomonas vaginalis* infection whereas a whitish discharge suggests *Candida albicans* (monilia, thrush) infection. A blood-stained discharge may occur with severe cervical erosions, polyps or carcinoma. A history of vaginal or perivaginal blisters or irritant vesicles suggests genital herpes.

Female genital tract

- Always ask less upsetting or less embarassing questions first.
- Pelvic inflammatory disease encompasses cervicitis, endometritis and/or salpingitis.
- Always consider whether a woman might be pregnant.
- Ectopic pregnancy may present with profuse haemorrhage and collapse.

FEMALE GENITAL TRACT (II)

GYNAECOLOGICAL EXAMINATION

Always explain why you need to perform a gynaecological 'internal' examination and always explain exactly what will happen. Be sure that a gynaecological internal examination is indicated especially if the patient is a virgin and, if she is, be very careful not to rupture an intact hymen. In such circumstances a rectal examination may be preferable.

The patient should have emptied her bladder prior to the examination unless testing for stress incontinence is a necessary part of the examination. A good light is essential.

After appropriate explanation (and in the presence of a chaperone for a male examiner), the patient is asked to lie on her back with the hips and knees flexed and her knees apart (Fig. 1).

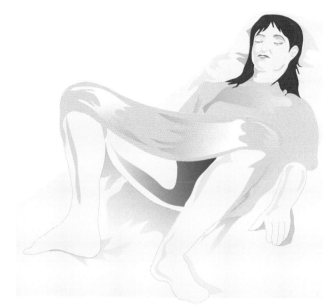

Fig. 1 **Position for gynaecological examination.**

Vulva, clitoris and urethra

The vulva, clitoris and urethra are inspected for abnormalities (Fig. 2) and the labia are gently separated and inspected. The labia majora are hair-lined skin folds and the labia minora are hairless skin folds interior to the labia majora. The index finger of the gloved right hand is then inserted a short way and the posterior part of each labium major palpated between the finger and thumb to detect any swelling of Bartholin's glands on each side. Normal Bartholin's glands are about 0.5 cm in diameter and become enlarged (usually unilaterally) if a cyst or abscess develops. A normal Bartholin's gland cannot be palpated.

Vaginal wall

Ask the patient to strain down 'as if constipated' and observe if the anterior wall of the vagina is weak and bulging (resulting in a cystocoele with the bladder prolapsing into the vagina), if the posterior wall is weak and bulging (resulting in a rectocoele with the rectum prolapsing into the vagina), or if weakness of the uterine supports allows the uterus to prolapse into the vagina. If the patient has stress incontinence and urine in her bladder, then such straining (or coughing) will cause leakage of urine.

Anterior fornix

The extended gloved and lubricated index finger, or the index and middle finger (Fig. 3) are then advanced into the anterior fornix (the small pouch in front of the cervix). The adequacy of the surrounding pelvic musculature can be assessed by asking the patient to squeeze the inserted fingers. The tip of the finger(s) should feel the cervix as a semi-soft disc with a dimple in the middle (Fig. 4). The normal cervix is slightly mobile and move-

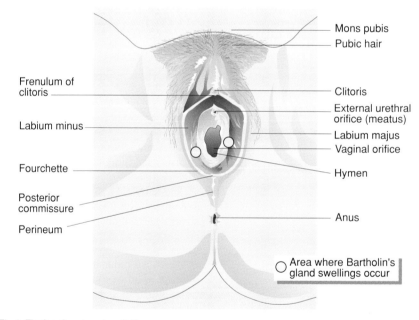

Fig. 2 **The female external genitalia.**

Mons pubis
Pubic hair
Frenulum of clitoris
Clitoris
External urethral orifice (meatus)
Labium minus
Labium majus
Vaginal orifice
Fourchette
Hymen
Posterior commissure
Anus
Perineum
○ Area where Bartholin's gland swellings occur

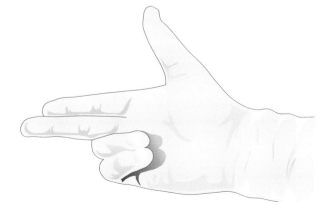

Fig. 3 **The position of the hand when used for vaginal examination.**

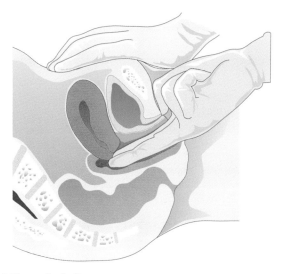

Fig. 4 **Bimanual palpation.**

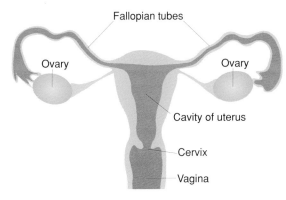

Fig. 5 **Female internal genitalia.**

ment does not cause pain unless an inflammatory lesion is present.

Adnexa uteri

The adnexa uteri (Fallopian tubes, ovaries and supporting tissues) should then be assessed. Normally the Fallopian tubes are impalpable whereas normal ovaries are smooth, firm, slightly tender and mobile. Each lateral fornix is palpated in turn and an attempt made to palpate for swellings of the ovaries or Fallopian tubes. The posterior fornix is then palpated; a retroverted uterus may be felt to be continuous with the cervix. If the free (left) hand palpates the lower abdomen an anteverted uterus may be felt between the two hands (bimanual palpation).

Ovaries and uterus (Fig. 5)

Ovarian and uterine swellings arise out of the pelvis and thus have a palpable upper border but an impalpable lower border. Uterine swellings, especially pedunculated fibroids, may be widely mobile. Ovarian swellings are less mobile and, if large, may appear to be midline, and large ovarian cysts containing fluid under low pressure may simulate ascites.

Rectum

On rectal examination the cervix will be palpable, as may intravaginal foreign bodies such as tampons. The normal cervix is firm and slightly mobile. A retroverted uterus may also be felt above and posterior to the cervix.

OBSTETRIC HISTORY

It is often useful to combine obstetric history taking with construction of a simplified family tree (p. 4).

Never assume that all women have had children; some women may have decided not to have children whilst other women may be distressed by their inability to have children. Also do not assume that women with children have borne them. I suggest the following order of questions to minimize possible distress:

- number of pregnancies ('How many times have you been pregnant?')
- number of full-term normal babies (do subtraction to determine whether there is need to enquire further into ectopic pregnancies, abortions, miscarriages, or still-births)
- when appropriate ask if there were any difficulties in conceiving
- birth weight of children if relevant (diabetic women tend to have heavier babies)
- complications of pregnancy, including hypertension or ankle oedema (both may be found in toxaemia of pregnancy)
- complications of labour
- complications occurring shortly after birth (the puer-perium).

Gynaecological examination and obstetric history

- Always explain why a gynaecological examination is necessary.
- Avoid a vaginal examination in a virgin if possible.
- Take great care to avoid rupturing the hymen if the patient is a virgin or does not use tampons.
- The Fallopian tubes are normally impalpable.
- Normal ovaries are smooth, firm and slightly tender.
- Large ovarian cysts may simulate ascites.
- Normally, movement of the cervix does not cause pain.

UROLOGICAL EXAMINATION

The urological system includes the kidneys, ureters, bladder, prostate in the male, and urethra. The following account commences with an analysis of urological symptoms and signs not detailed in the abdominal, genital or neurological sections. The neurological aspects of urinary function are detailed on page 95 and genital symptoms and signs on pages 60–65.

The questions relevant to the urological system that could be asked are summarized in Table 1.

Table 1 **Questions relevant to the urological examination**

Pain	Frequency
renal	Nocturia
ureteric	Urgency
bladder	Hesitancy
prostatic	Abnormal urinary stream
penile	Cloudy urine
urethrall	Discoloured urine
scrota	Haematuria
Urine output	Smelly urine
anuria	Enuresis
oliguria	Pneumaturia
polyuria	Incontinence

SYMPTOMS AND SIGNS

Anuria
Anuria is failure to pass any urine. In practice a urine flow of less that 100 ml daily has the same implications.

Bladder outflow obstruction
Bladder outflow obstruction, usually caused by prostatism in the male or severe urethral stenosis in the female, may cause:

- progressive urinary retention
- frequency
- urgency
- nocturia
- hesitancy
- intermittent urinary stream
- decreasing calibre and projection of the urinary stream
- a feeling of incomplete bladder emptying
- the need to strain to pass urine
- terminal dribbling
- complete urinary retention.

Decrease in calibre and force of the urinary stream is usually associated with hesitancy and straining at micturition, and the two in combination are highly suggestive of urinary tract obstruction distal to the bladder. In boys, urethral valves or congenital strictures may cause bladder outflow obstruction, whereas in older males prostatic obstructions or urethral strictures are often responsible.

Difficulty in passing urine may either be caused by compression of the urethra, urethral strictures, or urethral blockage by urinary stone or blood clots.

Acute retention of urine is painful and exacerbated by suprapubic palpation. Chronic retention of urine is often painless and a pathologically enlarged bladder may be missed unless routine palpation for the upper surface is performed (p. 54). An enlarged bladder may be palpated at the level of the umbilicus or even higher. A normal bladder in the absence of retention should empty on micturition such that it cannot be palpated or percussed above the pubic tubercles.

Cloudy urine
Cloudy urine may be caused by infection or excessive phosphates in the urine.

Discoloured urine
Yellowish brown urine may be caused by conjugated hyperbilirubinaemia which is found in obstructive pattern jaundice. Frothing on shaking the urine may also be evident. Red, brown or smokey urine suggests either haematuria or haemoglobinuria. Urine which turns red on standing may be caused by porphyria.

Certain drugs discolour the urine—notably rifampicin which usually reddens the urine (and tears and saliva) and this provides useful confirmation that the patient is taking the rifampicin. Phenolphthalein laxatives impart a bluish tinge to the urine.

Dysuria
Dysuria means either pain or difficulty in passing urine. As these two symptoms are very different the term dysuria should not be used without qualification. Urethral pain is usually well localized and worsens during micturition 'scalding' and is usually caused by urethral irritation, commonly in association with infection. Occasionally patients experience micturition-related back pain if there is reflux of urine up a ureter. Strangury is slow, painful micturition.

Enuresis
Enuresis, nocturnal bedwetting, is normal during the first 2-3 years of life. Primary enuresis occurs in older children who have never been continent and secondary enuresis occurs in children who had achieved continence. Enuresis may reflect an older age than normal for attaining nocturnal continence but may indicate pathology such as infection, urethral or bladder abnormalities, or neurological lesions affecting the bladder.

Frequency
Most people pass urine 4–6 times daily. Frequency may be caused by excessive urine production (polyuria), or by irritating lesions of the lower urinary tract including infections (particularly cystitis or urethritis). Nervousness or cold weather may cause frequency during the daytime but not at night.

Haematuria
Haematuria (blood in the urine) should only be attributed to uncomplicated urinary tract infection if there is a 'fullhouse' of other features of urinary infection. Otherwise full investigation is required as haematuria may be caused by glomerulonephritis or malignancies.

Incontinence
Incontinence is the inability to refrain from passing urine. Incontinence implies bladder dysfunction caused by:
- infection
- incompetent urinary sphincters
- foreign bodies
- urinary stones
- a small volume bladder
- a compressed bladder
- neurological problems
- tumours.

When relevant it is important that women are asked about incontinence as many will not volunteer incontinence. This questioning is important because the vast majority of patients with incontinence can be helped by treatment.

- *Stress incontinence* is associated with coughing, laughing or physical exertion and may be related to sphincter weakness or poor muscular support of the bladder. The latter may be confirmed by weakness of contraction of perivaginal muscles when the patient is asked to squeeze the examining finger on digital vaginal examination.
- *Urge incontinence* may be sensory in type with an urgent, often painful, desire to void caused by painful bladder disorders such as cystitis. Urinary frequency occurs but leakage is unusual. Urge incontinence of motor type is usually painless and occurs when detrusor muscle contraction cannot be inhibited.

- *Total incontinence* is perpetual leakage of urine. It occurs with extreme sphincter weakness and with chronic retention with overflow.
- *Overflow incontinence* occurs when the bladder becomes acutely or chronically overdistended and the resistance of the urinary sphincters is overcome resulting in constant dribbling. Patients usually have to strain to pass urine and may feel, correctly, that their bladder is still full after micturition.

Nocturia

Nocturia is interruption of sleep by frequent or excessive voiding during the night. Nocturia may indicate:

- decreased renal concentrating power in early renal failure, in heart or liver failure
- an irritable bladder (the vernacular for detrusor instability)
- a diminished bladder capacity.

Oliguria

Oliguria is passage of noticeably less urine than is normal, usually meaning less than 500 ml daily.

Pneumaturia

Pneumaturia is gas in the urine, which implies a fistula between the urinary tract and bowel, either benign (caused by diverticular diseases or Crohn's disease for example) or malignant (caused by tumour invasion).

Polyuria

Polyuria is passing of noticeably more urine than is normal, usually meaning in excess of 2500 ml daily.

Renal failure

The symptoms and signs of chronic renal failure are shown in Figure 1.

Smelly urine

Infection is suggested if the odour is marked or ammonia-like. Acetonuria in diabetic ketosis may impart a sweet smell to the urine.

Urgency

Urgency is a strong desire to void urine. Urge incontinence is leakage of urine despite conscious effort to avoid leakage whilst desperately searching for a lavatory. It is usually caused by infection, bladder wall muscle (detrusor) instability or a small volume bladder.

THE PROSTATE ON RECTAL EXAMINATION

The technique of rectal examination is detailed on page 55.

A normal prostate feels rubbery, smooth, and non-tender (a tender prostate implies prostatitis or abscess). An enlarged benign prostate is smooth, slightly mobile, possibly slightly asymmetrical, with a palpable median groove. A malignant prostate may be irregular, hard, fixed, and the median groove may be impalpable. The seminal vesicles may be felt laterally just above the prostate.

COMMON URINARY TRACT CONDITIONS

Cystitis

Cystitis is inflammation of the bladder which usually causes frequency, nocturia, painful micturition ('scalding'), cloudy and smelly urine, and occasionally haematuria. Unlike pyelonephritis, uncomplicated cystitis usually does not cause fever or unilateral back pain.

Pyelonephritis

Pyelonephritis is usually associated with symptoms of cystitis but with additional fever and lateralized back pain if pyelonephritis is unilateral. Rigors suggest pyelonephritis possibly with septicaemia. A useful sign of pyelonephritis is tenderness on percussion over the lower ribs posteriorly.

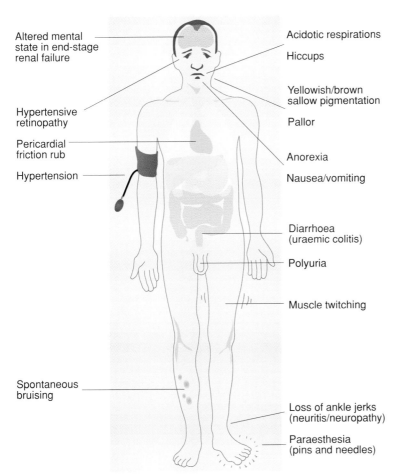

Altered mental state in end-stage renal failure

Hypertensive retinopathy

Pericardial friction rub

Hypertension

Spontaneous bruising

Acidotic respirations

Hiccups

Yellowish/brown sallow pigmentation

Pallor

Anorexia

Nausea/vomiting

Diarrhoea (uraemic colitis)

Polyuria

Muscle twitching

Loss of ankle jerks (neuritis/neuropathy)

Paraesthesia (pins and needles)

Fig. 1 **Signs of chronic renal failure.**

Urological examination

- After micturition the bladder should not normally be palpable or percussable.
- Always differentiate dysuria into painful or difficult micturition.
- Urinary frequency caused by 'nerves' or cold weather does not occur at night.
- Haematuria occurring without symptoms and signs of infection should always be investigated.
- Patients often do not volunteer incontinence—therefore you have to ask.

PITUITARY RELATED HORMONES (I)

INTRODUCTION

The hormone secreting systems are either:

- endocrine in which glands secrete internally, usually into the bloodstream
- exocrine in which glands secrete externally (the gut lumen being considered external to body tissue).

The major endocrine systems are detailed in Tables 1 and 2.

The hypothalamus exerts a major effect on pituitary function by sending blood (containing anterior pituitary hormone releasing factors) to the anterior pituitary, and by sending oxytocin and vasopressin via nervous tissue to the posterior pituitary. Thus, single or multiple endocrine dysfunctions may occur secondary to hypothalamic or pituitary gland dysfunctions.

This section will discuss:

- the effects of the hormones produced by the glands which interact with the pituitary (these glands may also hyperfunction or hypofunction independently of the pituitary)
- the effects of dysfunction of the pituitary or hypothalamus

- the effects of pituitary-independent hormones.

Table 2 **Autonomous glands**

Hormone	Gland	Effect
Catecholamines	Adrenal medulla	Sympathetic activity increased
Aldosterone	Adrenal cortex	Sodium retention
	Adrenal cortex	Virilization
Insulin	Pancreas	Glucose metabolism
Parathormone	Parathyroids	Calcium metabolism

Table 1 **The main actions and effects of the endocrine system**

Action in tissues	Hormones produced	Target glands	Anterior pituitary hormones	Hypothalamus Stimulating factors	Inhibiting factors
Carbohydrate, protein and fat metabolism	← Cortisol ←	Adrenal cortex ←	Adrenocorticotrophic hormone← (ACTH)	Cortisol releasing factor	
			Melanocyte stimulating hormone		
Maturation of follicles ← Feminization	Oestrogens and← progestogens	Ovaries ←	Follicle stimulating and luteinizing hormone (FSH and LH)	← Follicle stimulating and luteinizing hormone releasing factors (FSH-RF and LH-RF)	
Virilization ←	Testosterone ←	Testes ←			
Ovulation and development of corpus luteum	←	Corpus luteum ←			
Growth increase ← Glucose increase		Skeleton, connective tissue, ← viscera, glucose metabolism	Growth hormone (GH) ←	Growth hormone releasing factor (GH-RF)	Somatostatin
Lactation ←		Breast ←	Prolactin ←	Prolactin releasing factor	Prolactin inhibiting factor
Metabolic activities of most ← tissues increased	Thyroxine ← tri-iodothronine	Thyroid ←	Thyroid stimulating hormone ← (TSH)	Thyroid releasing factor (TRF)	

GLANDS WHICH INTERACT WITH THE PITUITARY

THE ADRENAL CORTEX

The adrenal cortex secretes three main classes of hormones (Fig. 1):

- Glucocorticoids (including cortisol) affect carbohydrate, protein and fat metabolism.
- Mineralocorticoids (including aldosterone) affect electrolyte and water regulation.
- Androgens are anabolic (building up) and virilizing in action.

Adrenal cortical hyperfunction

Excessive production of androgens causes adrenal virilism, whilst overproduction of cortisol causes Cushing's syndrome. Excessive aldosterone production causes

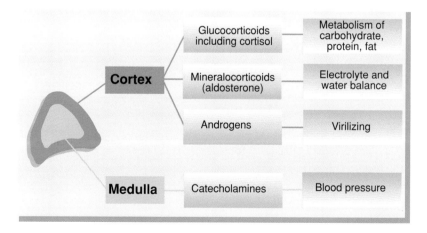

Fig. 1 **Hormones of the adrenals and their effects.**

hyperaldosteronism. Adrenal cortical hyperfunction may be caused by adrenal cortical hyperplasia, adenomas or adenocarcinomas. Cushing's syndrome may also

be caused by excessive pituitary production of adrenocorticotrophic hormone (ACTH). Certain non-pituitary tumours (e.g. in the lung) may secrete ACTH.

Cortisol overproduction (Cushing's syndrome)

Cushing's syndrome may be produced by endogenous cortisol overproduction or by therapeutic administration of gluco-corticoids. There is a rounded moon-shaped face, an obese body with thin limbs, skin striae, hirsutism, acne, a buffalo hump on the back of the neck and, occasionally, a proximal myopathy (Figs 2 & 3). Hypertension or diabetes mellitus may occur (the latter because cortisol antagonizes the action of insulin). Occasionally, chronic alcoholism produces appearances simulating Cushing's syndrome.

Adrenal virilism

Excessive production of androgens causes adrenal virilism, with manifestations more evident in females. Features include hirsutism (which may be the only feature), hair loss possibly with baldness, acne, a deep voice, cessation of periods, clitoral enlargement and decreased breast size. Other causes of hirsutism in the female include racial and familial predisposition, idiopathic factors, ovarian tumours, Cushing's syndrome, acromegaly, hypothyroidism and iatrogenic factors (including phenytoin therapy).

Deficiencies of adrenal androgens do not give rise to symptoms in the male (the testes compensate), but in the female, muscle weakness and loss of axillary hair may result.

Adrenal cortical hypofunction (Addison's disease)

Adrenal cortical hypofunction (Fig. 3) may be produced by atrophy or destruction of the cortex (usually by immune mechanisms or by tuberculosis).

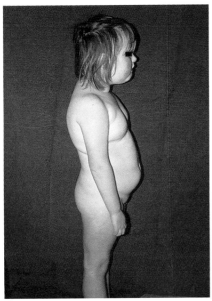

Fig. 2 **Cushing's syndrome.**

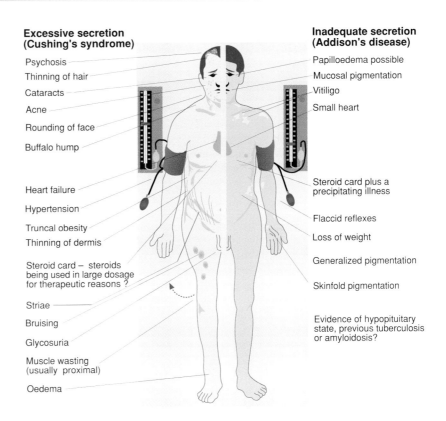

Excessive secretion (Cushing's syndrome)

- Psychosis
- Thinning of hair
- Cataracts
- Acne
- Rounding of face
- Buffalo hump
- Heart failure
- Hypertension
- Truncal obesity
- Thinning of dermis
- Steroid card – steroids being used in large dosage for therapeutic reasons ?
- Striae
- Bruising
- Glycosuria
- Muscle wasting (usually proximal)
- Oedema

Inadequate secretion (Addison's disease)

- Papilloedema possible
- Mucosal pigmentation
- Vitiligo
- Small heart
- Steroid card plus a precipitating illness
- Flaccid reflexes
- Loss of weight
- Generalized pigmentation
- Skinfold pigmentation
- Evidence of hypopituitary state, previous tuberculosis or amyloidosis?

Fig. 3 **The possible clinical signs of abnormal adrenal cortical function.**

Cortisol deficiency causes numerous metabolic dysfunctions including hypoglycaemia. In response to the lower levels of cortisol, the pituitary over-produces ACTH to stimulate the failing cortex. ACTH has a melanocyte stimulating hormone-like action and this causes pigmentation, particularly of palmar creases and skin folds.

The mineralocorticoids (notably aldosterone) are partially responsible for retention of sodium and excretion of potassium and thus with adrenal cortical hypofunction there is an increased excretion of sodium and retention of potassium which may lead to dehydration, hypotension (particularly postural hypotension), and circulatory collapse. A patient with Addison's disease may give a history of anorexia, weakness, weight loss, gastrointestinal disturbance, and postural hypotension.

On examination there may be diffuse tanning which is most marked on pressure points and mucous membranes: in contrast patients with pituitary-dependent cortical hypofunction (with low ACTH levels) do not develop such tanning. There may be pigmentation of the mucous membranes of the mouth. The heart is typically small (because of chronic hypotension). If the adrenal cortex hypofunction is of rapid onset (an adrenal crisis) there is profound weakness, circulatory failure with profound hypotension and pre-renal renal failure.

Congenital adrenal hyperplasia

In this condition cortisol production is defective leading to excessive pituitary production of ACTH and this causes adrenal cortical hyperplasia with accumulation of cortisol precursors and androgens. In female fetuses masculinization of the external genitalia results whereas in male fetuses the penis is enlarged. If the defect is severe babies may present after birth with acute adrenal failure but, if mild, children of both sexes grow rapidly with accelerated bodily development and premature fusion of bone epiphyses preventing linear bone growth.

Pituitary related hormones (I)

- Endocrine glands secrete internally, usually in the blood stream.
- The adrenals produce glucocorticoids, mineralocorticoids, androgens and adrenaline.
- Adrenaline secretion is effectively independent of the pituitary.
- The major glucocorticoid is cortisol.

PITUITARY RELATED HORMONES (II)

HYPOGONADISM

There are several syndromes which are associated with hypogonadism. The following account deals with the principal manifestations rather than their integration into syndromes. Hypogonadism may be the result of target organ, pituitary, or hypothalamic dysfunctions. Examination of the testes and ovaries are detailed on pages 61 and 65 respectively.

Male hypogonadism

Normally puberty begins between 10–15 years and involves increased release of luteinizing hormone (LH) and follicle stimulating hormone (FSH), the former stimulating testosterone or progesterone release. Testosterone is responsible for the pubertal secondary sexual characteristics, enlargement of gonads and penis, and accelerated growth. Lack of LH and FSH leads to gonadal atrophy and impaired reproductive functions.

Male hypogonadism, particularly if occurring before puberty, may result in an outstretched arm span greater than height, lack of bodily hair, an unbroken voice, small testes, poor muscle development, and a small penis and scrotum. In postpubertal males hypogonadism is usually of slow onset with decreased libido and, when severe, less need to shave and regression of secondary sexual characteristics.

Testicular feminization syndrome results if there is end-organ unresponsiveness to testosterone in the male. This syndrome usually presents with a genetically male patient of superficially female appearance but with sparse pubic hair, a normal vulva but with a 'blind-pouch' vagina without uterus or ovaries. Undeveloped testes may be felt in the labial folds or within the inguinal canal. The clinical presentation is usually with a history of primary amenorrhoea after the expected age of onset of menstruation has passed.

Female hypogonadism

The menopause is of course a physiological form of female hypogonadism: related symptoms are those of oestrogen deficiency and include vaginal dryness and loss of libido. Other manifestations include infertility and amenorrhoea.

EXCESSIVE GROWTH HORMONE (ACROMEGALY, GIANTISM)

Growth hormone hypersecretion prior to closure of the epiphyses (the growing areas of long bones) causes excessive linear and transverse bone growth resulting in giantism. After epiphyseal closure has occurred acromegaly results with

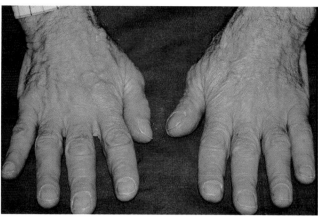

Fig.1 **The hands in acromegaly.**

thickening of the bones and, notably, a prominent protruded jaw (prognathism). The face appears coarse because of facial bone and soft tissue overgrowth (see p. 3). The hands become enlarged and spade-like (Fig. 1) and the feet become enlarged. Classically patients require larger gloves, hats, and shoes. Hypertension and

diabetes mellitus may result (the latter because growth hormone is an insulin antagonist).

PROLACTIN

Prolactin, the commonest hormone to be secreted by pituitary tumours, is

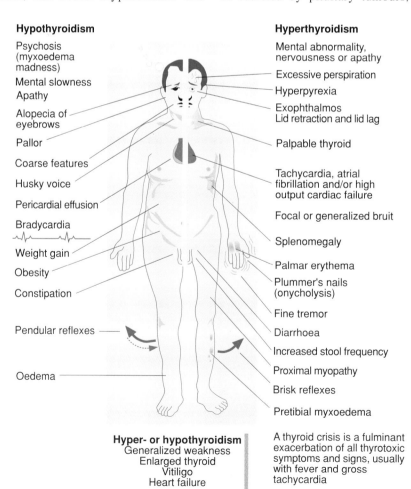

Hypothyroidism

Psychosis (myxoedema madness)
Mental slowness
Apathy
Alopecia of eyebrows
Pallor
Coarse features
Husky voice
Pericardial effusion
Bradycardia
Weight gain
Obesity
Constipation
Pendular reflexes
Oedema

Hyperthyroidism

Mental abnormality, nervousness or apathy
Excessive perspiration
Hyperpyrexia
Exophthalmos
Lid retraction and lid lag
Palpable thyroid
Tachycardia, atrial fibrillation and/or high output cardiac failure
Focal or generalized bruit
Splenomegaly
Palmar erythema
Plummer's nails (onycholysis)
Fine tremor
Diarrhoea
Increased stool frequency
Proximal myopathy
Brisk reflexes
Pretibial myxoedema

Hyper- or hypothyroidism
Generalized weakness
Enlarged thyroid
Vitiligo
Heart failure

A thyroid crisis is a fulminant exacerbation of all thyrotoxic symptoms and signs, usually with fever and gross tachycardia

Fig. 2 **The possible symptoms and signs of hyper- and hypothyroidism.**

responsible for lactation and plays a part in other 'feminine' functions.

Hyperprolactinaemia in females presents with inappropriate lactation, amenorrhoea, or infertility (because prolactin interferes with LH and FSH). In males hyperprolactinaemia may produce lactation, slight gynaecomastia, a low sperm count (and thus infertility), and impotence.

THYROID DYSFUNCTION

The thyroid gland produces thyroxine which acts as a 'general metabolic stimulant' for most tissues. Examination of the thyroid is detailed on page 15.

Hyperthyroidism

In cases of suspected hyperthyroidism (Fig. 2), ask about:

- changes in weight
- appetite (increased)
- stool frequency (increased)
- tolerance of heat (decreased)
- sweating (increased)
- mental changes (usually agitation although paradoxically apathy may occur).

Lid retraction and lid lag may both be found in hyperthyroidism. Lid retraction is elevation of the upper eyelid at rest above the normal position just below the top of the iris. Figure 3 shows lid retraction in

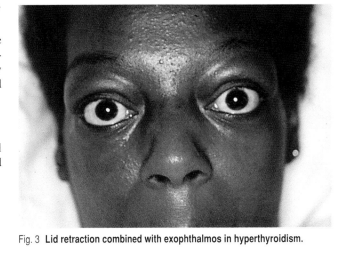

Fig. 3 **Lid retraction combined with exophthalmos in hyperthyroidism.**

combination with exophthalmos. Lid lag is best demonstrated by asking the patient to keep his head still and to look at the ceiling and then to glance downwards slowly towards the floor: normally the lid follows the iris downwards but in thyrotoxicosis the lid lags behind.

Exophthalmos is a pushing forward of the eyes by excessive tissue deposition behind the eyeball. It is best seen if the doctor looks vertically downward from above the patient's head or by looking at each eyeball from the side.

The tremor of thyrotoxicosis is very fine and best revealed by placing a sheet of paper across the patient's outstretched fingers.

Pretibial myxoedema (paradoxically found in thyrotoxicosis) is puffy tissue usually found on the anterior shin.

A thyroid crisis is a fulminant exacerbation of all thyrotoxic symptoms and signs with fever and gross tachycardia.

Hypothyroidism

In hypothyroidism (Fig. 2) there may be a history of predisposing factors including iodine deficiency, previous thyroid surgery, or over effective treatments for previous hyperthyroidism. The possible symptoms and signs of infantile hypothyroidism are detailed in Figure 4.

Delayed tendon reflexes found in hypothyroidism are best elicited by asking the patient to kneel on a chair with the ankles projecting: after eliciting the ankle jerk the return of the foot to its original position will be delayed (p. 93).

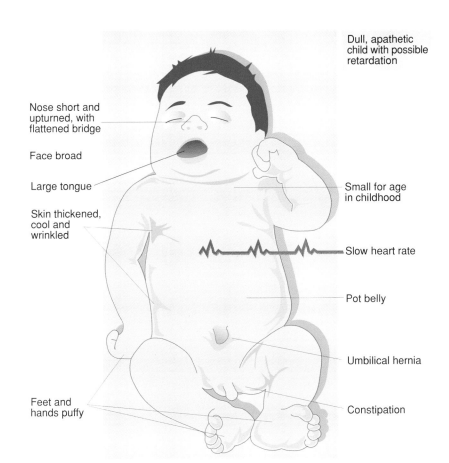

Dull, apathetic child with possible retardation

Nose short and upturned, with flattened bridge

Face broad

Large tongue

Skin thickened, cool and wrinkled

Small for age in childhood

Slow heart rate

Pot belly

Umbilical hernia

Feet and hands puffy

Constipation

Fig. 4 **Symptoms and signs of infantile hypothyroidism.**

Pituitary related hormones (II)

- The manifestations of male hypogonadism depend on whether puberty has occurred.
- The features of growth hormone excess depend on whether the epiphyses have fused.
- Thyroid hormones are general metabolic stimulants.

PITUITARY DYSFUNCTION / PITUITARY INDEPENDENT HORMONES

PITUITARY DYSFUNCTION

The effects of hyper- or hypopituitarism depend on the function of the target end-organs: symptoms suggesting that the primary pathology is in the pituitary includes headache or visual field defects, particularly bitemporal hemianopia if a pituitary tumour is compressing the optic chiasma.

ANTERIOR PITUITARY HYPOFUNCTION

Hypofunction of all or most of the anterior pituitary hormones (hypopituitarism) presents with a picture which, if complete, comprises hypothyroidism, signs of hypocortisolaemia, and signs of lack of FSH and LH. If hypopituitarism occurs in early childhood the stature is small (pituitary dwarfism).

Hypopituitarism may be caused by space occupying or infiltrative lesions of the pituitary, aneurysms, hypothalamic lesions, meningitic illnesses, by pituitary infarction after post-partum haemorrhage (Sheehan's syndrome) or after haemorrhage into a pituitary tumour.

With progressive hypopituitarism the anterior pituitary hormones usually fail sequentially, GH and LH first, then FSH, TSH, and then ACTH. Prolactin deficiency is rare.

POSTERIOR PITUITARY DYSFUNCTION

Diabetes insipidus

Diabetes insipidus (the passing of insipid urine rather than the sweet urine of diabetes mellitus) is caused by deficiency of vasopressin (antidiuretic hormone, ADH), which is necessary for water conservation by the kidney. Patients may give a history of excessive micturition (up to about 10 litres daily) and/or excessive thirst in association with a history of predisposing factors such as destructive operations on the pituitary, head injury, or symptoms suggesting tumour, infiltrations, or meningitis, all of which may affect the pituitary. A similar condition, renal diabetes insipidus, occurs if the kidneys do not respond to normal levels of ADH.

Oxytocin

Oxytocin has a role in parturition and in lactation.

PITUITARY INDEPENDENT HORMONES

HYPERALDOSTERONISM (CONN'S SYNDROME)

Hyperaldosteronism causes excessive sodium retention and excessive potassium loss by the kidneys. If severe there may be signs of hypokalaemic alkalosis with weakness, parasthesiae, and polyuria with secondary polydipsia. Often the only clinical manifestation is a raised blood pressure.

THE PARATHYROID GLANDS

Parathormone is secreted by the four small parathyroid glands which are situated behind the thyroid gland and are responsible for maintaining the blood calcium.

Hyperparathyroidism

Hyperparathyroidism (Fig. 1) and its associated hypercalcaemia are often asymptomatic but the hypercalcaemia may present with vague symptoms of weakness, anorexia, abdominal pain, constipation, renal stones, metabolic bone disease, polyuria and thirst. Psychiatric problems and conscious level disturbance are found in severe hypercalcaemia. The only physical sign of (chronic) hypercalcaemia is corneal calcification.

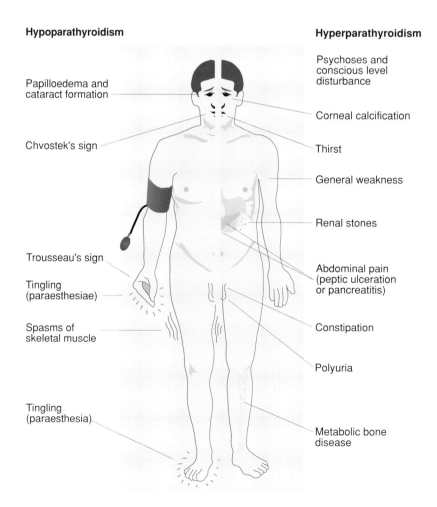

Fig. 1 **The symptoms and signs of hypo- and hyperparathyroidism.**

Hypoparathyroidism

With hypoparathyroidism (Fig. 1) there may be a history of previous thyroidectomy with inadvertent removal or damage to the parathyroid glands. In such cases symptoms typically present one day after the operation. Symptoms are caused by hypocalcaemia and include tingling (parasthesiae) affecting the lips, tongue, hands and feet, spasms of skeletal muscle (tetany), and there may be a history of facial or laryngeal muscle spasms: these signs are a result of increased neuromuscular excitability caused by hypocalcaemia. A low calcium or a rapid fall in calcium level may precipitate fits in children.

Chvostek's sign is facial muscle spasm elicited by tapping the parotid which irritates the facial nerve. Trousseau's sign is spasm of the muscle of the lower arm occurring when a blood pressure cuff is kept inflated above the systolic pressure for 3 minutes (Fig. 2). Papilloedema and cataract formation occur in chronic hypocalcaemia. Occasionally hypocalcaemia and associated signs are caused by metabolic unresponsiveness to parathormone (pseudohypoparathyroidism).

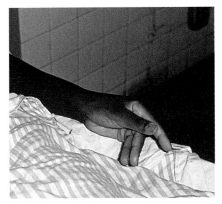

Fig 2 **Trousseau's sign: carpopedal spasm affecting the hand in hypoparathyroidism.**

THE ADRENAL MEDULLA

A phaeochromocytoma is a tumour of the adrenal medulla (in 20% the tumour is in an extra-adrenal situation) which produces intermittent or sustained excessive secretion of catecholamines. Patients may give a history of paroxysmal headaches, angina, or anxiety. On examination there may be paroxysmal or sustained hypertension. Occasionally the causative catecholamine secreting tumour may be palpable, and attempted palpation or abrupt changes in body posture may precipitate the patient's symptoms.

DIABETES MELLITUS

Diabetes mellitus is a clinical syndrome characterized by hyperglycaemia (Tables 1 and 2), which is usually associated with absolute or relative lack of insulin. Overproduction of antagonists to insulin, such as growth hormone or cortisol excess, may also produce or unmask diabetes.

Insulin is produced by the pancreas and there may thus be a history of pancreatitis, haemochromatosis 'bronze diabetes', pancreatic neoplasia, pancreatic surgery, or cystic fibrosis. Most cases of diabetes are of uncertain aetiology, however.

Insulin dependent diabetes mellitus (IDDM)
IDDM usually develops in patients under the age of 40 and there is usually a rapid development (over several days) of symptoms and signs.

Non-insulin dependent diabetes mellitus (NIDDM)
NIDDM usually presents in middle-aged or elderly patients who are often overweight. They do not usually present with rapid onset symptoms or signs unless illness is precipitated by the stress of infec-

tion or trauma. Diabetic retinopathy and chronic neurological changes such as peripheral neuropathy are more common in NIDDM diabetics.

In both IDDM and NIDDM there is a predisposition to infection which ranges from trivial fungal infection such as candida to more serious infections such as pneumonia.

Hypoglycaemia
Hypoglycaemia may be caused by excessive pancreatic insulin secretion or by excessive administration of exogenous insulin: chronic hypoglycaemia suggests insulinoma. Hypoglycaemia may also be caused by 'overshoot' hyperinsulinism occurring after a high blood glucose has stimulated and been 'over-rectified' by excessive insulin secretion.

Table 1 **Signs of chronic diabetes**

Diabetic retinopathy
Diabetic card in wallet
Lipodystrophy at possible injection sites (Fig. 3)
Neuropathy
Peripheral vascular disease

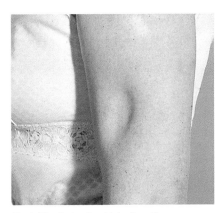

Fig. 3 **Lipodystrophy at injection site.**
Lipohypertrophy may also occur.

Table 2 **Possible signs of acute presentation diabetes**

Symptom	Hypoglycaemia	Hyperglycaemia
Drowsiness	+	+
Coma	+	+
Eyeballs soft	−	+
Hunger	+	Possible
Thirst	±	+
Dehydration	−	+
Acetone on breath	−	+
Acidotic respiration	−	+
Blood pressure	Non-specific	Usually low
Sweating	+	−
Tachycardia	+	Non-specific
Secondary focal neurological signs	Possible	Possible

Pituitary dysfunction/ pituitary independent hormones

- Headache and visual field defects, especially bitemporal hemianopia, suggest pituitary problems.
- The only sign of chronic hypercalcaemia is corneal calcification.
- Hypocalcaemia may cause Chvostek's and Trousseau's signs to be positive.
- Diabetes insipidus may be caused by posterior pituitary or hypothalamic dysfunction or renal insensitivity to antidiuretic hormone.
- Diabetes mellitus predisposes to infection (and vascular disease).

STRUCTURE AND FUNCTION

The design of the human nervous system is not renowned for simplicity, and almost all motor and sensory pathways cross the midline at some stage. The reason for this curious occurrence is almost certainly the overwhelming evolutionary advantages conferred by integrated binocular vision which involves crossing of the midline of the visual pathways and, consequently, most other pathways.

The following account is long but necessary to enable an adequate understanding of nervous system function so that history taking and examination can be approached in a rational way. The anatomical (Fig. 1) and physiological features of the nervous system are detailed, followed by the examination of the cranial nerves, trunk and limbs, and then the history and findings in various conditions.

THE CEREBRAL HEMISPHERES

The cortex caps the cerebral hemispheres and is responsible for interpretation and integration of sensory inputs, and for initiating motor output. The cortex is a multidimensional matrix of electrical activity in non-myelinated, and therefore grey-coloured, nervous tissue. The cerebral cortex is responsible for initiating movements of the opposite side by their downwardly projecting corticospinal (pyramidal) motor tracts. These comprise the myelinated (and therefore white-coloured) matter of the cerebral hemispheres, brainstem and spinal cord.

In addition, each hemisphere has extra distinctive functions. Those of the dominant (usually the left) hemisphere are detailed on page 94. The major distinctive function of the non-dominant hemisphere is the integration of visiospatial relationships.

THE EXTRAPYRAMIDAL SYSTEM

The extrapyramidal system comprises the basal ganglia and various tracts responsible for certain optic and auditory reflexes. Damage to the extrapyramidal system (Table 1) causes involuntary movements and abnormalities of muscle tone with tremor superimposed onto rigidity.

THE THALAMUS

The thalamus is a sensory relay station above the pons where (spinothalamic)

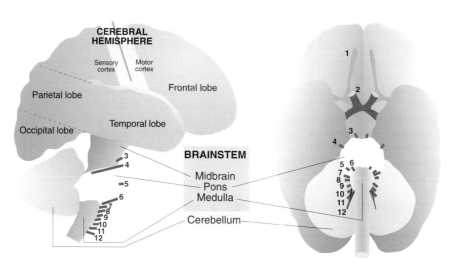

Fig. 1 **The anatomy of the brain and brainstem.** The cranial nerves are numbered.

sensory fibres synapse. If the thalamus is damaged, major disturbances occur in spinothalamic and posterior column sensations (joint position and vibration sense). If the damage is unilateral the signs will be on the opposite side because all ascending sensory pathways have crossed at lower levels.

THE HYPOTHALAMUS

The hypothalamus (which is just below the thalamus and just above the pituitary) and some parts of the cerebral cortex form the limbic system which integrates autonomic (non-consciously supervised) activity occurring in association with emotions. The hypothalamus is also involved with pituitary function.

THE ASCENDING RETICULAR FORMATION

The ascending reticular formation receives information derived from sensory nerves and also stimulates the cortex into activity, literally keeping the cortex awake. If the function of the ascending reticular formation is impaired a deep sleep results with unresponsiveness to pain.

THE DESCENDING RETICULAR FORMATION

The descending reticular formation, which extends throughout the brainstem from medulla to thalamus, ultimately inhibits various excitatory impulses in the spinal cord which would eventually affect

motor nerves. The muscle stretch (tendon) reflexes become exaggerated if this inhibitory influence is removed.

THE CEREBELLUM

The cerebellum has been termed the head ganglion of the proprioceptive system. It receives sensory input from muscles, tendons, joints, bones, and vestibular (balance) information from the ear. By processing this information the cerebellum controls and coordinates movement, predominantly by controlling muscle tone.

Unilateral damage to the cerebellum (Table 2) causes clinical signs on the *same* side of the body (unlike damage to the cerebral hemispheres).

Table 1 **The possible findings in extrapyramidal tract lesions including Parkinson's disease and phenothiazine overdosage**

Bradykinesia
Cogwheel rigidity
Tremor
Positive glabellar tap

Table 2 **The possible findings in cerebellar lesions**

Intention tremor	Pendular tendon reflexes
Scanning speech	Abnormalities of gait including typical cerebellar gait, dysmetria (inability to direct or limit movement), dyssynergia (muscular incoordination)
Nystagmus	
Hypotonia	

THE BRAINSTEM

The brainstem comprises the midbrain, pons and medulla. The cerebral cortex is connected to the midbrain by the cerebral peduncles; the cerebellum is connected to the brainstem by its peduncles. All cranial nerves except the first and second have stations in the brainstem. The brainstem functions like a 'spaghetti junction' for nervous pathways. Many moderating influences are exerted upon these pathways as they pass through the brainstem. All this is complicated enough, but the brainstem also contains many of the nerve fibres which cross the midline.

Impulses from the spinal cord

For reasons obscure, the sensory input derived from the peripheral nerves ascends via two separate pathways. Proprioception (joint position) and vibration senses ascend (without crossing the midline) in the posterior columns of the spinal cord to the lower medulla where they then cross the midline to form the medial lemniscus. Most touch sense ascends posteriorly in the spinal cord and crosses at a higher level. In contrast, pain, temperature, and some touch fibres cross the midline shortly after their entry into the spinal cord, thereafter ascending as the spinothalamic tract which, after relaying in the thalamus, becomes the spinal lemniscus which is contiguous with the medial lemniscus. The two lemnnisci ascend together to the sensory cortex – thus the two sensory inputs are eventually reunited.

Impulses to the spinal cord

The descending motor output for each side of the body forms a long tract, the upper motor neurone, which originates in the motor cortex, crosses the midline in the medullary (pyramidal) decussation and then travels down the spinal cord as the lateral corticospinal tract. It eventually connects with the anterior horn cells of the

Table 3 **The possible findings in brainstem lesions**

Nystagmus	Sweating
Vomiting	Horner's syndrome
Increased muscle tone	Rapid respirations
Hyperreflexia	Tachycardia
Opisthotonus	'Crossed' cranial nerve palsies
Extension of limbs	
Hyperpyrexia	Death

lower motor neurone. Table 3 details the possible clinical signs of brainstem dysfunction.

THE SPINAL CORD

Sensory impulses from the peripheral nerves relay in the posterior root ganglion and enter the spinal cord (Fig. 2).

Upper motor neurone impulses descend in the corticospinal tracts, connect with the anterior horn cells and thereafter travel in the lower motor neurone which leaves the spinal cord in the anterior root. The cause of upper motor neurone dysfunction may be anywhere between the cortex and the synapse with anterior horn cells of the lower motor neurone. The signs of upper and lower motor neurone lesions are shown in Table 4.

If the spinal cord is completely transected there are bilateral peripheral nerve symptoms or signs at the level of the lesion (almost as if the peripheral nerve had been cut) and complete loss of sensation and muscle control below on both sides.

PERIPHERAL NERVES

Peripheral nerves may carry sensory, motor and autonomic information. Each peripheral nerve has two roots:

- posterior sensory root
- anterior motor root.

Each posterior nerve root receives sensation from a limited area of skin (a dermatome or spinal segmental area). Root pain is usually lancinating and is often made worse by coughing or spinal movements. In posterior root lesions, cutaneous pain loss usually exceeds that of touch loss, whereas in peripheral nerve lesions, touch loss usually exceeds that of pain.

Complete interruption of a peripheral nerve causes total sensory loss, total loss of muscle power and autonomic function in areas supplied exclusively by that nerve.

Incomplete interruption of a peripheral nerve may reduce all forms of cutaneous sensation, although the reduced sensation and tingling may be experienced as being very unpleasant. There will be weakness of the muscles supplied, possibly with fasciculation (fine or coarse muscle contractions which ripple across the surface of a muscle).

If peripheral nerves (or their sensory part) are diffusely affected by metabolic or toxic illnesses (a peripheral neuropathy), the sensory loss does not restrict itself to any one nerve but rather causes 'glove and stocking' sensory loss.

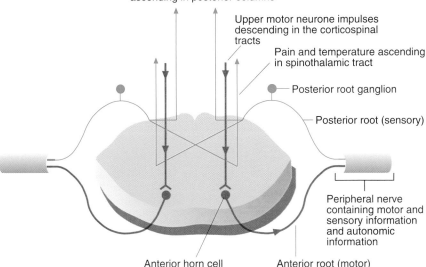

Vibration and joint position sense ascending in posterior columns

Upper motor neurone impulses descending in the corticospinal tracts

Pain and temperature ascending in spinothalamic tract

Posterior root ganglion

Posterior root (sensory)

Peripheral nerve containing motor and sensory information and autonomic information

Anterior horn cell

Anterior root (motor)

Fig. 2 **The peripheral nerves, nerve roots and spinal cord – simplified anatomy and function.**

Table 4 **Clinical signs of upper and lower motor neurone lesions**

Upper motor neurone lesions
Clonus
Abdominal reflexes absent unilaterally
Weakness
Spasticity (initially a flaccid paralysis may be present as in spinal shock)
Tendon reflexes increased
'Clasp knife' phenomenon present (on initial passive movement tone is increased but once movement occurs tone is reduced markedly)
Increased tone in anti-gravity muscles

Lower motor neurone lesions
Flaccid paralysis
Absent reflexes
Fasciculation (later signs include contractures and trophic changes)

1ST CRANIAL NERVE/ 2ND CRANIAL NERVE AND EYES (I)

Anatomical and functional considerations of the twelve cranial nerves will be considered on the following pages along with details of clinical examination. Non-neurological considerations are mentioned when these are usually assessed with the neurological examination.

THE OLFACTORY (I) NERVE

Nerve fibres responsible for the sense of smell (olfaction) originate in the nasal olfactory mucosa and penetrate the cribriform plate of the ethmoid bone at the apex of the nasal cavity to form the olfactory bulb. From here impulses are relayed to the hypothalamus and temporal lobes. The olfactory nerve is responsible only for smell sensation and *not* for the recognition of irritating or painful stimuli (which is a function performed by the trigeminal nerve).

Most causes of anosmia (absence of smell) are nasal and not neurological in aetiology. To test appreciation of smell, first ask the patient if there is any impairment of smell, and then exhibit various odorous substances to one nostril whilst occluding the other. It is simplest to offer the patient a bottle containing a specific odour and give him a choice of responses (including the actual odour). Floral or musky odours provide a more sensitive and specific assessment of olfactory acuity.

THE OPTIC (II) NERVE AND EXAMINATION OF THE EYES

Visual stimuli strike the retina of the eye (Fig. 1) and nervous impulses are

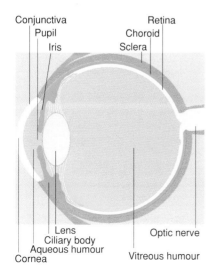

Fig. 1 **The anatomy of the eye.**

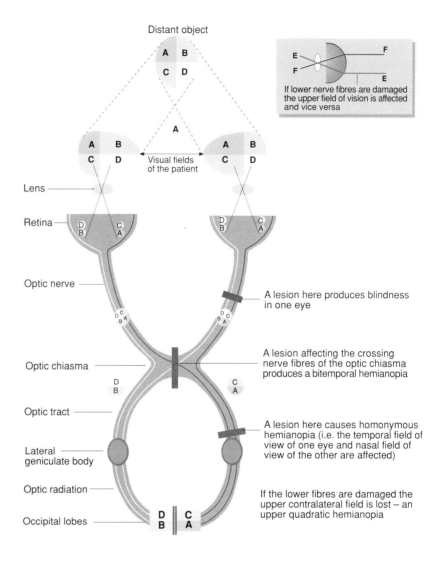

Fig. 2 **The visual losses produced by lesions at various sites of the optic pathways.**

generated which are relayed either to the occipital cortex for integration and onward transmission for conscious appreciation, or to the light reflex centres. The lateral geniculate bodies are synapse stations between the optic tracts and optic radiations.

To enable binocular vision, fibres from each retina have to cross the midline. This allows stimuli from one visual field (but derived from both eyes) to be reunited and processed in the occipital cortex of the opposite side. For a rapid response to occur to a one-sided stimulus the motor output has to cross the midline so that the limb of that side, which is nearer and thus more relevant to the stimulus than the limb of the other side, can respond rapidly (this probably is the fundamental reason why most other pathways cross).

Lesions affecting the crossing fibres of the optic chiasma produce a bitemporal hemianopia (Fig. 2) and lesions affecting the optic tract or radiation produce a contralateral homonymous hemianopia (homonymous means affecting the temporal half of one visual field and the nasal half of the other, and hemianopia means a blindness in one half of the visual field experienced by one or both eyes).

The upper parts of the retina are responsible for stimuli received from the lower visual fields and vice versa. When the upper fibres of the optic tract or radiation are involved, a lower quadrantic hemianopia affecting the contralateral side results. Conversely when the lower fibres are involved, there is a contralateral upper quadrantic defect.

Examination of the optic nerve involves assessing:

- visual acuity
- visual fields
- light reflexes
- eye tissues with an ophthalmoscope
- pupil characteristics.

VISUAL ACUITY

Visual acuity is tested by occluding the eye not under test and ascertaining whether the patient can read various sizes of print. More formally, a Snellen chart at a distance of 6 metres can be used to test each eye in turn (Fig. 3). If at 6 metres, the patient can only just read print that a normal person could read at 60 metres, the visual acuity is recorded as 6/60.

Severe lesions of one eye or its optic nerve produce blindness of that eye.

VISUAL FIELDS

A useful, but occasionally fallible, screening test of visual fields is to ask the patient (with both eyes open) to look at your face, and for you to move the index fingers of both your hands which are held laterally midway between you and the patient (Fig. 4). Ask the patient how many fingers he sees moving. Repeat this in both upper and lower halves of your (and thus the patient's) visual fields. If, on each occasion, the patient has not seen both fingers moving then suspect a homonymous hemianopia, a quadrantic hemianopia or an inattention defect affecting one visual field.

A warning: patients, especially those with optic radiation damage, may be unaware of gross defects of vision.

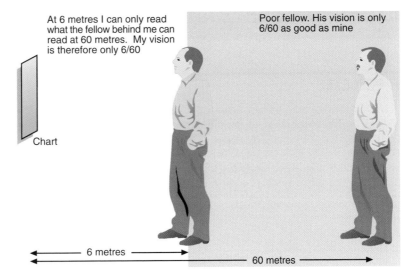

At 6 metres I can only read what the fellow behind me can read at 60 metres. My vision is therefore only 6/60

Chart

Poor fellow. His vision is only 6/60 as good as mine

6 metres

60 metres

Fig. 3 **Snellen chart interpretation.**

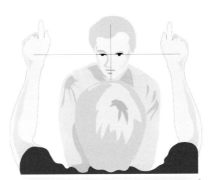

Move each finger in turn, then both together, in each quadrant of the patient's (binocular) visual field. On each occasion ask 'Which finger do you see moving ?'

Fig. 4 **Confrontation as a screening test to detect abnormalities in visual fields.**

More detailed testing of visual fields involves testing each eye in turn with the patient sitting in front of the examiner (Fig. 5). One of the patient's eyes and the examiner's opposing eye are closed or shielded. The examiner's eye should be about 2 feet from the patient so that the examiner's (normal) visual field corresponds to that of the patient. Both the patient and examiner should look directly at each other's opposing eye so that visual fields can be compared. The examiner then advances a hat pin slowly above and to the sides of the eye being tested, midway between the patient's and the examiner's eye. The patient is asked to say yes as soon as the hatpin bobble is seen.

Each quadrant should be tested in turn and then the extent of the central scotoma (blind spot) estimated. In each instance the comparison with normal is provided by the examiner's visual fields. Accurate perimetry requires specialized ophthalmological equipment.

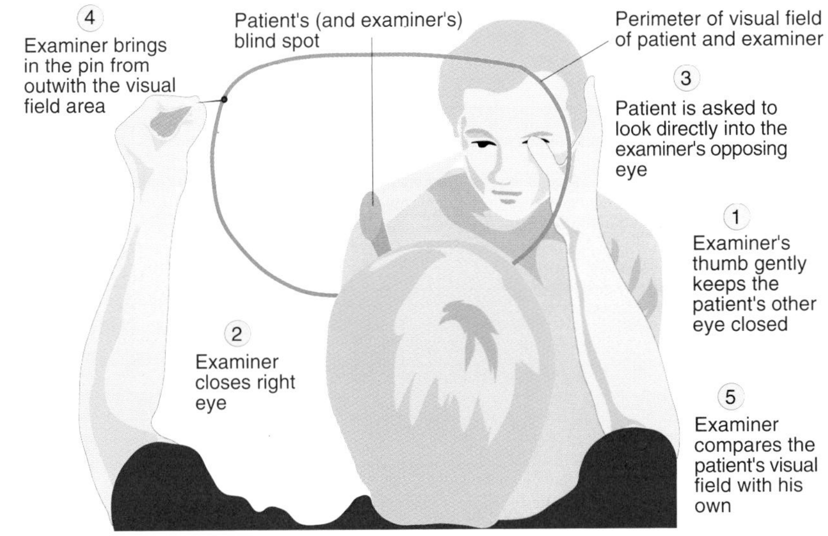

④
Examiner brings in the pin from outwith the visual field area

Patient's (and examiner's) blind spot

Perimeter of visual field of patient and examiner

③
Patient is asked to look directly into the examiner's opposing eye

①
Examiner's thumb gently keeps the patient's other eye closed

②
Examiner closes right eye

⑤
Examiner compares the patient's visual field with his own

1st cranial nerve / 2nd cranial nerve and eyes (I)

- Most causes of anosmia are nasal and not neurological in aetiology.
- Lesions affecting the optic chiasma produce a bitemporal hemianopia.
- Lesions affecting the optic tract and radiation produce a contralateral homonymous hemianopia.
- Never test visual acuity if both of the patient's eyes are open: vision will be reported as normal even if the patient has one glass eye.

Fig. 5 **Testing of individual eye visual fields by confrontation.**

2ND CRANIAL NERVE AND EYES (II)

LIGHT REFLEXES

If one eye is exposed to a bright light, constriction of both pupils occurs (Fig. 1). The constriction of the illuminated eye is the *direct* reflex and that of the non-illuminated eye the *consensual* reflex (Fig. 2).

Loss of pupillary constriction implies a lesion affecting a site or sites in the reflex pathway which comprises (Fig. 2):

- the retina
- the optic nerve
- the optic chiasma
- a small portion of the optic tract
- the superior corpora quadrigemina and the Edinger–Westphal

nuclei (where information crosses the midline, explaining the consensual reflexes)

- the pupilloconstrictor part of the oculomotor nuclei
- the oculomotor nerve supplying the circular constrictor muscle of the pupil.

Predictably, it is possible to have total blindness in one visual field and intact light reflexes with light shone in from that visual field if there is damage just anterior to the lateral geniculate body (Fig. 2).

To test the light reflexes the patient should be asked to look into the distance and not at the light (to avoid the accommodation reflex). A small beam of bright light is shone into the eye under the test *from the side* to avoid eliciting an accommodation reflex.

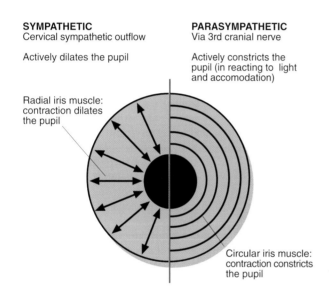

Fig. 1 **Physiology and anatomy of pupilloconstriction and pupillodilation.**

Fig. 2 **The anatomy of the pupillary light reflexes.**

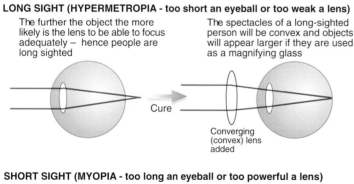

LONG SIGHT (HYPERMETROPIA - too short an eyeball or too weak a lens)

The further the object the more likely is the lens to be able to focus adequately – hence people are long sighted

The spectacles of a long-sighted person will be convex and objects will appear larger if they are used as a magnifying glass

Cure

Converging (convex) lens added

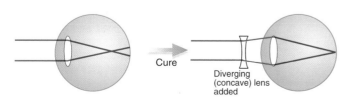

SHORT SIGHT (MYOPIA - too long an eyeball or too powerful a lens)

The nearer the object the more likely is the lens to be able to focus adequately – hence people are short sighted

The spectacles of a short-sighted person will be concave and objects will appear smaller if they are used as a magnifying glass

Cure

Diverging (concave) lens added

OPHTHALMOSCOPY

Ophthalmoscopy is best done in a darkened room. If mydriatics are used always record this in the notes. There is no substitute for experience combined with pictorial knowledge of possible abnormalities.

Most ophthalmoscopes (Fig. 4) have plus lenses (convex, usually red on the dial) and minus lenses (concave, usually marked in white). With a long-sighted patient (who has an inappropriately short eyeball or a too weakly converging ocular lens) a plus lens will need to be used. Conversely, with a short-sighted patient (with an inappropriately long eyeball or a too strongly converging ocular lens), a minus lens should be used (Fig. 3).

Fig. 3 **Use of the ophthalmoscope in long and short sight.** The ophthalmoscope can add in a variety of converging (red or +) and diverging (white or –)lenses.

The examiner should train himself to examine the patient's right eye with his right eye, and the patient's left eye with his left eye (Fig. 4). This enables the examiner to request that the patient look into the distance without the examiner's head being interposed.

For the initial approach a markedly plus lens should be selected as this will allow inspection of the cornea and iris, and thereafter progressive selection of a 'less plus' lens will allow the structure of the eye to be examined from front to back.

An important practical point. Do not breathe, or allow the patient to breathe, on the ophthalmoscope head. The lens being used will always become unusable because of condensation.

ASSESSING THE PUPILS

Observe whether:

- the pupils are of equal size
- they are regular
- they are centrally placed
- their size is normal, abnormal or asymmetrical
- they react normally to light and accommodation.

An Argyll Robertson pupil is an abnormal pupil usually caused by syphilis. It is:

- small
- constant in size
- does not react to light
- pupilloconstriction occurs with accommodation to near vision
- the iris usually has a patchy depigmentation and reacts only slowly to pupillodilator drugs (mydriatics).

A Holmes–Adie pupil is probably caused by a denervation hypersensitivity of the iris muscle. It is:

- usually slightly dilated
- minimally reactive to light
- the pupil constricts very slowly to light but may subsequently over-constrict (so that it becomes smaller than its fellow)
- unilateral in 80% of cases
- may be associated with absence of some of the tendon reflexes.

THE ACCOMMODATION REFLEX

The accommodation reflex is included in the examination of the optic nerve because it is invariably tested along with the light reflexes. On looking from a far object to an object within a few inches of the eyes the pupils normally constrict. The probable mechanism is that the oculomotor nerves, which supply the medial recti, are active to obtain convergency. As part of this activity, parasympathetic pupilloconstrictor activity is also evoked.

CATARACTS

Cataract is the term used to describe any lens opacity. The signs are:

- impairment of visual acuity
- a diminished redness of the retina on ophthalmoscopy
- change in appearance of the lens – usually opacity.

Cataracts are associated with:

- age
- diabetes
- steroid therapy
- inflammatory lesions affecting the lens
- trauma.

After using a plus 20 or plus 15 lens to inspect the cornea, iris and the lens for possible opacities, focus onto the retina and bring the vessels into sharp focus. Follow these towards the centre to locate the optic disc (Fig. 5).

2nd cranial nerve and eyes (II)

- Shine a beam of light in from the side when testing light reflexes.
- Do not breathe or allow the patient to breathe on the ophthalmoscope.
- If the retina cannot be visualized suspect cataract.
- Plus lenses are convex (usually red on the dial) and converge.
- Minus lenses are concave (usually white on the dial) and diverge.

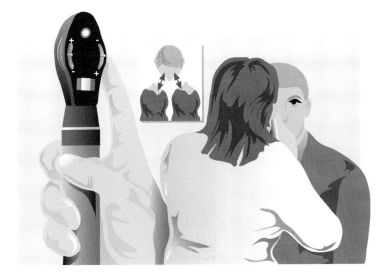

Fig. 4 **Examination with an ophthalmoscope.**

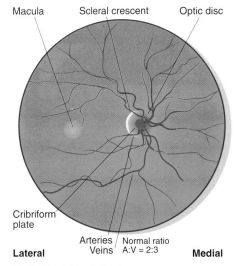

Fig. 5 **The right optic fundus.**

2ND CRANIAL NERVE AND EYES (III)

OPTIC DISC

The optic disc is normally whitish with slight temporal pallor and the circumference is usually well defined, but focusing on the nasal edges may require special care. The optic cup is a concave surface at the middle of the disc.

The rest of the fundus should then be inspected systematically, usually in a clockwise or anticlockwise fashion, using the disc at the centre as the reference point.

MACULA

The macula, which is the area of greatest visual sensitivity, should be inspected with care because even small lesions at the macula can cause profound visual impairment. If your ophthalmoscope can provide a narrow beam of light this is ideal as the macula can be brought into sight by asking the patient to look into the beam of light.

In the centre of the macula there may be a glistening whitish dot, the fovea. Star-shaped lesions tend to occur around the macula because there is a radial pattern of nerve fibres away from it.

THE BLOOD VESSELS

Normally the arteries are slightly tortuous and the ratio of the width of the arteries to the width of the veins is 2:3. The arteries usually cross over the veins without compressing them.

Haemorrhages

Haemorrhages (Fig. 1) are initially reddish and darken as they become old. Causes of haemorrhage include:

- hypertension
- diabetes mellitus
- papilloedema

- vascular occlusions
- arteritic illnesses.

Subhyaloid haemorrhages usually occur adjacent to the optic disc and bulge forward in front of the retina. They usually glisten because the inner membrane of the retina (the hyaloid) covers the haemorrhage. Haemorrhages are initially blob-shaped but later the blood cells sediment downwards to give a horizontal level. Occasionally the haemorrhages break through into the vitreous humour. Subhyaloid haemorrhages may be found in association with subarachnoid haemorrhage.

EXUDATES

Exudates (Fig. 2) are whitish/yellow patches, and if confined to the choroid do not usually disrupt blood vessels (because blood vessels do not run in the choroid). In contrast, retinal lesions may well disrupt the blood vessels as the vessels run in the retinal tissue. The situation of exudates is important because, in general, choroiditis is usually inflammatory in nature (causes include sarcoidosis, syphilis, tuberculosis and toxoplasmosis), whereas retinitis is often degenerative or metabolic in nature (causes include hypertension, diabetes mellitus and certain blood diseases).

Soft exudates are fluffy, ill-defined, superficial and are caused by small infarcts consequent to arteriolar occlusion: they thus may disrupt the blood vessels. Causes include hypertension, diabetes mellitus and vasculitis.

Hard exudates are small, dense, well-defined spots which occasionally may coalesce to form larger patches. They are caused by lipid deposits, often as part of a diabetic retinopathy.

Other fundal appearances to be noted are microaneurysms, new vessel formation or myopic crescents which are white crescentic patches contiguous to the disc edge, usually on the temporal side.

FUNDAL APPEARANCES IN CERTAIN CONDITIONS

Arteriosclerotic retinopathy

The retinal arterioles become thickened and there is an increased width of the reflected light therefrom. Nipping of the veins by arteries may occur.

Diabetic retinopathy

Diabetes mellitus, being a metabolic disease, produces approximately similar appearances in both eyes. There may be roundish 'dot or blot' haemorrhages (Fig. 3) or hard exudates which may coalesce. Modern views of diabetic retinopathy almost always include the well-defined circular white lesions of laser photocoagulation scars. Small aneurysms may be seen pouching off blood vessels. Retinitis proliferans, with marked proliferation of blood vessels often with evidence of a fibrous reaction, is almost always diagnostic of diabetes mellitus.

Glaucoma

Glaucoma is associated with raised intraocular pressure. With established glaucoma there is enlargement and deepening of the optic cup. An approximate (and occasionally fallible) guide to the intraocular pressure can be gained by gently assessing the hardness of each eye by minimal variation of soft pressure on the patient's closed eyes exerted by the index fingers, with the fingers being placed on the brow to steady the hand (Fig. 4). If

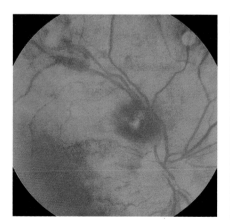

Fig. 1 **Retinal haemorrhages.**

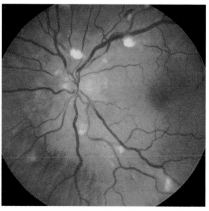

Fig. 2 **Retinal exudates (in this case caused by uncomplicated HIV infection).**

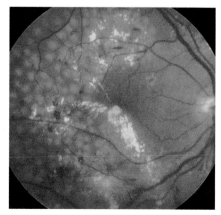

Fig. 3 **Diabetic retinopathy.**

glaucoma is a possibility, specialist advice should be sought.

Hypertensive retinopathy

Hypertensive retinopathy (Fig. 5) may be associated with arteriosclerotic changes. There may be linear, fan or flame-shaped haemorrhages. Although accurate description is preferable to numbers, the enumerators seem to predominate and four grades of hypertensive retinopathy have been defined.

- **Grade 1:** Increased tortuosity of the arteries
- **Grade 2:** Grade 1 changes plus arteriovenous nipping
- **Grade 3:** Grade 2 changes plus haemorrhages and/or exudates
- **Grade 4:** Grade 3 changes plus papilloedema.

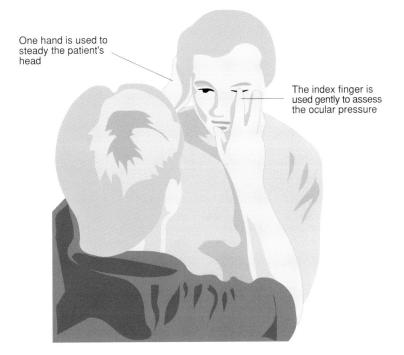

One hand is used to steady the patient's head

The index finger is used gently to assess the ocular pressure

Fig. 4 **Testing for glaucoma.**

Papilloedema

In papilloedema (Fig. 6) the retinal veins become engorged, the disc becomes reddened with a blurred contour, the optic cup becomes filled in, the blind spot becomes enlarged and visual acuity diminishes. Causes of papilloedema include raised intracranial pressure, hypertension and central retinal vein occlusion. Impaired vision is usually a late feature of papilloedema.

Optic atrophy

The disc becomes paler than normal and visual acuity is diminished. Optic atrophy may occur:

- secondary to retrobulbar neuritis
- secondary to retinal artery occlusion
- as a response to direct invasion or pressure effects by tumours
- as part of certain degenerative diseases.

Retinitis pigmentosa

Retinitis pigmentosa is a degenerative disease with bilateral spidery pigment patches in the retina. It is associated with progressive optic atrophy with visual impairment inexorably leading to blindness.

Retrobulbar neuritis

Retrobulbar neuritis is a disorder affecting the optic nerve between the eyeball and optic chiasma. Usually there is central scotoma (a blind spot in the centre of the visual field of the eye involved). If the retrobulbar neuritis is unilateral, the pupil of the eye affected may be larger than its fellow (in response to diminished light appreciation). The direct light reflex will be impaired, but there will be a consensual response to light shone in the other eye. If the nerve head is affected, papilloedema may result. Causes of retrobulbar neuritis include multiple sclerosis, syphilis and various poisons. Retrobulbar neuritis either improves or optic atrophy develops.

Retinal artery occlusion

Retinal artery occlusion is usually of a rapid and painless onset. The retina is anaemic and pale, being 'empty' of blood. The macula is often spared because it receives its blood supply independently from the rest of the retina.

Retinal vein occlusion

In retinal vein occlusion papilloedema results and, predictably, there is impressive venous congestion with haemorrhages into the retina.

2nd cranial nerve and eyes (III)

- The retinal artery to vein width is 2:3.
- The major blood vessels run through retinal tissue.
- Choroiditis is usually caused by inflammatory disorders.
- Soft exudates are caused by small infarcts.
- Hard exudates are caused by lipid deposits.
- Retinal vein occlusions tend to be haemorrhagic.
- Retinal artery occlusions tend to be anaemic.

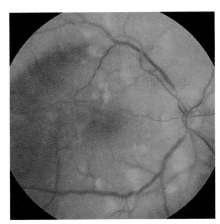

Fig. 5 **Hypertensive retinopathy.**

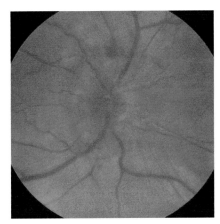

Fig. 6 **Papilloedema.**

CRANIAL NERVES OF EYE MOVEMENT

The cranial nerves responsible for eye movement are the oculomotor (III), trochlear (IV) and abducent (VI) cranial nerves. Eye movements depend on the coordinated function of these nerves and of the muscles they supply. Damage to either nerves or muscles allows unopposed action of the unaffected muscles that move the eye.

All three nerves responsible for eye movements proceed from the brainstem and pass in relation to the cavernous sinus to the eye. Damage in this area may produce a complete external ophthalmoplegia (paralysis of eye movements) and may also cause blindness if the optic nerve is also damaged.

The **oculomotor nerve** supplies the striated elevating muscles of the eyelids, the superior, medial and inferior recti, the inferior obliques, the (non-striated) ciliary muscles and the (parasympathetically innervated) constrictor muscles of the pupil. The upper eyelid has both 'strong' striated muscle, innervated by the oculomotor nerve, and 'weak' smooth muscle, innervated by the sympathetic system. Damage to either causes a ptosis, but an oculomotor lesion may produce a complete ptosis whereas a sympathetic lesion only produces a slight drooping of the eyelid. As might be anticipated, an oculomotor lesion also usually disrupts parasympathetic pupilloconstrictor function which then allows sympathetic activity to dilate the pupil. The **trochlear nerve** supplies the superior oblique muscles. The **abducent nerve** supplies the lateral rectus muscles.

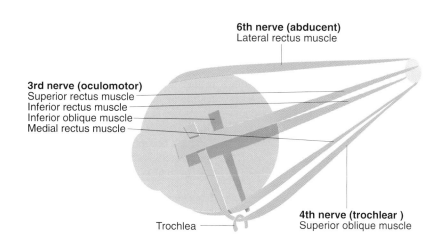

Fig. 1 **Innervation of the eye muscles.** The patient's right eye is viewed from above.

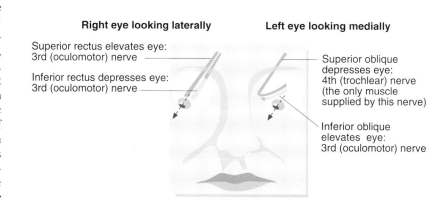

Fig. 2 **Extrinsic eye muscles and their actions.**

EXTRINSIC EYE MUSCLES

All muscles are inserted into the more distant half of the eyeball as judged from the direction from which they pull the eyeball (Figs 1 and 2). It is important to note:

- When the eye is looking straight ahead the lateral rectus muscle abducts the eye and the medial rectus adducts the eye.
- When the eye is looking laterally the superior rectus rotates the eye upwards.
- When the eye is looking laterally the inferior rectus rotates the eye downwards.
- When the eye is looking medially the superior oblique rotates the eye downwards.

- When the eye is looking medially the inferior oblique rotates the eye upwards.

If there is a paralysis of a particular muscle then obviously diplopia will be most marked when the muscle is the major mover for that particular eye movement. Therefore, for example, a superior oblique paralysis (or a trochlear nerve lesion) will cause maximum diplopia when the patient is trying to look inwards and downwards, and with a lateral rectus paralysis (or an abducent nerve lesion) maximum diplopia will occur when the patient affected is attempting to look laterally.

If diplopia is evident the examiner has to determine which eye is at fault. Consideration of the physiology illustrates how this can be achieved (Fig. 3). In practice

the examiner finds the position of maximum diplopia and then shields each eye in turn to determine which image disappears.

None but a genius would pretend that eye movements are easy to understand and even the above is a simple account. Most students start (and not a few doctors end up) by remembering the end results of the nerve lesions! For example, a complete oculomotor nerve lesion causes a complete ptosis (which masks the diplopia), a dilated pupil which does not constrict to light and accommodation and the eye looks downwards and outwards. A trochlear nerve lesion causes paralysis of downward gaze whilst the patient looks inwards ('double vision whilst walking down the stairs, doctor'). An abducent nerve lesion causes loss of abduction.

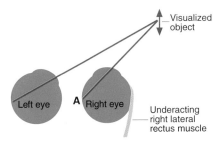

Fig. 3 Identification of the eye at fault if there is diplopia. Because one eye is malpositioned the brain receives two images. Point A in the right eye usually receives light from more peripheral objects. This causes the brain to interpret the right eye's image as being the peripheral image. The false image is always the more peripheral image and, by obscuring each eye in turn, the eye at fault can be identified.

Examination

Eye movements are best tested by asking the patient to follow an 'H' drawn in the air by the index finger of one hand of the examiner in front of the patient's head (the patient's head may need to be held still by the examiner's other hand). Before this is performed the patient should be asked to report if double vision occurs at any time. Provided that the vertical columns of the 'H' are not drawn too laterally, each column will test the superior and inferior recti of the nearer eye and the superior and inferior oblique muscles of the further eye.

EYE MOVEMENT DYSFUNCTION

Strabismus

Apart from extreme near vision the eyes move in concert as if they were parallel. If the eyes are not parallel then there is a squint (a strabismus).

A squint may be classified on anatomical grounds as either *convergent* or *divergent*, depending on whether the eyes appear to be 'crossed' or one or both eyes appear to be looking outwards. A squint may also be classified on functional grounds as either:

- *paralytic*, in which there is a weakness of one or more muscles usually affecting one eye only
- *concomitant* (non-paralytic) in which the movements of the squinting eye are all normal on testing.

In other words, with a ·concomitant squint the muscles are working well but there is a neurological imbalance of some sort affecting integration of movement of both eyes.

Use the cover test to confirm strabismus. Arrange for the patient to fixate upon an object and then briefly cover the eye

that appears to be the major fixator: if the other eye has to change its position in order to become the fixator, then there is a strabismus.

Ophthalmoplegia

Ophthalmoplegia is a paralysis of eye muscles. External ophthalmoplegia is of the muscles which move the eye, whereas internal ophthalmoplegia is a paralysis of pupillary reaction to light and/or accommodation.

Conjugate ophthalmoplegia (conjugate = moving together). Extensive lesions, often vascular, below the cerebral cortex of one side may damage the centre for conjugate *contraversive* movements. Thus there will be conjugate deviation of the eyes to the side of the lesion and failure of conjugate gaze to the opposite side. In unconscious patients the head, as well as the eyes, may be turned towards the site of the lesion. Pontine lesions may occasionally cause conjugate ophthalmoplegia but in this case other cranial nerves are usually involved.

Internuclear ophthalmoplegia. Eye movements of both eyes are adequate when tested individually, but on attempted conjugate lateral gaze in either direction the medial recti do not adduct the adducting eye adequately. Internuclear ophthalmoplegia is almost pathognomic of multiple sclerosis affecting the medial longitudinal bundle in the pons. *Nuclear ophthalmoplegia* refers to damage to the nuclei of cranial nerves supplying eye movements.

Nystagmus

The normal stability of eye posture is influenced by the visual input, by the labyrinthine (vestibular) apparatus and by the cerebellum or its connections. Nystagmus is a rhythmical oscillation of eye position. It may be horizontal, vertical or rotatory in nature. Nystagmus may occur at rest, with movement or in some positions of the head (positional nystagmus). If there is a difference in oscillation the direction of the nystagmus is defined as the direction of the quicker component.

To test for horizontal nystagmus the examiner's finger must be 10 inches in front of and level with the patient's eyes, and should be moved to about 30° to the right and to the left of the midline. Normal people have a transient mild nystagmus on extremes of lateral gaze.

Nystagmus on upward or downward gaze is highly suggestive of a brainstem lesion. Congenital or familial nystagmus is usually present at rest, pendular, and increased on lateral gaze. Problems with vision are often notable by their complete absence.

Visual input ('retinal') nystagmus. Impaired vision, especially when occurring early in life may cause a horizontal pendular nystagmus with oscillations of approximately equal rate and amplitude in each direction of gaze.

Labyrinthine nystagmus. Labyrinthine lesions may produce a horizontal nystagmus which is worse on looking in the direction of the quick component. Labyrinthine nystagmus may be precipitated by head movements, and may be associated with vertigo or deafness.

Cerebellar nystagmus. Unilateral lesions of the cerebellum may produce nystagmus affecting both eyes which is coarser than that of labyrinthine nystagmus. The nystagmus is most marked on gazing towards the side of the lesion.

Ptosis

Ptosis is a drooping of the upper eyelid with inability to elevate it completely. The condition is caused by a weakness of levator muscles which can be caused by dysfunction of the cervical sympathetic or the oculomotor nerve. A sympathetic ptosis will usually be unilateral, slight and unassociated with compensatory frontalis overaction. An oculomotor ptosis will usually be unilateral, often marked and associated with compensatory frontalis overaction. A 'muscle disease ptosis' is usually bilateral (see Fig. 2, p. 104) and symmetrical, and unassociated with frontalis overaction (frontalis often being involved with the same disease). A congenital ptosis is often bilateral and associated with frontalis overaction. A hysterical ptosis is usually unilateral, marked, unassociated with frontalis overaction, but associated with spasm of orbicularis oculi so that the eye cannot be opened passively by the examiner.

Cranial nerves of eye movement

- A complete third nerve lesion causes ptosis and a dilated pupil which looks downwards and outwards.
- A fourth nerve lesion causes problems looking downwards and inwards.
- A sixth nerve lesion causes problems in looking laterally.
- An intranuclear ophthalmoplegia is almost always caused by multiple sclerosis.

8TH CRANIAL NERVE

The eighth cranial (auditory) nerve has two components, the cochlear (responsible for hearing) and the vestibular (labyrinthine) responsible for balance and appreciation of movement (Fig. 1).

COCHLEAR ASPECTS

Nerve fibres from the Organ of Corti are rapidly joined by the vestibular nerve, travel through the facial canal, pass via the internal auditory meatus into the cerebellopontine angle, and the cochlear fibres then enter the pons. Within the pons, fibres cross the midline so that hearing from both ears can be integrated.

Ward testing of hearing should be carried out in a quiet room and after inspection of the ear drum. Each ear is tested separately whilst the other auditory meatus is occluded by a fingertip. Classically a ticking watch was used for this test despite the fact that the pitch was higher than ideal, but because of the epidemic of digital watches, some other stimulus such as the whispered voice has to be used. If a patient is deaf, and if the tympanic membrane is normal and unobstructed by wax, then tuning fork tests are useful.

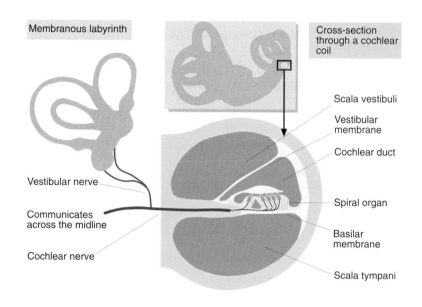

Fig. 1   **The anatomy and simplified neurological connections of the ear.**

THE RINNE TEST

If the conduction of sound impulses through the external or middle ear is decreased (by about 30 decibels or more) then the normal advantage of air conduction is lost and bone conduction becomes better than air. The Rinne test is performed to compare air conduction with bone conduction. To perform the test (Fig. 2), the base of a (512 vibrations per second) tuning fork is set vibrating and placed upon the patient's mastoid process. The patient is then asked to say when the (bone conducted) tuning fork vibrations cease. When this point has been reached, the distal (vibrating end) of the fork is held about 1 cm from the external auditory meatus to test air conduction.

Normally air conduction is better than bone — Rinne positive. If bone conduction is better than air conduction unilaterally, the Rinne test is negative indicating a conductive deafness.

When testing a totally deaf ear it would (spuriously) appear that bone conduction was better than air conduction — a false negative Rinne test. This is because bone conduction to the ear *not* under test is better than air conduction to the ear under test. This false negative Rinne test should not cause confusion because severe deafness should have already been discovered.

WEBER'S TEST

In Weber's test (Fig. 3) the tuning fork base is placed on the vertex of the skull and the patient asked in which ear the sound is best heard. Normally, the sound is heard in the centre. In conductive deafness the sound is heard in the ear most affected by the deafness (as if the cochlea on that side is perpetually straining to hear and becomes hypersensitive as a result). In sensineural deafness, the tuning fork will be heard best in the unaffected ear.

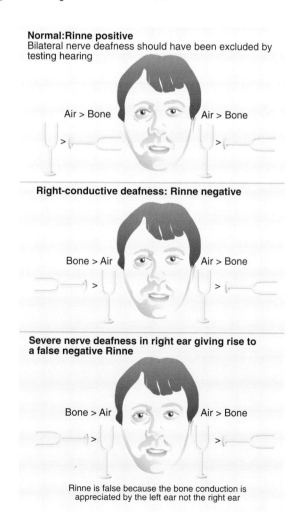

Normal:Rinne positive
Bilateral nerve deafness should have been excluded by testing hearing

Air > Bone   Air > Bone

Right-conductive deafness: Rinne negative

Bone > Air   Air > Bone

Severe nerve deafness in right ear giving rise to a false negative Rinne

Bone > Air   Air > Bone

Rinne is false because the bone conduction is appreciated by the left ear not the right ear

Fig. 2   **The Rinne test.**

THE VESTIBULAR APPARATUS

The vestibular apparatus gives the brain information about head position and head movement. After emerging from the internal auditory meatus, the vestibular fibres enter the brainstem and relay with other nervous elements, including structures relevant to eye movements and the vagus nerve.

TINNITUS

Tinnitus is a buzzing, ringing or hissing sound heard by the sufferer. The commonest types of tinnitus are those associated with cochlear dysfunction with sensorineural deafness, especially presbyacusis (poor hearing associated with age).

VERTIGO

Vertigo is a false impression of rotation (not dizziness or swimminess) of either the patient or the surroundings. Vertigo may result from vestibular nerve lesions, lesions of the brainstem connections or lesions of 'brainstem associated' tissues —especially the cerebellum. Balance may be impossible and the patient may become ataxic or unable to stand. Vertigo, unless trivial, is almost always associated with nystagmus and because of the numerous connections within the brainstem, nausea, vomiting and sweating may be associated.

Several well recognized vertiginous syndromes exist, with suggestive findings on history or examination.

Benign positional vertigo

Patients with benign positional vertigo are usually middle aged and have sudden onset of vertigo whilst changing position. To test for this the patient is positioned sitting up so that the head, held by the examiner, can be quickly lowered over the end of the couch below the horizontal, with one ear downwards (Fig. 4). The examiner should look for nystagmus (the patient will surely tell the examiner if vertigo results!). After a resting period this manoeuvre can be repeated with the other ear downwards. Vertigo plus nystagmus tends to occur when the dysfunctioning vestibular apparatus is in the 'underneath' position.

In 'benign' positional vertigo there is a delay of several seconds before nystagmus, directed towards the lower ear, occurs. On repetition the response is less marked.

In 'malignant' positional vertigo there is no delay in onset of nystagmus, and the nystagmus persists as long as precipitating position is maintained. On repetition the response persists unchanged. Such a response may be indicative of a posterior fossa space-occupying lesion.

Vestibular neuronitis

In vestibular neuronitis the patient experiences variable vertigo which is independent of head position. Recovery occurs over several weeks.

Menière's syndrome

Menière's syndrome is characterized by episodes of sudden onset severe vertigo with prostration lasting up to 24 hours. There is tinnitus and usually subsequent nerve deafness.

Migraine

Migraine may cause vertigo. The clues are the characteristic features of the associated headache.

Multiple sclerosis (MS)

Vertigo is a possible feature of MS. There may be other brainstem signs including diplopia, numbness of the face, dysarthria, or limb ataxia.

Brainstem ischaemia or temporal lobe epilepsy

Both brainstem ischaemia or temporal lobe epilepsy may cause vertigo.

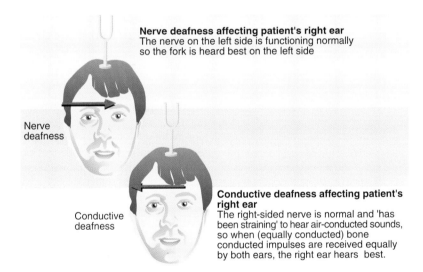

Nerve deafness affecting patient's right ear
The nerve on the left side is functioning normally so the fork is heard best on the left side

Nerve deafness

Conductive deafness

Conductive deafness affecting patient's right ear
The right-sided nerve is normal and 'has been straining' to hear air-conducted sounds, so when (equally conducted) bone conducted impulses are received equally by both ears, the right ear hears best.

Fig. 3 **Weber's test.**

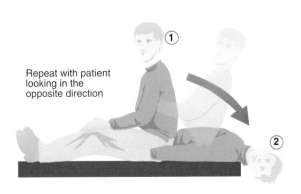

Repeat with patient looking in the opposite direction

8th cranial nerve

- Air conduction is normally better than bone conduction
- Air conduction is normally better then bone conduction in sensineural deafness, but the Weber response will lateralize to the unaffected side.
- If patients can report the direction of rotation then they certainly have had vertigo.

Fig. 4 **Positional testing in cases of vertigo.** Nystagmus which appears with about 15 seconds of this manoeuvre and which subsides spontaneously indicates a problem in the lower-most ear.

OTHER CRANIAL NERVES

THE TRIGEMINAL (V) NERVE

The large sensory and a smaller motor root pass forward from the lateral pons to enter a cavity in the dura mater overlying the apex of the petrous temporal bone. There the gasserian ganglion is formed which gives rise to three divisions of the trigeminal nerve — the ophthalmic, the maxillary and the mandibular. The sensory distribution of trigeminal nerve innervation is shown in Figure 1.

Internal sensation is also provided by the trigeminal nerve for the nasal mucosa, the hard and soft palate, teeth, anterior two-thirds of the tongue (via the chorda tympani of the facial nerve) and the buccal mucosa.

After entry to the brainstem trigeminal pain and temperature appreciation fibres descend and may reach the second cervical segment of the spinal cord. There they cross the midline, eventually uniting with the pain and temperature sensory input from the trunk and limbs. Touch sensation crosses at a higher level, and thus dissociated sensory loss may be found if these lower midline-crossing pain and temperature fibres are damaged. This results in trigeminal pain and temperature impairment, whilst touch appreciation is retained.

Examination of trigeminal nerve function

The touch, pain and temperature cutaneous sensation of the three divisions can be tested separately. The corneal blink reflex is in many ways the most crucial sensory function of the trigeminal nerve because an impaired corneal reflex leaves the eye vulnerable to injury by trauma. To test the corneal reflex, a thin wisp of cotton wool should be introduced from the side (so that the patient cannot see the wool) and be stroked gently across the cornea. A blink (of both eyes) is normally elicited.

To test the motor trigeminal function, the temporalis, masseter and pterygoid muscles are assessed. To test the temporalis and masseter muscles the patient should be asked to clench his teeth so that these two muscles can be seen (or palpated) to be contracting normally (Fig. 2). To test the pterygoids the patient should be asked to protrude the jaw or open the mouth against slight resistance. The jaw will deviate towards the paralysed side (Fig. 3).

The jaw jerk reflex should also be elicited. Like all routinely tested reflexes,

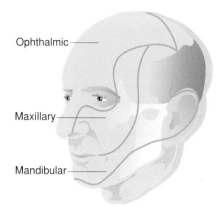

Fig. 1 **Trigeminal nerve sensory distribution.**

Ophthalmic

Maxillary

Mandibular

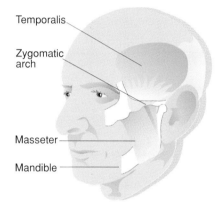

Fig. 2 **Masseter and temporalis muscle action.**

Temporalis

Zygomatic arch

Masseter

Mandible

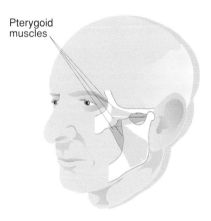

Fig. 3 **Pterygoid muscle action.** When the mouth is being opened against resistance the pterygoids usually prevent the jaw from moving over. If one pterygoid is weak the jaw moves *towards* that side.

Pterygoid muscles

the jaw jerk is a muscle stretch reflex. The patient lets the jaw flop open and the examiner puts a finger horizontally across the chin and taps the finger with a patellar hammer (it helps if the patient has the eyes shut). If the response is brisker than normal this, like any other abnormally brisk muscle stretch reflex, implies upper motor

neurone damage. This reflex has localization value.

If the jaw jerk is pathologically brisk in the presence of bilateral upper motor neurone signs in the limbs, the lesion should be above the pons, whereas if the limb reflexes are brisk but the jaw jerk is normal, the lesion should be below the pons.

THE FACIAL (VII) NERVE

The facial nerve is mostly motor, although for part of its course it carries along with it taste sensation from the anterior two-thirds of the tongue, and some fibres which stimulate salivary secretion. The nucleus of the facial nerve is in the pons. The facial nerve supplies motor impulses to the stapedius muscle, stylohyoid, posterior belly of the digastric, and to the muscles of facial expression.

The forehead muscles are represented bilaterally in the cerebral cortex. Because of this, unilateral cerebral damage does not cause an upper motor neurone type weakness of the forehead muscles of that side. A lower motor neurone lesion of the facial nerve causes weakness of *all* facial nerve innervated muscles on that side of the face. Thus, there is a paradox in terminology — an *upper* motor neurone lesion only affects the *lower* half of the face. Because the orbicularis oculi is weak, overaction of the other eyelid muscles means that the eyelid cannot close. This leads to the possibility of corneal damage.

Testing facial nerve function

Ask the patient to wrinkle the forehead. This will be unilaterally impaired with a unilateral lower motor neurone lesion.

Ask the patient to close his eyes tightly. With a lower motor neurone lesion this is difficult and in the attempt the eyeball also rolls upwards.

Test taste sensation of the anterior two-thirds of the tongue. Place small quantities of the substance under test (traditionally sugar for sweet, quinine for bitter, vinegar for sour and table salt for salt) onto the patient's protruded tongue. The patient should be asked by the examiner to nod his head slightly to indicate a positive reply during the examiner's serial questions: 'Is this sweet? Bitter? Sour? Salty?'. The patient obviously cannot speak his reply!

Ask the patient to wrinkle his nose, show his teeth and blow out the cheeks whilst trying to keep the mouth shut ('pretending to play the trumpet'). An upper or a lower motor neurone lesion impairs the performance for all three and, in particular, blowing out the cheeks results in leakage from the corner of the mouth on the affected side.

With an upper motor neurone lesion, emotionally induced movements are usually only slightly impaired.

THE GLOSSOPHARYNGEAL (IX) NERVE

The glossopharyngeal nerve gathers sensation from the back third of the tongue, the fauces, the palate and the upper pharynx, and provides secretory fibres to the parotid gland. It also transmits impulses from the chemoreceptors and baroreceptors of the carotid body and sinus. In addition the glossopharyngeal nerve also supplies the stylopharyngeus muscle which, together with the palatopharyngeus muscle (X nerve), elevates the palate.

To test for pharyngeal sensation, gently touch the soft palate on each side with an orange stick, and then the posterior pharyngeal wall on each side (Fig. 4). After withdrawal of the orange stick the patient should be asked if all four stimuli were similar. If it is deemed necessary to elicit the gag reflex these stimuli should be evoked with a spatula. The gag reflex tests both IX (sensory) and X (motor) functions. It is almost impossible to assess differential taste discrimination on the posterior third of the tongue.

THE VAGUS (X) NERVE

The vagus nerve contributes to various autonomic plexuses. Motor fibres drive the muscles of the palate, larynx, pharynx and also gather a small sensory input from around the external auditory meatus. The recurrent laryngeal nerve (a branch of the vagus) *on the right* winds posteriorly around the subclavian artery, whereas *on the left* the recurrent laryngeal nerve winds around the arch of the aorta. Both drive the intrinsic muscles of the larynx: unilateral laryngeal nerve palsies cause dysphonia (impairment of voice production), whilst bilateral palsies cause stridor (p. 145).

Examination of the vagus nerve includes observation of palatal movements, assessment of the patient's voice and the ability to cough. Weakness of the palate may cause nasal speech and/or regurgitation of food into the nose. If one side of the palate is paralysed, the uvula is pulled over to the intact side when the patient says 'Aah'.

Weakness of one vocal cord caused by lack of vagal innervation leads to a weak, sometimes hoarse, voice and an inability to cough explosively.

THE ACCESSORY (XI) NERVE

The accessory nerve drives the upper part of the trapezius and the sternomastoid muscle. An accessory nerve lesion causes weakness and wasting of these muscles with impairment of lateral rotation of the head to the opposite side (Fig. 5). Shoulder shrugging is also impaired.

THE HYPOGLOSSAL (XII) NERVE

The hypoglossal nerve is the motor nerve to the tongue. Unilateral lower motor neurone type damage causes weakness, wasting and often unilateral fasciculation of tongue muscle. Weakness of one side enables the muscle component responsible for protrusion of the other side to push over the weak side. Therefore, the protruded tongue deviates *towards* the weak side (Fig. 6). Upper motor neurone type damage causes a stiff, non-wasted tongue which may be hyperreflexic if percussed.

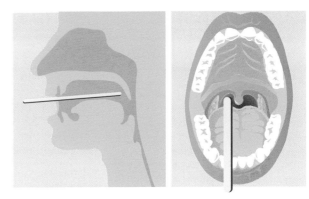

Fig. 4 **Testing pharyngeal sensation.**

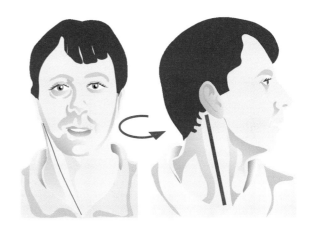

Fig. 5 **Accessory nerve paralysis results in impaired rotation to the opposite side.**

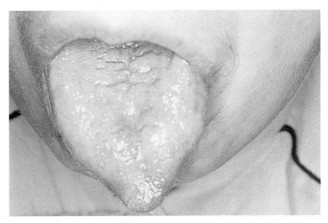

Fig. 6 **Unilateral wasting of the tongue.**

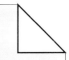

Other cranial nerves

- An absent corneal reflex predisposes to corneal injury.
- An upper motor neurone facial palsy only affects the lower face.
- With a lower motor neurone facial palsy the upper eyelid cannot be closed because the orbicularis oculi muscle that arches over the eye cannot contract normally.
- A lower motor neurone facial palsy predisposes to corneal injury.

EXAMINATION OF LIMBS AND TRUNK — TONE AND POWER

BASIC PRINCIPLES

Neurological examination can be incredibly complex but in an account written for students of medicine more simple screening schemes are more appropriate. This section will therefore concentrate on such techniques before dealing with specific neurological manifestations.

The more complex a screening neurological test requested of a patient, the more likely it is to reveal an abnormality. However, the precise identification of the underlying abnormality almost invariably requires more specific testing.

Testing at the periphery of limbs rather than centrally is more likely to reveal a neurological defect. For example, if the patient can maintain the position of an outstretched upper limb whilst the examiner presses down upon the outstretched fingers, muscle weakness in shoulder, elbow and wrist muscles is unlikely.

Screening for sensation defects is best performed at the peripheries, because the nerves supplying the peripheries are longer and thus more vulnerable to diffuse pathologies such as polyneuritis or neuropathies (which often first manifest by changes in the feet).

Diffuse metabolic or degenerative nervous system pathologies usually produce symmetrical signs rather than isolated or unilateral signs.

When testing sensation move from areas of normal sensation to areas of reduced sensation as patients find it easier to be precise about boundary definition.

The five neurological elements of limb and trunk examination are:

- tone
- power
- sensation
- coordination
- reflexes.

Abnormalities of one or more of these elements may be integrated to produce clinical signs. For example, normal coordination may require integration of proprioception, muscle power, intact higher mental function and vision.

TONE

Clinical assessment of tone

Before assessing tone by means of passive limb movements it is important to ensure that the patient does not have joint immobility or arthritis. Over vigorous passive movements may cause pain or fractures!

In the upper limb the most useful screening test involves holding hands with the patient, flexing and extending the wrist joints, and then flexing and extending the elbow joint whilst simultaneously rotating the forearm gently.

In the lower limb, the hip joint, the knee joint and the ankle joint can be passively flexed and extended. The lower limb can be 'rolled' on the bed and, in the absence of arthritis of the hip, stiffness will be caused by increased tone. A useful technique is to place your hand beneath the patient's relaxed and extended knee and then lift up the knee. Normally the patient's heel will almost come to touch the buttocks as the legs 'fold up'. However, if there is hypertonia this folding-up' will not occur and the whole lower limb will remain more or less straight. If the knee lifting is performed rapidly, the abrupt stretching of the quadriceps may elicit a pathological knee jerk reflex which results in a kicking-like action (Fig. 1).

Normal muscle tone is maintained by negative and positive feedback mechanisms.

Hypotonia

Hypotonia is produced by:

- *lower motor neurone lesions* leading to lack of motor input to the muscles
- *acute neurological lesions* affecting the spine 'spinal shock'
- *lesions of the cerebellum*
- *chorea* which may be caused by degenerative lesions or by neurological toxins
- *intrinsic muscle disease*
- *some conditions such as tabes dorsalis* in which sensory impulses derived from the muscles are lacking.

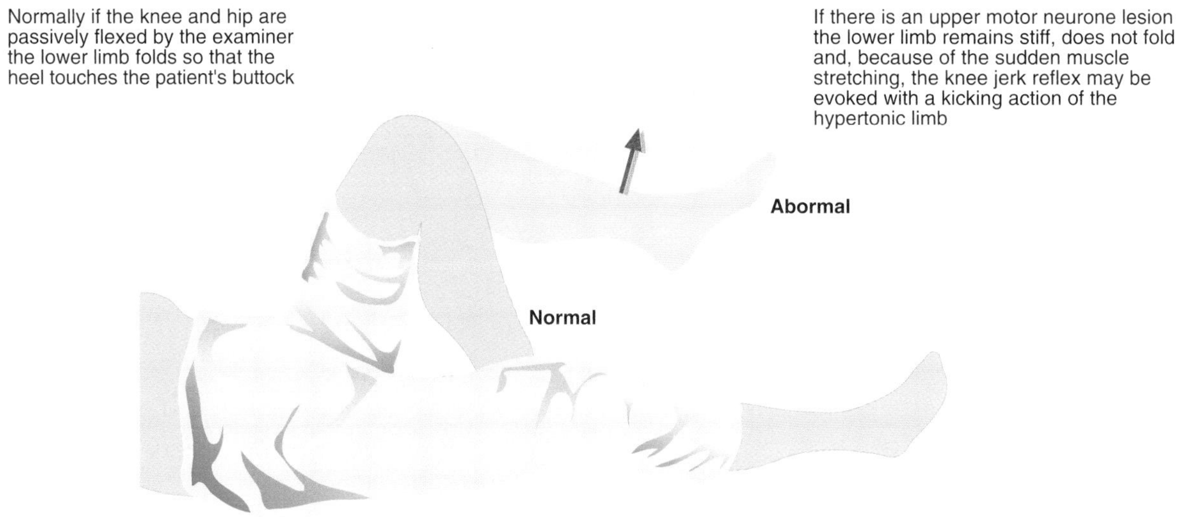

Normally if the knee and hip are passively flexed by the examiner the lower limb folds so that the heel touches the patient's buttock

If there is an upper motor neurone lesion the lower limb remains stiff, does not fold and, because of the sudden muscle stretching, the knee jerk reflex may be evoked with a kicking action of the hypertonic limb

Abormal

Normal

Fig. 1 **Testing for hypertonicity in the lower limb.** Ensure that there is no arthritis of hip or knee joint before performing this test.

Hypertonia

Hypertonia is produced in muscles from which the higher neurological 'relaxatory' influences have been removed.

With upper motor neurone type rigidity there is 'lead-pipe' type spastic rigidity, often with rigidity predominantly manifest in either the agonist or antagonist muscles. There may also be sudden reduction of hypertonia on passive movements — the 'clasp-knife phenomenon'.

Damage to extrapyramidal pathways causes a persisting hypertonia which affects agonist and antagonist muscles equally: this often causes difficulties in initiating bodily movement. Additionally, there may be a typical coarse compound tremor superimposed to give a 'cog-wheel' type rigidity.

Rarely, hypertonia may be caused by certain intrinsic muscle disease (e.g. dystrophia myotonica), anxiety, lack of patient cooperation or hysteria.

Clonus

Clonus is usually tested at the same time as tone. Clonus is a rhythmical involuntary contraction of a muscle placed under tension. Pathological clonus (which implies damage to the corticospinal tract relevant to the affected side) increases with increased tension of the muscle concerned, whereas normal 'physiological' clonus is abolished with persistent or increased muscle tension. Pathological clonus is often associated with upper motor neurone type hypertonia and hyperreflexia. Quadriceps clonus is best elicited by a firm and rapid distal displacement of the patella, whilst ankle clonus is best elicited by a firm dorsiflexion of the ankle (Fig. 2).

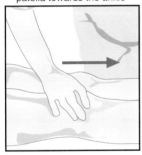
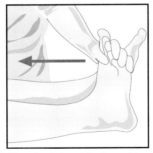

1. Examiner's hand firmly displacing patella towards the ankle

2. Examiner's hand firmly pushing toes towards the pelvis

Fig. 2 **Testing for clonus.**

MUSCLE POWER

Muscle power is graded on an MRC (Medical Research Council) scale of 0 – 5.

0 = no visible contraction
1 = visible contraction without active movement
2 = movement possible, but not against gravity
3 = movement possible against gravity
4 = movement possible against gravity and resistance, but weaker than normal
5 = normal power.

Marked muscle weakness should be initially apparent from the patient's gait, posture or limb movements.

Formal testing of muscle power

Ask the patient to extend forwards the whole of both upper limbs symmetrically with the palms upwards. Ask the patient to close both eyes (to abolish visually initiated compensation for muscle weakness) and then ask the patient to maintain the position of the limbs. A weak arm will drift downwards under its own weight. If the drift downwards is corrected when the patient's eyes are open then this implies that there was also some impairment of joint position sense. There is often a slow pronation of the hand if the weakness is due to an upper motor neurone lesion (Fig. 3). Ask the patient to maintain gently the position of his outstretched arms whilst you push both hands upwards, downwards, medially and laterally to assess and compare the power which the patient can utilize in each upper limb to maintain the original position. Hypotonia can also be assessed at the same time by tapping the hand upwards, downwards or sideways (in the presence of hypotonia there tends to be excessive excursion of the pushed limb with 'overshoot' when the patient attempts to return the limb to the original position).

In the lower limbs, similar principles apply. Ask the patient to keep his legs straight and lift each ankle in turn off the bed and assess the strength of each leg by pressing downwards at the base of the toes.

If a weakness is demonstrated, determine whether it is a global or localized weakness. A global weakness affect all muscles to a greater or lesser extent and usually indicates an upper motor neurone type weakness. A localized weakness confined to an individual muscle or groups of muscles sharing common innervations usually indicates a lower motor neurone lesion. If a lower motor neurone is partially damaged there may be fasciculation, a visible 'wriggling' of muscles, either spontaneously or induced by gentle tapping of the muscle.

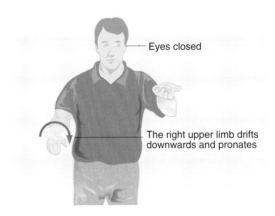

Eyes closed

The right upper limb drifts downwards and pronates

Fig. 3 **Upper motor neurone weakness of the upper limb.**

Tone and power

- Test power at the periphery when screening for reduced power.

- Test sensation at the periphery when screening for sensory defects.

- The more complex an activity the patient can perform, the less likely is there to be a significant neurological problem.

- Do not undertake passive movements unless you are sure the patient does not have a painful limb or arthritis.

EXAMINATION OF LIMBS AND TRUNK — SENSATION AND COORDINATION

SENSATION

There are five cutaneous sensory modalities which can usefully be tested (Fig. 1):

- pain
- temperature (both pain and temperature cross the midline soon after entry into the spinal cord)
- touch (most often crosses the midline at higher levels than pain or temperature)
- joint position sense
- vibration sense.

Patients use many colloquial descriptions of their sensory experiences. Always be sure you derive correctly the medical definition of the patient's symptoms. Pain due to neuritis or nerve irritation is often described as 'burning' or 'stabbing'. Some patients often describe total loss of sensation as 'numbness' but for others numbness is reduced but abnormal sensation.

The purpose of testing cutaneous sensation is to determine whether dysfunction is caused by peripheral nerve dysfunction (either focal or generalized), or by upper motor neurone damage (caused by spinal or more highly situated neurological damage). A dermatome pattern of sensory loss usually occurs in spinal cord lesions, or in nerve root lesions just after the nerves have left the spinal cord, but injury distal to this causes sensory impairment of peripheral nerve distribution (Fig. 2).

Pain

Superficial pain is tested by pin-prick and deep pain by deep muscle or tendon pressure. When testing by pin-prick *never use the same pin on different patients as this constitutes a definite infection risk*. Always ask if the pin-prick feels like a pin-prick should (to avoid testing for touch — a different sensation). An opened out paper clip for pin-prick sensation is recommended. The point is not too sharp, the convex ends can be used for bluntness appreciation and the two ends can be used for two point discrimination. They are also cheap, safe and disposable.

Deep pain is tested (only if indicated) by firm squeezing of muscles or tendons. Assessment of response is rather subjective, but asymmetry of response is likely to be significant.

Temperature

Temperature appreciation is assessed by using warm and cool tubes of water applied to the skin in random sequence. This test is usually only employed if dissociated sensory loss is suspected (touch and pain intact but with loss of hot and cold appreciation). This situation occurs if the pain and temperature fibres, which cross soon after entry into the spinal cord, are damaged by lesions in the centre of the spinal cord, with the touch fibres (which do not cross until they have ascended) intact. Affected patients typically burn themselves on hot objects. Syringomyelia, in which expanding cavities destroy the centre of the spinal cord, is a common cause.

Touch

Touch is usually tested by using a small point of cotton wool which is gently dabbed onto the skin. Stroking the skin, the neurological appreciation of which utilizes different spinal pathways, may provide misleading information. Always ask the patient if the cotton wool feels like cotton wool should feel and not just 'can you feel this?'. It is also useful to request the patient to close his eyes to avoid vision-related positive responses.

Joint position sense

Joint position sense, if intact at the peripheries, is almost always intact proximally. Grip the innermost and outermost surfaces of the end of the big toe between your thumb and first finger. Show the patient, by moving the toe, which is 'up' and which is 'down'.

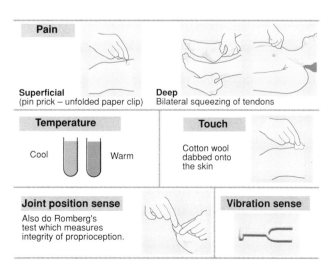

Fig. 1 **Testing for sensation.**

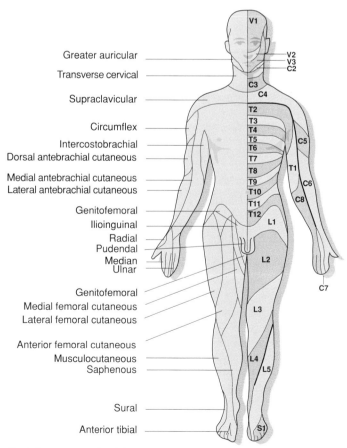

Fig. 2 **Dermatome and peripheral nerve innervation.**

Then ask the patient, with eyes closed, to report the direction of your random movements of the toe (remember that a guessing patient will achieve a 50% success rate). A similar technique can be used on the thumb and other peripheral joints. If there is peripheral impairment proceed to test more proximal joints.

'Internal' position sense is tested by Romberg's test in which a patient (who can stand securely with feet together when the eyes are open) sways or falls when the eyes are shut — thus demonstrating that equilibrium is dependent on vision and there is inadequate input from the internal position sensors. Always stand by the patient and terminate the test if the patient sways such that he/she might fall. Patients will fail Romberg's test if there is cerebellar incoordination but in this case visual input will not steady the patient.

Vibration sense

Vibration sense, if intact at the peripheries, is almost always intact proximally. To test vibration sense, place the base of a large 128 cycle per second tuning fork on a bony prominence (the medial malleolus is the traditional site although the base of the big toe is more peripheral). The patient should be told that it is *not* the sensation of touch that is being tested but rather the 'buzzing' feeling of vibration. The patient is then asked to close the eyes and the tuning fork is removed, tapped briskly (and preferably silently). The base is replaced on the bony prominence and the patient is asked if the buzzing can be felt, and when the buzzing ceases to be appreciated. In theory when this occurs, place the base of the (still vibrating) tuning fork on the corresponding part of your body. If you can appreciate vibration, the patient's vibration sense is worse than yours.

Vibration sense impairment is an early sign of neuropathy —

the nerve is unable to conduct sufficient numbers of discrete impulses. Vibration sense, like joint position sense, is also impaired with posterior column damage.

COORDINATION

Coordination is best assessed by observing the patient's everyday movements including walking, eating and writing. When examining coordination be aware that any previously detected deficit in tone, power or certain types of sensation may affect your assessment of coordination. This is the reason why coordination should only be assessed after evaluating tone, power and sensation. However if complex coordination is normal the tone, power and sensation are very likely to be normal.

To test coordination it is important that the patient performs the requested action with eyes open and then with the eyes closed.

To test coordination ask the patient to tap the back of one hand rapidly with the fingers of the other hand (dysdiadochokinesis). Other ways of assessing coordination include the successive touching of the thumb tip with each of the fingers of the same hand. Another easily understood request is to ask the patient to 'play the piano' with outstretched fingers of both hands.

Then there is the famous finger nose test which is one of the more idiotic requests that doctors make of their patients! If the patient is incoordinated or has a tremor he may well miss the nose and poke himself in the eye! (The fact that this does not feature in the medical insurance company's annual reports is testimony to the integrity of patients' blink reflexes.) It is more sensible to ask the patient to touch the point of the jaw. With the patient's eyes closed, move one of his hands to various positions and ask the patient to put the index finger onto the point of the jaw.

The heel-shin test of coordination requires that the patient strokes the heel of one foot up the shin of the other leg. Patients often find difficulty in understanding the instructions about this test. It is far easier to ask the patient to draw a circle or a square in the air with the big toe of each outstretched lower limb (firstly with the eyes open and then with the eyes shut).

Incoordination due to impaired joint position sense will be minimized when the patient's eyes are open because the patient will be able to compensate for the defect by using vision. When the eyes are closed incoordination will be revealed.

Cerebellar incoordination cannot be usefully compensated for by vision, although incoordination caused by pure muscle hypotonia or weakness may be compensated to some extent. Incoordination must be distinguished from visiospatial impairment. In the latter, coordination may be normal but the patient cannot draw a clock, or lay a table or draw a star.

Greater occipital
Lesser occipital
Greater auricular
Posterior divisions of cervical nerves
Supraclavicular
Circumflex
Dorsal brachial cutaneous
Intercostobrachial
Dorsal antebrachial cutaneous
Lateral antebrachial cutaneous
Medial antebrachial cutaneous
Ilohypogastric
Radial
Median
Ulnar
Lateral femoral cutaneous
Medial femoral cutaneous
Posterior femoral cutaneous
Musculocutaneous
Sural
Saphenous
Calcaneal and plantar

Sensation and coordination

- Always ensure that you interpret the patient's description of sensory symptoms correctly.

- Pain and temperature fibres cross soon after entry into the spinal cord.

- Touch fibres ascend the spinal cord and cross later.

- Incoordination caused by impaired joint position sense will be minimized if the patient has his eyes open.

- Cerebellar incoordination is not helped by vision.

EXAMINATION OF LIMBS AND TRUNK — REFLEXES

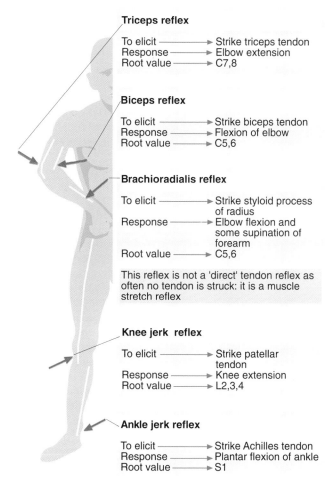

Triceps reflex

To elicit ⟶ Strike triceps tendon
Response ⟶ Elbow extension
Root value ⟶ C7,8

Biceps reflex

To elicit ⟶ Strike biceps tendon
Response ⟶ Flexion of elbow
Root value ⟶ C5,6

Brachioradialis reflex

To elicit ⟶ Strike styloid process
of radius
Response ⟶ Elbow flexion and
some supination of
forearm
Root value ⟶ C5,6

This reflex is not a 'direct' tendon reflex as
often no tendon is struck: it is a muscle
stretch reflex

Knee jerk reflex

To elicit ⟶ Strike patellar
tendon
Response ⟶ Knee extension
Root value ⟶ L2,3,4

Ankle jerk reflex

To elicit ⟶ Strike Achilles tendon
Response ⟶ Plantar flexion of ankle
Root value ⟶ S1

Fig. 1 **The five routinely tested tendon reflexes.**

TENDON (MUSCLE STRETCH) REFLEXES

Despite the fact that any striated muscle rapidly stretched will give a reflex, only five muscle stretch reflexes are usually tested routinely (Fig. 1).

To elicit muscle stretch reflexes the patient must be relaxed, with attention distracted from the fact that you are about to strike, albeit gently, with a hammer! If necessary, the patient should close the eyes to abolish visually initiated involuntary muscle tensing.

The tendon should be struck firmly with the head of a 12-inch length patellar hammer (the miniaturized versions are not adequate) so that maximum stretching of the muscle is elicited (Fig. 2). It is important to provide identical stimuli to each side when comparing the reflexes. A useful technique to confirm asymmetry of reflexes is to diminish progressively a stimulus on one side until there is no response. If an identical stimulus provokes a response on the other side then there is asymmetry of the reflexes (either hyporeflexia on one side or hyperreflexia on

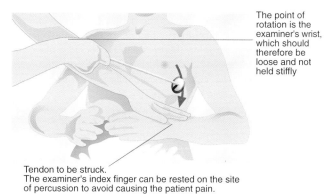

The point of rotation is the examiner's wrist, which should therefore be loose and not held stiffly

Tendon to be struck.
The examiner's index finger can be rested on the site of percussion to avoid causing the patient pain.

Fig. 2 **Use of the patellar hammer.**

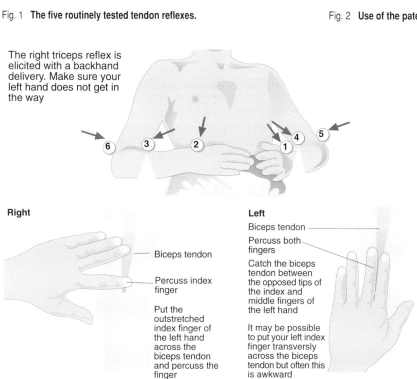

The right triceps reflex is elicited with a backhand delivery. Make sure your left hand does not get in the way

Right

Biceps tendon

Percuss index finger

Put the outstretched index finger of the left hand across the biceps tendon and percuss the finger

Left

Biceps tendon

Percuss both fingers

Catch the biceps tendon between the opposed tips of the index and middle fingers of the left hand

It may be possible to put your left index finger transversly across the biceps tendon but often this is awkward

Fig. 3 **Suggested order of percussion of the upper limb reflexes.** The patellar hammer is held in the right hand.

the other). When percussing a tendon it is helpful to have the hammer head at right angles to the tendon. Figure 3 details the practical order of percussion of the upper limb reflexes.

Hyperreflexia

Pathologically brisk reflexes occur with upper motor neurone lesions or in patients with painful limbs. Anxiety may cause brisk reflexes. There is a well-recognized syndrome (to the author at least) of symmetrical markedly brisk reflexes, normal plantar responses and bitten finger nails which signifies an anxiety state.

Hyporeflexia

Hyporeflexia is found if either sensation or motor innervation is defective, or if there is spinal cord dysfunction at the level of the reflex concerned. If the defect is motor, there will usually be muscle wasting, but if the hyporeflexia is caused by sensory impairment, muscle wasting is unusual.

Points to note

The gracilis reflex (L2, 3) is useful in collapsed patients, or in patients who cannot flex their knees. A finger or thumb is placed transversely across the gracilis muscle just above the knee and percussed with a patellar hammer. The gracilis contraction even if not visible, can be felt by the finger or thumb (Fig. 4).

Lesions at C7, 8 sometimes cause inversion of the triceps reflex — which is a flexion rather than extension of the elbow joint — almost as if the absent triceps response allows the transmitted stretching stimulus to be transmitted to the biceps which then contracts.

In hypothyroidism, reflex contractions may be sustained with a slow relaxation phase (Fig. 5).

THE ABDOMINAL REFLEXES

The normal abdominal reflexes (Fig. 6) consist of a contraction of the relevant quadrant muscles when the skin of that quadrant is gently scratched with a pointed object. A normal response requires an intact upper motor neurone relevant to the affected side, intact cutaneous sensation and lower motor neurone supply to the contracting muscles. This reflex may be absent in old people and in some normal individuals, but any asymmetry of response would be significant.

THE PLANTAR RESPONSES

The most useful way of eliciting the plantar response is to use the prongs of a tuning fork which provide two stimuli for the price of one. The prongs should be gently drawn along the lateral border of the foot from the heel towards the little toe (S1 cutaneous

innervation). It is important that the toes are in the resting position at the start of the test. A normal response is flexor with plantar flexion of the big toe. A pathological response is extensor with extension of the big toe (often with a fanning of the other four toes).

An extensor response is found in lesions of the upper motor neurone relevant to that foot. In comatose patients both plantar responses may be extensor and of no diagnostic significance, but any asymmetry of response would imply an asymmetrical causative lesion. Absent plantar response may be also found in peripheral neuropathy. Equivocal responses are found in infants under the age of 12 months.

A convenient method of recording the findings on examination of the reflexes and plantar responses is shown in Figure 7.

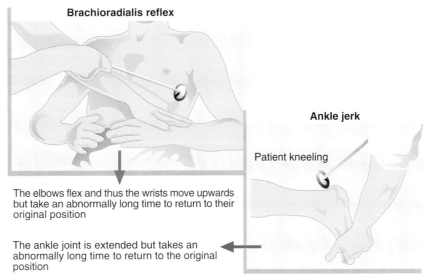

Brachioradialis reflex

Ankle jerk

Patient kneeling

The elbows flex and thus the wrists move upwards but take an abnormally long time to return to their original position

The ankle joint is extended but takes an abnormally long time to return to the original position

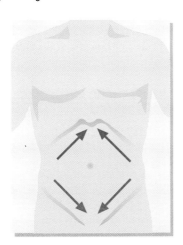

Put the index finger of your right hand on the tendon of the right gracilis (or your thumb on the tendon of the left gracilis) and percuss with a patellar hammer. You can feel (if not see) the reflex muscle contraction (L2, 3)

Fig. 4 **The gracilis reflex.**

Fig. 5 **The muscle stretch reflexes in hypothyroidism.**

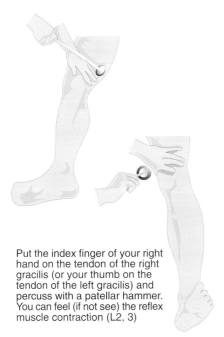

Fig. 6 **The abdominal reflexes.** Scratch gently with the proximal tip of the patellar hammer handle. A normal response is a contraction of the underlying muscle.

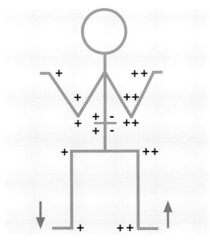

Fig. 7 **A method of recording findings on examination of limb reflexes and plantar responses.** The findings illustrated here are typical of left hemiparesis.

Reflexes

- Aiming the patellar hammer with the head at right angles to a tendon enhances the chances of hitting the tendon.

- Asymmetry of reflexes has lateralizing value.

- Asymmetry of the plantar responses has lateralizing value.

- Having the patient subtract serial sevens and/or close the eyes often makes the reflexes easier to elicit (reinforcement).

THE CORTEX AND AUTONOMIC NERVOUS SYSTEM

CORTICAL SENSORY FUNCTIONS

Cortical sensory function depends upon sophisticated interpretation of the multiple sensory modalities reaching the cortex. Before cortical sensory function can be assessed the patient must be fully conscious, have intact peripheral sensory modalities, be cooperative and fully aware of what is being asked.

To test for cortical sensory function ascertain that the patient can:

- Appreciate shape, weight, size, and texture of various objects placed (usually) in the hand.
- Identify certain common objects by palpation alone (stereognosis).
- Recognize numbers drawn on the palms.
- Discriminate between two points which can be tested by using dividers, or an opened out paper clip. Normally separation of 2–3 mm can be appreciated by the finger tips, whereas only separations of 0.5–1.0 cm or more can be appreciated on the legs. Two-point discrimination is also impaired if there is sensory nerve damage.

Also test for sensory extinction, a 'perceptual rivalry' in which unilateral stimuli are appreciated normally, but when identical stimuli are present bilaterally only one is appreciated.

DOMINANT HEMISPHERE DYSFUNCTIONS

There are several clinical syndromes which localize dysfunction to the dominant hemisphere (Table 1).

Table 1 **Dominant hemisphere lesions**

Hemiplegia

Focal or generalized seizures

Dysphasia (difficulty with words) – expressive (motor) and receptive (sensory)

Dyslexia (difficulty with words)

Dysgraphia (difficulty with drawing)

Dyscalculia (difficulty with calculations)

Dyspraxia (difficulty with movement)

Agnosia (failure of recognition)

Dysphasia

Dysphasia is specific difficulty with words in the absence of defects of articulation or dysfunctions of the vocalizing apparatus.

Dysphasia can be motor (expressive) or sensory (receptive), or a mixed motor and sensory pattern may be found. A patient with motor dysphasia understands what is being asked of him, knows what he wants to say but cannot say it. A patient with sensory dysphasia has impaired comprehension of words (either spoken or written). Frequently comprehension loss is only partial with the patient appreciating basic but not complex instructions. With damage to the temporal lobe, dysphasia is motor in type, but with damage to the posterior parietal lobe sensory dysphasia results. The important feature differentiating motor from sensory dysphasia is that in the former the patient is often able to indicate comprehension of what has been requested (showing that there is no sensory dysphasia) and, indeed, can often manage very basic spoken responses such as 'yes' or 'no'.

Dyslexia

Dyslexia is a specific type of dysphasia which causes difficulty with words, including spelling, reading and writing.

Nominal dysphasia

Nominal dysphasia is a specific variety of motor dysphasia in which the patient is unable to name specific objects, although the use of the object may be described. When testing for nominal dysphasia show the patient an object such as a pen and ask the patient to name the object, *but say you are testing vision*. This avoids irritating patients by asking them to do such superficially silly tests.

Dyspraxia

Dyspraxia is an impaired ability to perform familiar purposeful acts.

Dysgraphia and dyscalculia

Dysgraphia is an impaired writing ability. Dyscalculia is an impaired calculating ability. Dysgraphia and dyscalculia, if associated with inability to differentiate between right and left, constitute Gerstmann's syndrome.

NON-DOMINANT HEMISPHERE DYSFUNCTIONS

The major function of the non-dominant hemisphere is the integration of visiospatial relationships. Non-dominant hemisphere dysfunction can be more disabling than dominant hemisphere lesion because it is difficult to learn compensatory techniques to compensate for visiospatial impairment (Table 2).

Table 2 **Non-dominant hemisphere lesions**

Visiospatial impairment

Focal or generalized seizures

Hemiplegia

THE AUTONOMIC NERVOUS SYSTEM

The autonomic (self-controlling) nervous system supplies involuntary muscles, secretory glands and the heart (Fig. 1). There are two divisions of the autonomic nervous system, the sympathetic and the parasympathetic.

Certain tissues have combined sympathetic and parasympathetic innervation which function in an integrated reciprocal fashion. Sensory receptors for the autonomic nervous system include baroreceptors, chemoreceptors and smooth muscle stretch receptors, which provide the stimuli for reflex 'motor' activity of the sympathetic and parasympathetic nervous systems. All autonomic reflexes are influenced by the hypothalamus which in turn receives inputs from other parts of the brain. Diffuse damage to the autonomic nervous system causes impotence, disturbances of bowel and bladder function and postural hypotension.

THE SYMPATHETIC AUTONOMIC NERVOUS SYSTEM

The spinal sympathetic outflow is derived from the thoracic and upper lumbar spinal cord segments.

Activity of the sympathetic nervous system, usually in response to stress, induces a fast heart rate, dilatation of the pupils, sweating, piloerection and cessation of digestion. The adrenal medulla is also innervated by the sympathetic system and its hormonal output usually augments the effect of the sympathetic nervous system.

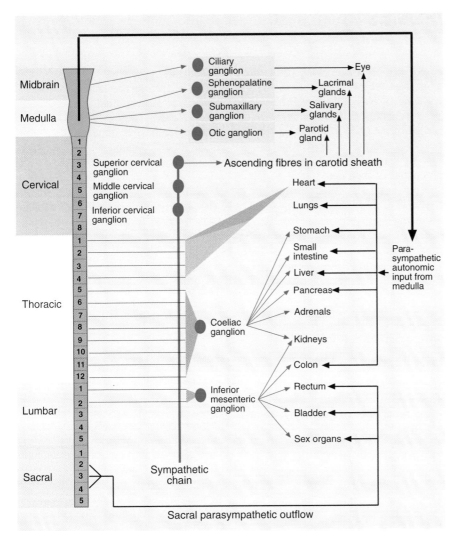

Fig. 1 **The autonomic nervous system.**

THE PARASYMPATHETIC AUTONOMIC NERVOUS SYSTEM

The parasympathetic outflow travels with the third cranial nerve (causing pupilloconstriction), the seventh cranial nerve (secretomotor to the lachrymal and salivary glands) and with the 9th and 10th cranial nerves (to the thorax and abdomen). The parasympathetic nervous system provides the emptying impulses of the body (in particular to the gut and bladder), stimulates secretion of certain gut glandular tissues and contributes to sexual function.

Bladder function
Micturition normally requires integration of the autonomic and voluntary nervous systems (Fig. 2). Contraction of the smooth muscle of the bladder (the detrusor muscle) is initiated by parasympathetic activity, whilst the internal sphincter mechanism (which is normally kept closed by sympathetic activity) is allowed to open by decreased sympathetic activity. The external sphincter mechanism, which can be voluntarily relaxed to allow micturition, is controlled by the pudendal nerves (S2, S3, S4). Perianal sensation is also mediated by these nerve roots so that intact perianal sensation usually implies intact external sphincter innervation.

There is a reciprocal relationship (coordinated in the pons) between external sphincter relaxation and detrusor contraction, the former preceding the latter by a few moments. Micturition may be assisted by expiration against a closed glottis which, in association with abdominal muscle contraction, raises the intra-abdominal pressure. As should be predicted, micturition becomes an autonomic spinal reflex if the spinal cord is transected above S2 level.

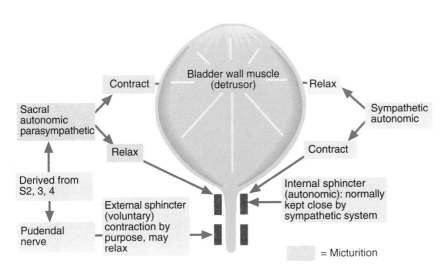

Fig. 2 **Physiological and neurological principles of bladder function.**

The cortex and autonomic nervous system

- Cortical sensory function depends on intact peripheral sensory input.

- Dysphasia may be motor (expressive) or sensory (receptive) or mixed.

- Autonomic dysfunction may cause impotence, disturbances of bowel and bladder, and postural hypotension.

- In a patient with urinary dysfunction, intact perianal sensation usually implies intact external sphincter innervation.

NEUROLOGICAL SYNDROMES (I)

The following five pages will discuss some important specific neurological syndromes which a clinician may come across in the course of a routine examination.

ABNORMAL GAITS (Fig. 1)

Basal ganglia gait (Parkinson's disease type)

Basal ganglia gait is characterized by slow movement with impaired initiation, a forward flexed posture and shuffling of the feet. This leads to a hurrying (festinant) gait, as if the patient is trying to catch-up with his/her centre of gravity.

Cerebellar gait

Cerebellar dysfunction causes difficulty in standing. The feet are placed well apart and the patient sways from side to side but usually does not fall. On being asked to walk in a straight line the patient may veer off towards the side of the lesion. Mild degrees of cerebellar gait can be revealed by asking the patient to walk 'heel to toe'.

Foot drop gait

In foot drop gait there is inability to dorsiflex the foot, necessitating a high-stepping gait with extra flexion of the hips and knees. The foot is then kicked forward and may slap onto the ground.

Hemiplegic gait

In hemiplegic gait there may be leg stiffness with particular difficulty with stairs if clonus of the calf muscles is produced by forced flexion of the foot as the stairs are mounted. The hip may be adducted, the knee extended and the foot plantar flexed, resulting in dragging of the foot with the toes being scraped along the ground.

Paraplegic gait

Paraplegic gait is really a bilateral hemiplegic gait affecting both legs with a slow, stiff, jerking gait, a dragging of the feet and scraping of the toes. A tendency to bilateral hip adduction may cause a scissors type gait.

Vestibular gait

Patients with unilateral vestibular dysfunction tend to veer off to the side of the lesion.

Waddling gait

Waddling gait is usually caused by muscular dysfunction affecting the trunk and pelvic girdle muscles. The gait is wide based with a marked swing of the body from side to side with each step and reciprocal movements of the trunk because the pelvis cannot be held horizontal when the weight of the body is supported by only one leg. For the same (compensatory) reasons there is often a lumbar lordosis and a protuberant abdomen.

ABNORMAL MOVEMENTS

Asterixis

Asterixis is a flapping tremor which may develop in metabolic failures including liver failure, uraemia, carbon dioxide retention or diabetic coma. The patient's outstretched fingers are separated and the wrist is extended. Alternate flexion and extension of the wrist occurs so that the hand flaps.

Tremor

Tremor may be caused by:

- congenital factors
- cerebellar or basal ganglia dysfunction
- fatigue
- anxiety
- emotion
- thyrotoxicosis
- drug side-effects
- drug withdrawal (including from alcohol).

Chorea

Chorea is an involuntary abrupt, jerking, short duration movement, whereas athetoid movements are slower, more sinuous, and writhing in nature. Huntingdon's chorea is an autosomal dominant inherited disease in which either dementia or abnormal movements may be the presenting feature. A family history is obviously important, although spontaneous cases may occur.

Dyskinesia

These are brief involuntary movements which are slower than tics with each spasm lasting longer. Drugs (including phenothiazines, L-dopa and metoclopramide) are common causes.

Tics

Tics are frequent, compulsive, involuntary, stereotyped and predictable repetitions of the same movement. Usually no organic pathology can be demonstrated. In contrast, myoclonic jerks are sudden, brief, unpredictable shock-like contractions of muscle groups. The causes of myoclonic jerks include epilepsy and certain metabolic or infective diseases.

PARKINSON'S DISEASE

In Parkinson's disease, bradykinesia (a slowness in initiating movements) is often evident and blinking is often infrequent. Paradoxically when the bridge of the nose is repeatedly tapped (from above to avoid eliciting a visual threat response) unremitting involuntary blinking is found constituting a positive glabellar tap (in normal people the automatic blinking fades out after the first few taps). The gait is also abnormal (see above). Whilst testing eye movements a normal patient's jaw usually has to be restrained with one hand (to prevent spontaneous head movements), but typically in a patient with basal ganglia dysfunction such restraint is unnecessary because the patient's head remains still whilst the eyes move. The face is often expressionless, caused by a combination of rigidity and bradykinesia.

The tremor of basal ganglia dysfunction is coarse and not restricted to muscle

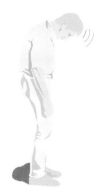

Basal ganglia gait
- slow shuffle
- forward flexed
- impaired initiation

Fig. 1 **Abnormal gaits.**

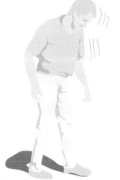

Cerebellar gait
- patient sways from side to side
- veers off to side of lesion

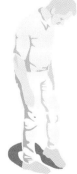

Foot drop gait
- impaired dorsiflexion of foot
- high-stepping gait

groups supplied by root or peripheral nerves. Cogwheel rigidity (a resistance to passive movement subject to rapid fluctuations) is found which, unlike upper motor neurone type rigidity, tends to affect all points in the range of movement. The muscle stretch reflexes are usually normal.

BULBAR PALSY

Bulbar palsy is produced by lower motor neurone dysfunction affecting the lower cranial nerves. Predictably there is dysarthria, difficulty in swallowing, and a bilaterally weak, wasted tongue which may show fasciculation. Motor neurone disease is a notable cause of bulbar palsy in Britain, but in world terms polio ranks high.

COMA

The signs and classification of coma are detailed on page 140.

DYSARTHRIA

Dysarthria is a failure of proper articulation of words despite anatomical integrity of the lips, tongue and palate. There is usually no dysphasia. Various tongue-twisting phrases are used to elicit dysarthria, particularly those that bring out difficult consonant sounds—'The Royal Irish Constabulary' or 'The Leith Police dismisseth us'. Dysarthria may be caused by muscle disorders (myopathy), myasthenia, bulbar palsy, pseudobulbar palsy, basal ganglia dysfunction, certain upper motor neurone lesions or cerebellar dysfunction.

DYSPHONIA

Dysphonia, an abnormal quality or volume of the voice, is usually caused by pathologies which affect the vocal cords.

FRONTAL LOBE DYSFUNCTION

In frontal lobe dysfunction there may be uninhibited behaviour and an involuntary grasping of fingers placed in the patient's palm.

OCCIPITAL LOBE DYSFUNCTIONS

If unilateral there may be a contralateral homonymous hemianopia but if bilateral there may be cortical blindness — failure to appreciate visual stimuli but with intact pupillary light reflexes.

PARIETAL LOBE DYSFUNCTION

Apraxia is the main manifestation – the patient's ability to construct is impaired. This is usually tested by asking the patient to lay a table place setting or draw a clock face.

TEMPORAL LOBE DYSFUNCTION

Dysphasia results if the dominant hemisphere is damaged. A homonymous hemianopia may be produced if damage is extensive but a contralateral upper quadrantic defect may be produced if only the lower fibres of the optic radiation are affected.

PSEUDOBULBAR PALSY

In pseudobulbar palsy there is bilateral upper motor neurone type weakness of the lower cranial nerves, usually caused by vascular-related cerebral infarcts or by multiple sclerosis. This bulbar palsy is called 'pseudo' because the bulbar part of the brainstem (the bulb is the medulla of the brainstem) is intact, although the signs appear on superficial evaluation to be caused by bulbar dysfunction alone.

Predictably there is usually also limb spasticity and hyperreflexia with extensor plantar responses. The (pseudo) bulbar signs include dysarthria and a spastic tongue with tongue muscle wasting being minimal compared to that of bulbar palsy. Because the muscles of the jaw are hyperreflexic, the jaw jerk is increased. Inappropriate emotional responses (include crying and laughing for no reasonable cause) are often seen and are caused by lack of inhibition resulting from diffuse cortical damage.

TENTORIAL HERNIATION (CONING)

The tentorium is a sheet of dura separating the lower lobes of the brain from the cerebellum. The upper brainstem passes through the tentorium, which has a fixed size. It is *not* the tentorium which herniates, rather the brainstem which is forced downwards.

Tentorial herniation is often a pre-terminal condition in which there is expansion of brain tissue above the tentorium which may compress the temporal lobe against the tentorium, displacing the brainstem, and often results in early damage to the oculomotor nerve (particularly the pupilloconstrictor fibres). Diagnosis and urgent treatment is mandatory. Usually there is:

- a deteriorating conscious level
- initially a unilateral dilating pupil
- later a complete third nerve palsy
- hemiplegia if either cerebral peduncle is compressed against the edge of the tentorium
- quadriplegia and decerebrate posturing occur if coning is unchecked.

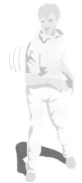

Hemiplegic gait
- leg stiffness
- forced flexion of foot
- hip adduction
- knee extension

Vestibular gait
- tendency to veer off to side of lesion

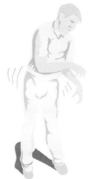

Waddling gait
- wide based gait
- body sway
- lumbar lordosis and protuberant abdomen

Neurological syndromes (I)

- Asterixis, a flapping tremor of the outstretched hand, is not specific for liver failure.
- Cogwheel rigidity in Parkinson's disease may be brought out by active movements of the contralateral limb.
- Bulbar palsy is lower motor neurone in origin.
- Pseudobulbar palsy is upper motor neurone in origin.
- Tentorial herniation demands urgent intervention.

NEUROLOGICAL SYNDROMES (II)

SEIZURES

Seizures (epilepsy) are the clinical manifestations of abnormal electrical activity in the brain. There are four basic types of epilepsy:

- grand mal
- Jacksonian (focal)
- petit mal
- temporal lobe.

Grand mal epilepsy

In grand mal epilepsy the patient may experience premonitory symptoms which usually reflect the initiating site of the seizure in the brain. The patient becomes unconscious and falls to the ground. Generalized sustained non-jerking muscle contraction occurs (the tonic phase). The associated respiratory muscle contraction initiates the 'epileptic cry' as air is rapidly forced out through the larynx. The tonic stage usually lasts for less than 30 seconds and is followed by rhythmical generalized muscle jerking (the clonic phase). The patient may become cyanosed, froth at the mouth, bite the tongue and be incontinent of urine. The seizure may last a variable period of time, usually a few minutes. After cessation of the clonic phase the patient usually remains unconscious or confused for a brief time.

Jacksonian (focal) epilepsy

The focus for Jacksonian epilepsy is in the precentral motor cortex. A seizure usually commences with clonic (regular repetitive) jerking, usually of the thumb and fingers of one hand. Such jerking may spread proximally and occasionally progress to grand mal epilepsy. There may be transient paralysis of the parts affected after the seizure.

Petit mal epilepsy

In petit mal epilepsy there are recurrent brief losses of full awareness which usually start in early childhood. Typically patients appear dazed or 'distant' for a few seconds. There is no abnormality of muscle tone and thus patients do not fall to the ground. With the advent of adolescence petit mal usually ceases or progresses to grand mal epilepsy.

Temporal lobe epilepsy (psychomotor epilepsy)

Temporal lobe epilepsy is characterized by subjective, stereotyped phenomena, usually comprising sensory hallucinations which may be auditory, visual or olfactory. Déjà vu (a feeling that visualized objects have been seen before) may occur. The patient appears to be detached from environmental occurrences and automatic behaviour may occur without the patient being aware of, or able to control, his/her actions.

STROKES

A stroke (a sudden onset of focal neurological signs) is a useful descriptive term because it does not imply any particular causative pathology.

A *monoplegia* is paralysis of one limb whereas a *paraplegia* is paralysis of both lower limbs which is usually caused by bilateral damage to the corticospinal tracts in the spinal cord. *Hemiplegia* is unilateral paralysis of the arm and leg (and perhaps the face) and is usually caused by upper motor neurone dysfunction. A brainstem dysfunction is implied if there is a crossed paralysis—paralysis of the limbs of one side of the body with a cranial nerve lesion of the other side. *Quadriplegia* is paralysis of all four limbs: if there are lower neurone signs of any cranial nerve in a quadriplegic patient, suspect a high spinal cord or brainstem lesion.

HEADACHE

Most headaches are caused by migraine or muscular tension, or by a combination of both. Mentioned below are a few causes of headache of particular neurological relevance.

Cerebral space-occupying lesions

Cerebral space-occupying lesions including neoplasms may present with headaches, especially early morning headache, associated with vomiting (sometimes with effortless regurgitation). Later papilloedema, mental confusion and drowsiness develop. Sixth nerve lesions may occur because of pressure during its long intracranial course. The headache may be posture related.

Meningitis

The meninges surround and support the brain and spinal cord. The cerebrospinal fluid lies between the innermost and middle of the three meningeal membranes. Meningeal infections are usually associated with headache, vomiting, neck stiffness and an abnormal mental state (particularly in bacterial meningitis).

Test for meningeal irritation by ascertaining if there is neck stiffness by gently flexing the neck, and test for back and neck stiffness by seeing whether the patient can 'kiss the knees'. Further evidence of meningeal irritation is provided if pain results on attempted knee extension of an initially flexed hip and knee (a positive Kernig's sign). Patients may have an arched back (Fig. 1).

Meningeal irritation is usually caused by meningitis, but posterior fossa neoplasms or subarachnoid haemorrhage can also be responsible. Occasionally, meningismus (signs of meningeal irritation with no cerebrospinal fluid abnormalities) occurs in response to infection outwith the nervous system (renal and pulmonary infections are notable in this respect).

Migraine (Fig. 2)

Almost invariably in patients with migraine there will have been a history of previous headaches of a similar if not identical pattern. Classical migraine usually occurs in paroxysms with symptom-free periods. Symptoms usually commence with visual disturbance (the aura), typically including misting or shimmering of part of the visual fields 'flashing lights'. The edge of visualized objects may have a glittering or jagged 'zig-zag' outline (fortification spectra). Blind spots (defects in the visual fields) may occur as may focal neurological symptoms or signs. The headache, which is unilateral in about 50% of attacks, typically starts as the aura fades, with boring or throbbing pain. The headache, which may last for several hours, may be associated with nausea, and is made worse by exertion or light and patients prefer to lie down in a darkened room. The patient is often aware that the headache is a deep throbbing pain, whereas in tension headaches the patient often localizes the pain as being exclusively external to, or around the skull, 'like a tight band'.

Migraine can, on occasion, cause cutaneous sensory symptoms, dysphasia or even transient focal neurological signs.

Variations of migraine occur, including headaches with an occipital dull ache extending anteriorly to a retro-orbital position. Migranous neuralgia is a severe, retro-orbital and stabbing or 'bursting' headache, or a continually fluctuating retro-orbital pain.

Cluster headaches are another migraine variant. Patients are usually male, middle-aged and without a history of classical migraine. Headache is severe, and if periorbital pain is produced the affected

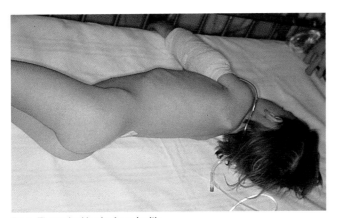

Fig 1 **The arched back of meningitis.**

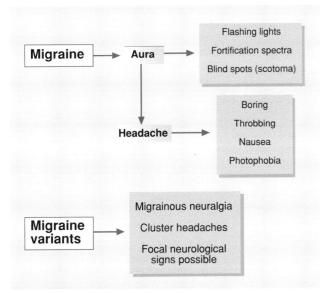

Fig. 2 **Migraines—symptoms and variants.**

eye becomes suffused, the nose congested and attacks are often nocturnal. Attacks cluster over about 6 – 8 weeks and then remit only to appear again in clusters some time later.

Migraine is a dangerous diagnosis to entertain if headaches are of recent onset in the middle-aged or elderly, especially if effortless vomiting is associated (think of posterior fossa neoplasms in this situation).

Raised intracranial pressure headaches

Raised intracranial pressure headache is often worse on lying down, coughing or straining and may be associated with vomiting (which may not be associated with nausea). Papilloedema may be a late sign. Suspect neoplasms or abscess if the onset of symptoms was gradual, or intracranial haemorrhage if symptoms were of rapid onset.

Tension headaches

Tension headaches do not exclude coincidental migraine. Indeed one may cause or perpetuate the other. Patients with tension headaches typically complain of a 'tight' headache spreading from the occiput to the forehead.

Temporal arteritis

Temporal arteritis is a variant of giant cell arteritis. Patients are usually over 60 years of age, and have a painful, often palpable, swollen temporal artery. Often there is vague generalized headache. Patients often feel ill, and look unwell — whereas those with tension headache often look well.

Intracerebral haemorrhage

Intracerebral haemorrhage may present with severe headache and rapid development of focal neurological signs.

Subarachnoid haemorrhage

Subarachnoid haemorrhage usually presents with an abrupt onset severe headache which may be followed by loss of consciousness. Usually the neurological findings are the same on both sides (i.e. there are no lateralizing signs) because the blood is present diffusely in the cerebrospinal fluid (CSF). However spasm in the vessel that has leaked may occur (presumably a protective reflex to minimize further bleeding) and lateralizing signs may be produced by ischaemia. Because blood in the CSF irritates the meninges there are signs of meningeal irritation with a stiff neck and a positive Kernig's sign (see above). Papilloedema may develop as may subhyaloid haemorrhages (the hyaloid is the innermost layer of the retina).

Other causes

Other causes of headache include trigeminal neuralgia, trigeminal nerve lesions or postherpetic neuralgia. Toothache, sinusitis, or ear problems occasionally present as headaches with minimal symptoms or signs relevant to the site of the initiating problem.

HORNER'S SYNDROME

Horner's syndrome comprises a unilateral constricted pupil, a slight ptosis (a complete ptosis suggests an oculomotor lesion) and lack of facial sweating on the side affected (Fig. 3). The affected eye is slightly sunken. The cause of Horner's syndrome is an interruption of sympathetic pupillodilator supply to the iris. The relevant sympathetic impulses descend from the hypothalamus in the brainstem and emerge by the anterior roots of C8, T1 and T2, passing into the cranial sympathetic nerve trunk and thereafter ascending on the internal carotid artery and thence to the eye. Damage anywhere on this pathway may produce Horner's syndrome.

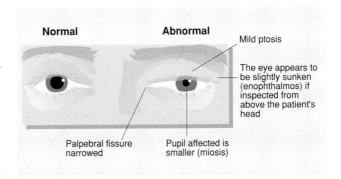

Fig. 3 **Horner's syndrome.**

Neurological syndromes (II)

- Hemiplegia and a cranial nerve lesion affecting the opposite side localizes the lesion to the brainstem.
- Signs of meningeal irritation occur in meningitis, subarachnoid haemorrhage, posterior fossa neoplasms or, occasionally, in patients with non-meningitis infections.
- The headache in migraine is not confined to one side in about 50% of attacks.
- A throbbing headache implies a vascular involvement.

NEUROLOGICAL SYNDROMES (III)

ALCOHOL-RELATED CONDITIONS

Alcohol intoxication causes cortical and cerebellar dysfunction, release of inhibitions and, if profound, dysarthria, hypotonia and ataxia leading to coma. Patients with alcohol-related hallucinations are fully conscious but have illusions (p. 133) and hallucinations (p. 133), often with paranoid features.

Korsakoff's psychosis is classically associated with chronic alcoholism and may persist after abstinence. There is a gross defect in the patient's memory for recent events and compensatory confabulation is often florid. Such patients are often generally well unless they also have Wernicke's encephalopathy.

Alcohol-related cerebellar degeneration is caused by damage to midline cerebellar structures which govern the lower trunk and lower limbs. There is incoordination of the trunk and lower limbs with an ataxic gait. Often there are no other cerebellar signs elsewhere.

Alcohol-withdrawl syndrome usually commences with unease after about eight hours, hence the need for 'a morning drink to steady the nerves'. Serious manifestations ('Delerium tremens') may commence 24–48 hours later but on occasion may develop a week or two later. There is anxiety, confusion, poor sleep, sweating and tachycardia. The pupils are dilated and there is a coarse tremor and ataxia. Hallucinations and illusions may occur and patients characteristically misinterpret sensory stimuli. Seizures, which are generalized rather than focal, may occur.

MOTOR NEURONE DISEASE

Motor neurone disease is caused by degeneration of upper motor neurones and their final common pathways in the central nervous system. Those affected are usually over the age of 50 and the male to female ratio is 2:1. There are several patterns of illness. In *progressive muscular atrophy* (associated with lower motor neurone degeneration) there is muscle atrophy and weakness, with fasciculation on gentle percussion of affected muscles. The onset is usually in the hands but later other muscles, notably those of respiration, become involved. In *amyotropic lateral sclerosis* (associated with upper motor neurone degeneration) there is weakness and spasticity (which, if

added to lower motor neurone involvement, may give rise to the surprising—and thus diagnostically suggestive—increase in muscle stretch reflexes in the presence of wasted muscles. Plantar responses are usually extensor. *Bulbar palsy* (p.97) or *pseudobulbar palsy* may occur.

GUILLAIN–BARRÉ SYNDROME

Guillain–Barré syndrome is an acute onset of peripheral nerve impairment with flaccid muscle weakness (which ascends from the peripheries), often with mild sensory loss perhaps preceded by tingling. The automatic nervous system can be affected as may the muscles of respiration. It is often preceded by a mild febrile illness.

MULTIPLE SCLEROSIS

In multiple sclerosis demyelination (damage to the white conducting nervous tissues) occurs in the brain and spinal cord, but not in the peripheral nerves. The onset may be acute or insidious with single focal lesions, a succession of lesions, or multiple lesions. There is a slow accumulation of neurological defecits with clinical manifestations caused by damage to nervous tissue occurring at different times and/or caused by damage to anatomically separated nervous tissues. The possible symptoms and signs are thus multiple. Symptoms include numbness, visual problems, areas of impaired sensation, leakage of urine and vertigo. On examination there may be upper motor neurone type weaknesses, intranuclear ophthalmoplegia (p. 83) which is almost diagnostic, ataxia and intention tremor, nystagmus, absent abdominal reflexes (p. 93), increased muscle stretch reflexes, and extensor plantar responses. Patients may eventually become bedridden, paralysed, with impaired eye movements and muscle spasms. Emotional changes may occur with depression or euphoria — often patients seem less concerned about their disabilities than would be anticipated.

VITAMIN DEFICIENCIES

Vitamin deficiencies affecting the nervous system, as might be anticipated, almost invariably give rise to bilateral symmetrical symptoms and signs.

Vitamin B_1 (thiamine) deficiencies are usually caused by inadequate intake in alcoholics or in those who survive on polished rice. Beriberi results which may

be 'wet' with heart failure and oedema, or 'dry' (i.e. neurological) with tingling of the feet, loss of vibration and joint position sense, and foot drop. Wernicke's encephalopathy often occurs in association with chronic alcoholism and there is difficulty in concentration progressing to confusion, collapse and coma. Nystagmus, impaired eye movements and ataxia may be evident as may signs of peripheral neuropathy.

Vitamin B_6 (pyridoxine) deficiency is usually associated with malabsorption, alcoholism or as a side effect to certain drugs, notably isoniazid. There is often painful sensory neuropathy—'burning feet' and optic neuropathy. There may be associated glossitis or cheilosis.

Vitamin B_{12} (cyanocobalmin) deficiency is usually associated with pernicious anaemia and causes subacute combined degeneration of the spinal cord with changes in the posterior and lateral columns and the peripheral nerves. The signs are those of peripheral nerve damage and spinal cord degeneration. Symptoms include tingling of the extremities (feet before fingers), sensory loss of glove and stocking type occurring later, weakness with or without spasticity (caused by corticospinal pathway damage) and loss of vibration sense and joint position sense leading to ataxia (caused by posterior column damage). In late cases the ankle jerks are lost but the plantar responses are extensor—the latter suggests upper motor neurone damage and the former suggests peripheral nerve damage, and this is an unusual and therefore diagnostically suggestive combination.

Nicotinic acid deficiency (pellagra) is usually only found in those who live almost exclusively off maize. In severe cases there is dermatitis, diarrhoea and dementia.

Neurological syndromes (III)

- Alcohol withdrawl symptoms occur after 8 hours but serious symptoms ('delerium tremens') usually occur after 24–28 hours.
- Motor neurone disease usually affects patients over the age of 50, with a male to female ratio of 2:1.
- Intranuclear ophthalmoplegia is almost diagnostic of MS.

SCREENING HISTORY AND EXAMINATION

The previous pages have given a detailed account of history and examination of the nervous system. In real life and in the absence of specific complaints, patients have to be screened for nervous system disorders.

What follows is a personal opinion of what is required when a patient presents with symptoms not obviously related to the nervous system, but in whom it is necessary to exclude nervous system disorders. It is not infallible but is highly relevant to busy medical practice.

If the patient has not given any neurological symptoms in the general history then it is unnecessary to inquire about every possible neurological symptom. Ask if the patient has experienced:

- headaches
- loss of consciousness
- muscle weaknesses
- previous head injuries
- any other 'nervous problems' (this usefully covers possible mental problems).

It is also important to:

- observe the patient's gait
- assess the patient's mental state (intelligence, mood, and content of conversation)
- assess the patient's facial appearance. Does it suggest thyrotoxicosis, myxoedema, acromegaly, alcoholism, myopathy or other condition?

EXAMINING THE CRANIAL NERVES

The cranial nerves are usually overexamined in neurologically asymptomatic patients.

Cranial nerve I

Unless there has been a head injury it is probably unnecessary to ask if the sense of smell is normal.

Cranial nerve II

Testing visual acuity and visual fields is probably unnecessary if the patient replies that the eyesight is normal. A quick screening test of visual fields is to ask the patient to close one eye and to look at your nose with the other (from a distance of about 12 inches), and report if there are any areas of your face not seen. Assess the light and accommodation reflexes routinely, and perform an ophthalmoscopy (for hypertensive or diabetic changes or early papilloedema).

Cranial nerves III, IV, VI

Assess eye movements and ask if the patient has diplopia. Look for nystagmus (which may be asymptomatic).

Cranial nerves V and VII

Ask the patient to open the mouth (testing the pterygoids) and then clench the teeth (feel the masseter). As patients invariably show their teeth when clenching, this effectively tests VII nerve function (if there is no mouth weakness there is most unlikely to be any forehead muscle weakness). Facial sensation, the jaw jerk or corneal reflex are unlikely to be abnormal in the neurologically asymptomatic patient.

Cranial nerve VIII

Occlude each ear in turn and test hearing by whispering questions for the patient to answer (by asking appropriate questions this can also be a subtle way to test for orientation, time, place and person).

Cranial nerves IX, X and XII

Test these together by noting the patient's articulation and phonation. The gag reflex is not likely to be abnormal if swallowing is normal and should probably be omitted. In any case the throat should have been inspected as part of the general examination and the centrality of the uvula will have previously been noted as will the neurological state of the tongue.

Cranial nerve XI

Rotation of the head can also usefully be tested at the time that the throat is examined.

THE LIMBS

The upper limb tone and power can be assessed by asking the patient to keep the arms outstretched for about 20 seconds or so. Then asking the patient to 'stop me pressing downwards or upwards', whilst the examiner presses on the finger tips of outstretched hands (to test power) and then the examiner can unexpectedly remove his restraining hands to see if there is overshoot suggesting hypotonia.

Complex coordination can be assessed by looking at the patient's handwriting. If there are muscle power or sensory abnormalities these will show up on complex coordination testing or on examination of the reflexes.

The 'routine five' muscle stretch reflexes should be elicited.

A vibrating tuning fork can be placed on an extremity to test for neuropathy and posterior column function, and then a prong can be laid on the skin and the patient asked if it feels cold (as it usually does) and the plantar responses elicited. Test coordination in the lower limbs by asking the patient to draw a triangle in the air with the big toes. Again if such complex coordination is normal then tone and power are also likely to be normal.

If any abnormalities are detected then a more rigorous examination will be necessary.

Screening history and examination

- Screening tests are quick means of excluding a nervous system disorder in diagnosis.

- The five standard muscle stretch reflexes, if normal, imply an intact senory nerve–spinal cord–motor nerve neurological arc.

- If abnormalities are detected on screening, then a more detailed analytical examination is required.

BASIC PRINCIPLES / JOINT DYSFUNCTIONS

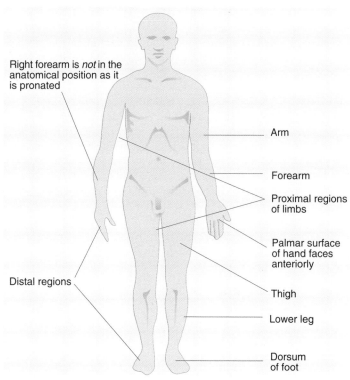

Right forearm is *not* in the anatomical position as it is pronated

Arm

Forearm

Proximal regions of limbs

Palmar surface of hand faces anteriorly

Distal regions

Thigh

Lower leg

Dorsum of foot

Fig. 1 **The 'neutral' anatomical position.**

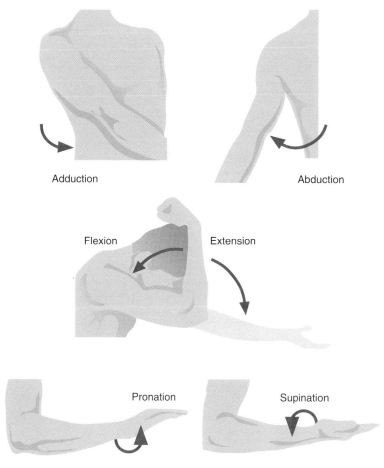

Adduction

Abduction

Flexion

Extension

Pronation

Supination

Fig. 2 **Main anatomical movements.**

For ease of presentation, the 'musculo-skeletal neurology' of the arms and legs are included in this section. Attention is restricted to aspects of common or important conditions relevant to a non-specialist.

BASIC PRINCIPLES

The history should be taken along general lines, with particular attention to the characteristics of pain (p. 3), weakness, stiffness, swellings (p. 6), duration of symptoms and their progression.

Examination of the locomotor system comprises:

- inspection
- palpation
- movement.

Movements of the affected limb should be those by the patient (active movements), or by the examiner (passive movements). Assess active movements first to avoid 'forcing the issue' by passive movements which may hurt the patient.

Always expose fully the part to be examined. Inspect for musculoskeletal abnormalities or tissue swellings, then palpate the affected part noting the temperature and whether there is local tenderness. Assess joint movements, their range and whether there is pain or crepitus. Assess muscle power (using Medical Research Council (MRC) grades p. 89); the stability of joints and the total function of the part under examination. Always assess how various abnormalities affect the patient's day-to-day life.

The 'neutral' reference anatomical positions are detailed in Figure 1. Note that the hands face forward and the feet point forward at right angles to the lower leg. The following definitions (Fig. 2) are relevant:

- *Adduction* is movement of a distal part of the body (compared to the contiguous proximal part) towards the centre or midline of the body
- *Abduction* is movement away from the centre or midline
- *Flexion* is the act of bending a joint
- *Extension* is the act of straightening a joint to the neutral position
- *Hyperextension* occurs when a joint can be extended beyond the normal limit
- *Pronation* is rotation of the forearm so that the palm faces forward
- *Supination* is rotation of the forearm so that the palm faces backwards.

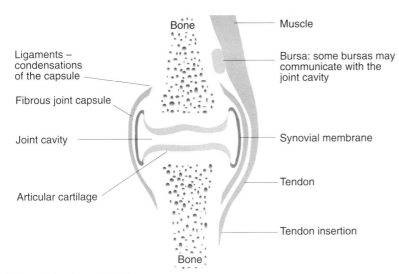

Fig. 3 **An archetypal synovial joint.**

JOINT DYSFUNCTIONS

Joints may be fibrous, cartilagenous or synovial. An archetypal synovial joint is illustrated in Figure 3. Abnormalities can arise in any of the structures illustrated.

Ankylosis

Ankylosis is abnormal immobility of a joint with restriction or abolition of movement. This restriction of movement is usually caused by bony fusion rather than by pain.

Bursitis

Muscles and tendons passing superficial to joints may be protected by a bursa (a synovial sac) which cushions excessive friction. Bursitis is usually caused by gout or repeated minor trauma.

Acute bursitis causes pain. On inspection there is swelling due to fluid accumulation, and on palpation there is localized tenderness with some associated limitation of movement.

Chronic bursitis occurs after repeated (usually minor) attacks of acute bursitis. On inspection there is swelling of the bursa. On palpation there is thickening of the bursa wall, tenderness and limitation of movement, perhaps with secondary muscle weakness.

Cartilage problems

Cartilage problems typically affect the knee joint. There is usually a history of twisting the knee at a time of weightbearing. Movement of joints exacerbates pain if displaced or torn cartilages are compressed, whereas decompressing movements relieve pain. Effusions usually develop after acute injury to cartilages. Joints which suddenly lock, often do so because of cartilage damage or loose bodies (which

are often flakes of cartilage) within the joint.

Dislocations

A dislocation occurs when all opposition between articular surfaces is lost. A subluxation is a partial dislocation in which some contact is retained.

Fractures

After an acute fracture there is almost always severe pain, local tenderness and reluctance to move the affected part.

Joint capsule damage

Damage to the joint capsule will cause pain particularly exacerbated by movement which places the affected part of the capsule under tension. Joint effusions may occur.

Joint movement restriction

Restriction of joint movement may be caused by:

- mechanical defects
- soft tissue contractures
- joint effusions
- muscle pain
- muscle spasm
- muscle paralysis.

Joint inflammations

Arthralgia is a pain in a joint, where arthritis is inflammation within a joint. Acute inflammatory joint lesions may show all the characteristics of inflammation:

- pain (which is often described as throbbing)
- redness
- swelling
- local heat
- loss of function.

Arthritis affecting one joint only is usually caused by infection, metabolic abnormalities (including gout), haemorrhage, mechanical lesions or, rarely, by tumour.

Diseases which cause chronic inflammation of joints tend not to cause heat or redness (unless the chronic process is in an acute exacerbation) but rather cause swelling, deformity or muscular wasting around the joint concerned.

Joint swelling

If a joint is swollen there may be a joint effusion (excess synovial fluid within the joint). Firm palpation with a finger will reveal a boggy feeling, and there may be displacement of fluid which causes extra swelling to develop elsewhere in relation to the joint. This can be detected by a clear sense of fluctuation between two palpating fingers. Joint swelling can also be caused by pus or haemorrhage in a joint.

Loose bodies within joints

Loose bodies within the joint can cause sudden but transient locking of a joint, usually followed by signs of joint fluid.

Ligament strain or rupture

Ligaments are tough bands of tissue within the fibrous capsule of joints. After acute ligament strain, pain may be severe and constant, but later only occurs on movements which stretch the ligament concerned. On palpation there may be superficial tenderness over involved ligaments. Chronic ligament strain becomes worse as the day progresses, and repeated minor strains have a cumulative effect. Rest relieves the pain.

Rupture of a ligament is initially painful and joints may become unstable. There may be swelling and bruising if, along with ligament rupture, joint fluid escapes into the tissues.

Basic principles / joint dysfunctions

- Examination of the locomotor system is by
  - looking
  - feeling
  - moving the part in question.
- Always expose fully the part to be examined.
- Joints which lock suddenly have damaged cartilage or loose bodies within the joint.

MUSCLE AND NECK PROBLEMS

MUSCLE DYSFUNCTIONS

Rupture of a muscle or its tendon results in inability to move the distal part of the affected joint on active muscle contraction, but passive movements will be normal. Lack of muscle restraint may cause an abnormal range of movement.

Myositis, inflammation of muscle, is usually associated with pain on contraction or squeezing of affected muscles. Any movement which stretches muscle will be painful, with active movements tending to be more painful than passive movements.

Neuritis or neuropathy may simulate muscle-type pain, but cutaneous sensory impairment is not found in myositis. Muscles which are malfunctioning because of lower motor neurone pathology may fasciculate with numerous visible 'minicontractions' which persist for several seconds after the muscle is gently percussed.

A *myopathy* is metabolically-induced muscle malfunction. Because there is no inflammation there is no muscle pain or tenderness, and muscle weakness is the main manifestation. Proximal myopathies usually have metabolic causes including thyrotoxicosis, corticosteroid excess or occult neoplasia.

Tendinitis / Tenosynovitis

Tendons are fibrous cords by which a muscle is attached to bone (or occasionally to other muscles). On inspection of suspected tendinitis, tendon sheaths may be visibly or palpably swollen by exudation of fluid from inflammatory lesions, or there may be no swelling but a dry 'sandpaper-like' crepitus or friction rub on movement. Tenderness is usually localized and severe pain may interfere with movement.

MUSCULAR DYSTROPHIES

Muscular dystrophies are caused by an inherited degeneration of various muscle groups. Muscle weakness usually antedates the wasting.

Duchenne (pseudohypertrophic) dystrophy

Duchenne muscular dystrophy usually:

- affects males
- starts between 3 to 10 years of age

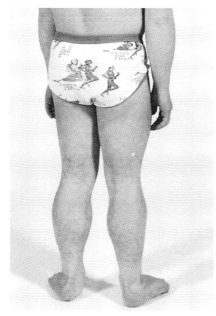

Fig.1 **Duchenne muscular dystrophy.**

- is usually inherited as a sex-linked recessive trait
- affects proximal muscle groups early
- is characterized by excessively developed calf muscles (Fig. 1).

Heart muscle may also be involved in Duchenne dystrophy.

Dystrophia myotonica

Inheritance is mostly autosomal dominant in dystrophia myotonica (Fig. 2). Onset can be at any age, but usually is in young adults. It presents with either weakness or myotonia (a sustained involuntary contraction of muscle), or both. Classically, the patients are slow to release a handshake. Associated features also include:

- frontal baldness
- bilateral ptosis
- a thin face caused by muscle wasting
- cataracts
- sternomastoid wasting.

Facioscapulohumeral dystrophy

Inheritance is also usually autosomal dominant in facioscapulohumeral dystrophy. Onset is usually between 10–40 years. There is facial and shoulder-girdle weakness. The progression is very slow, and the life span is unaffected.

Limb girdle dystrophy

Inheritance in limb girdle dystrophy is usually autosomal recessive. Symptoms of weakness usually develop in the

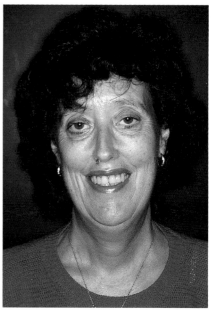

Fig. 2 **Dystrophia myotonica.**

second and third decade. Progression is slow, and the life span is usually unaffected.

Myotonia congenita (Thomsen's disease)

Inheritance in myotonia congenita is autosomal dominant. Myotonia is present from birth, and movements are slow and stiff but this may improve on sustained activity. Muscle hypertrophy may occur because of perpetual muscle tension. The life span is unaffected.

Other causes of muscle disease

Other causes of muscle disease include periodic paralysis caused by a metabolic error involving potassium, and endocrine diseases (usually causing a proximal myopathy). Myasthenia gravis is caused by failure of neuromuscular conduction which leads to weakness on continued contraction of affected striated muscles. Ptosis, dysphagia and limb weakness may result, as may respiratory muscle weakness. The Eaton–Lambert syndrome causes muscle weakness which *improves* after exercise; it is commonly a marker of internal malignancy.

NECK PROBLEMS

Because a nerve root comes out *above* C1, the cervical roots take their number from the vertebra *below*. The root which comes out between the seventh cervical and the first thoracic vertebra is called the C8 root,

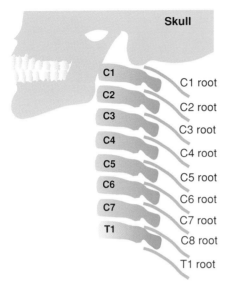

Skull

C1 — C1 root
C2 — C2 root
C3 — C3 root
C4 — C4 root
C5 — C5 root
C6 — C6 root
C7 — C7 root
T1 — C8 root
— T1 root

Fig. 3 **Diagram of labelling of upper nerve roots.**

so that all other roots below can take their number from the vertebra *above* (Fig. 3).

CERVICAL SPINE EXAMINATION

Note the relative posture of the head neck and shoulders. Normally, there is a cervical lordosis, a curvature of the spine convex anteriorly as viewed from the side; a *kyphosis* is a curvature convex posteriorly. Palpate for bony or muscle tenderness and swellings. Ask the patient to:

- put the chin on his/her chest
- arch the neck backwards
- put the left ear on the left shoulder
- put the right ear on the right shoulder
- rotate the head to the left and then to the right.

Note any restriction, pain or crepitus.

SPECIFIC CONDITIONS
Brachial neuritis

Brachial neuritis is an uncommon syndrome thought to be caused by 'allergic' nerve root inflammation of uncertain aetiology. It may follow immunizations. Pain, usually in C5 distribution, is followed by weakness predominantly of C5 and C6 distribution. Always beware of a similar pain caused by a carcinoma of the apex of the lung infiltrating the nerve trunks.

Brachial plexus lesions

Brachial plexus lesions are usually caused by trauma, either at birth or in road traffic accidents.

Cervical spondylitis

Spondylitis is inflammation of one or more vertebrae (usually caused by osteoarthritis), tending towards ankylosis. This leads to loss of flexibility which increases vulnerability to sudden movements or jolts.

Cervical spondylitis may cause problems by three mechanisms:

- Bony outgrowths (osteophytes) may impinge upon nerve roots.
- Large osteophytes may affect the spinal cord, either by causing narrowing of the bony spinal canal or by interfering with the cord blood supply.
- Extensive osteophytes involving the upper six vertebral foramina may impede ascending blood flow in the vertebral arteries. The brainstem and brain may then be starved of blood and symptoms and signs may result.

It is possible to attribute (wrongly) almost any neurological problem affecting the arm, vascular problem affecting the brain, or upper motor neurone signs affecting the legs to an arthritic neck X-ray.

C5 and C6 roots are the roots most commonly affected by cervical spondylitis. Symptoms may develop before signs, and include paresthesia which usually affects C5 and C6 dermatomes (p. 90). In late cases, the biceps jerk may be diminished because of interruption of the reflex arc or damage to the spinal cord at C5, C6 level, but the triceps jerk may be increased (as part of the upper motor neurone signs just below the level of the lesion). If severe, cervical spondylitis can produce upper motor neurone signs in the legs.

Cervical rib syndromes

An extra cervical rib, or a relatively prominent normal first rib, may produce problems by impinging on either the lower trunk of the brachial plexus or the subclavian artery. There is usually axillary pain, and pain in the ulnar side of the hand. Associated weakness particularly affects the abductor pollicis brevis.

Prolapse of cervical intervertebral discs

Prolapse of cervical intervertebral discs (Fig. 4) may cause pain. The onset may be abrupt or gradual. Typically, pain is exacerbated by head movement and by bodily pressure changes such as result from coughing or straining at stool. Lateral prolapse causes root compression which is usually unilateral, whereas posterior protrusion of a cervical (or less commonly a thoracic) disc may compress the spinal cord to cause sensory or lower motor neurone signs at

Spinal cord   Nerve roots

Posterior protrusion of disc   Lateral protrusion of disc

Fig. 4 **The ways in which protrusion of a cervical disc can cause neurological problems.** Cervical spondylosis can cause pressure on the spinal cord, nerve roots, nerves or their blood supply.

the site of the compression. There may be depression of the tendon reflexes of the affected root, with upper motor neurone signs below the site of compression. The pain of root compression is often felt in muscle–myotome groups, whereas other sensory symptoms are often felt in the relevant dermatome.

C6/C7 is the commonest site of an acute cervical disc, and the presence of an anatomically narrowed spinal canal makes such compressions more likely.

In patients with pre-existent cervical spondylosis, sudden anterior–posterior neck movements (such as occur in whiplash injuries) may cause acute root signs with possible additional cord damage. The neck will be stiff with muscle spasm causing loss of the normal cervical lordosis.

Muscle and neck problems

- Myositis may produce tender or painful muscles; myopathies are painless.
- Patients with muscular dystrophy should be asked if there is a family history.
- C5 and C6 are the roots most commonly affected by cervical spondylitis.
- C6/C7 is the commonest site of an acute cervical disc.

EXAMINATION OF THE UPPER LIMBS

THE HAND

Assessment of hand and finger functions is complex because neurological problems may be caused by lesions of the brain, spinal cord, nerve roots or peripheral nerves. Additionally, mechanical lesions may affect bones, joints, muscles or tendons.

Finger and thumb movements (Fig.1)

Thumb abduction is movement of the thumb upwards to a position at right angles to the index finger and palm, and adduction is moving it back again. Thumb extension is movement of the thumb from the anatomical position to a position at right angles to the index finger but in the plane of the palm. Thumb flexion returns the thumb to lie alongside the index finger.

The dorsal interossei (C8, T1, ulnar nerve) abduct the fingers away from the middle finger. The palmar interossei (Fig. 2) (C8, T1, ulnar nerve) adduct the fingers in conjunction with the lumbricals (lateral two lumbrical C8, T1, median nerve; medial two lumbricals C8, T1, ulnar nerve). Test for abduction by asking the patient to fan out the fingers against resistance and test for adduction by asking the patient to compress a card between the fingers. Figure 3 details the innervation of muscles and relevant movement.

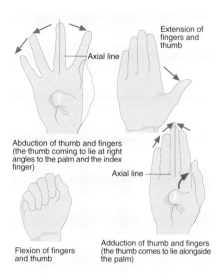

Extension of fingers and thumb

Axial line

Abduction of thumb and fingers (the thumb coming to lie at right angles to the palm and the index finger)

Axial line

Flexion of fingers and thumb

Adduction of thumb and fingers (the thumb comes to lie alongside the palm)

Fig. 1 **Finger and thumb movements.**

LARGE JOINTS OF THE UPPER LIMB

To examine the shoulder, note the contour of bones and muscles, and the posture of arm and scapula. Palpate to assess tenderness, but be aware that shoulder joint effusions are difficult to detect clinically. Assess active and passive movements in all three dimensions, noting restriction and whether restriction is caused by pain or stiffness. Test rotation by positioning the patient's forearm at right angles to the upper arm and

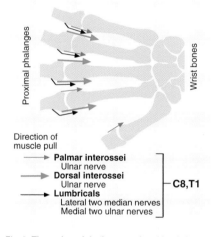

Proximal phalanges

Wrist bones

Direction of muscle pull

→ **Palmar interossei**
    Ulnar nerve
→ **Dorsal interossei**
    Ulnar nerve
→ **Lumbricals**
    Lateral two median nerves
    Medial two ulnar nerves

} **C8,T1**

Fig. 2 **The action of the interossei and lumbricals (the left hand viewed from in front).**

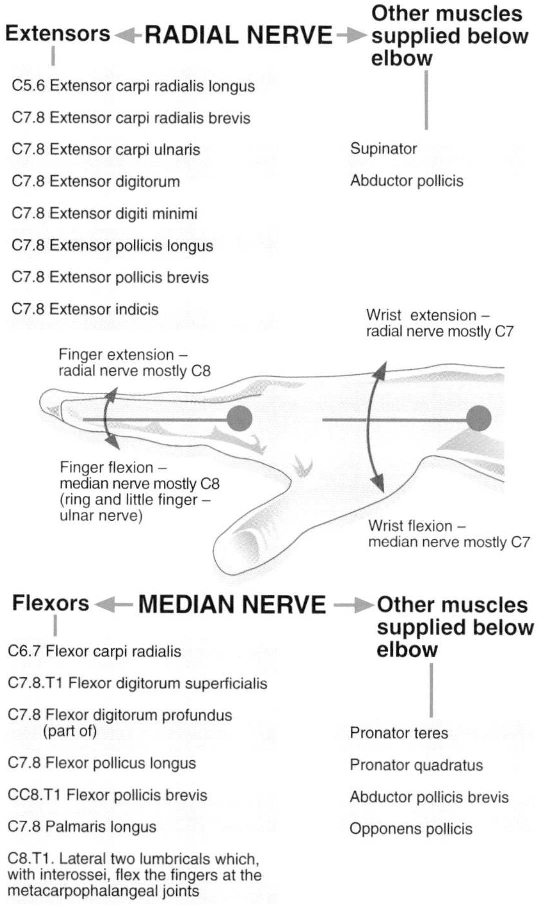

use movements of the lower arm to produce shoulder joint rotation. In all these movements hold the scapula with your other hand to ensure that shoulder joint movement, and not movement of the shoulder–scapula unit, is being assessed.

To examine the elbow joint, note any valgus or varus deformity. A varus deformity is one in which the angulation of the joint points away from the midline, whereas a valgus deformity points towards the midline. Assess joint temperature, swelling or tenderness. Synovial swelling may be palpable, and rheumatoid nodules may be felt around the joint. Compare flexion and extension on both sides.

COMMON UPPER LIMB DYSFUNCTIONS

Common causes of sensory symptoms or weakness in the arm include cervical spondylosis, nerve root lesions or compression of peripheral nerves. Trauma is relatively uncommon. In practice, the usual problem is to decide whether abnormalities detected are caused by a lesion of nerve roots or of a single peripheral nerve. The difference between nerve root lesions and peripheral nerve lesions are detailed

Extensors ◄ **RADIAL NERVE** ► Other muscles supplied below elbow

C5.6 Extensor carpi radialis longus

C7.8 Extensor carpi radialis brevis

C7.8 Extensor carpi ulnaris

C7.8 Extensor digitorum

C7.8 Extensor digiti minimi

C7.8 Extensor pollicis longus

C7.8 Extensor pollicis brevis

C7.8 Extensor indicis

Supinator

Abductor pollicis

Wrist extension – radial nerve mostly C7

Finger extension – radial nerve mostly C8

Finger flexion – median nerve mostly C8 (ring and little finger – ulnar nerve)

Wrist flexion – median nerve mostly C7

Flexors ◄ **MEDIAN NERVE** ► Other muscles supplied below elbow

C6.7 Flexor carpi radialis

C7.8.T1 Flexor digitorum superficialis

C7.8 Flexor digitorum profundus (part of)

C7.8 Flexor pollicus longus

CC8.T1 Flexor pollicis brevis

C7.8 Palmaris longus

C8.T1. Lateral two lumbricals which, with interossei, flex the fingers at the metacarpophalangeal joints

Pronator teres

Pronator quadratus

Abductor pollicis brevis

Opponens pollicis

Fig. 3 **Hand movements and associated nerves.**

on page 75. The differences between upper and lower motor neurone lesions are also detailed on page 75.

The usual sites of various pathologies which cause neurological problems in the upper limb are detailed in Figure 4.

The area of *pain* caused by neurological dysfunction may reflect the total area of sensory innervation, but cutaneous sensory *loss* may be much less than the area of pain because of overlapping innervation from normally functioning nerves. The dermatome and peripheral nerve innervation of the upper limb have been detailed on pages 90 and 91. Because of sensory overlapping, major sensory loss is

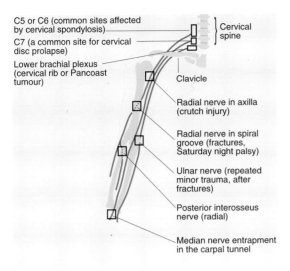

C5 or C6 (common sites affected by cervical spondylosis)

C7 (a common site for cervical disc prolapse)

Lower brachial plexus (cervical rib or Pancoast tumour)

Cervical spine

Clavicle

Radial nerve in axilla (crutch injury)

Radial nerve in spiral groove (fractures, Saturday night palsy)

Ulnar nerve (repeated minor trauma, after fractures)

Posterior interosseus nerve (radial)

Median nerve entrapment in the carpal tunnel

Fig.4 **The major sites of nerve problems affecting the upper limb.**

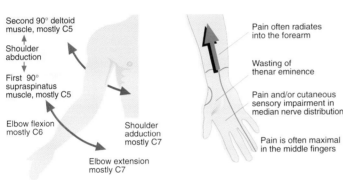

Second 90° deltoid muscle, mostly C5

Shoulder abduction

First 90° supraspinatus muscle, mostly C5

Elbow flexion mostly C6

Shoulder adduction mostly C7

Elbow extension mostly C7

Fig. 5 **Movements of the upper limb in terms of nerve root values.**

Pain often radiates into the forearm

Wasting of thenar eminence

Pain and/or cutaneous sensory impairment in median nerve distribution

Pain is often maximal in the middle fingers

Fig. 6 **Median nerve lesions.** Possible findings, particularly in compression in the carpal tunnel.

rare in radial nerve lesions, whereas more predictable sensory losses occur in lesions of the median and ulnar nerves.

There are certain movements of the upper limb which provide useful information concerning nerve root function (Fig. 5). Each movement illustrated is predominantly controlled by a single root. As an *aide memoire*, remember that the root values of the reflexes also give the value of the movements performed by the relevant muscles.

Median, radial and ulnar nerve lesions

Muscle weakness caused by damage to the median, radial or ulnar nerves causes 'negative' (weakness) manifestations but also positive manifestations (such as the claw hand of ulnar palsy) by allowing unopposed action of muscles driven by one or both of the other two nerves.

Median nerve lesions: root value C6–T1, mostly C8 and T1

The median nerve is particularly vulnerable to compression at the wrist in the carpal tunnel (Fig. 6). Symptoms (comprising paresthesiae or loss of cutaneous sensation in median nerve distribution) may be precipitated by hard manual work, are often worse at night and may be relieved by swinging the hand around.

Two point discrimination (affecting the palmar aspect of the thumb, index and middle fingers) is often impaired early (as in most incomplete sensory nerve entrapments or compressions). In late cases there is wasting of the lateral thenar eminence. The median nerve supplies most of the forearm flexor muscles and small muscles of the thumb, and the lumbricals to the index and middle fingers. Abductor pollicis brevis is often weak and is the most useful muscle to test if the carpal tunnel syndrome is suspected.

Radial nerve lesions: root value C5–C8, mostly C6 and C7

Incorrect use of a crutch may cause damage to the radial nerve in the axilla, causing weakness of all distally supplied muscles, whereas radial nerve damage at the middle of the humerus may spare the triceps and the brachioradialis. More distally, the radial nerve becomes the posterior interosseous nerve, damage to which causes weakness of the wrist extensors (Fig. 7). Sensory loss is variable as there is much sensory overlap and any loss is usually confined to a small patch on the dorsum of the hand between thumb and index finger.

Ulnar nerve lesions: root value C7–T1, mostly C8 and T1

We are all familiar with the effects of acute trauma to the ulnar nerve at the elbow ('knocking the funny bone'), but long-term, low-grade trauma may also cause problems with sensory and motor losses. At the wrist, the ulnar nerve divides into a sensory and a motor component. Damage to the motor part produces weakness of all the small muscles of the hand except flexor digitorum brevis, abductor and opponens of the thumb, and the lumbricals to the index and middle finger. If the ulnar nerve is damaged, the unopposed action of the metacarpophalangeal extensors and interphalangeal flexors causes the claw hand of ulnar palsy (the index and middle fingers are less clawed because the lumbricals to these fingers are supplied by the median nerve) (Fig. 8).

A T1 root lesion may cause weakness and wasting of all small hand muscles. An ulnar nerve lesion may do likewise, but abductor pollicis brevis and opponens pollicis (which are driven by the median nerve) will be unaffected.

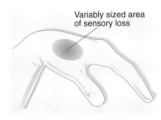

Variably sized area of sensory loss

Fig. 7 **Radial nerve lesions.** Wrist drop caused by weakness of extensors of the wrist, particularly extensors of the index finger and thumb.

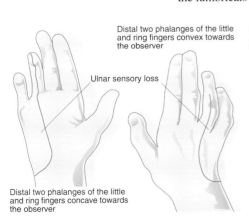

Distal two phalanges of the little and ring fingers convex towards the observer

Ulnar sensory loss

Distal two phalanges of the little and ring fingers concave towards the observer

Fig. 8 **Ulnar nerve lesions 'claw hand' sensory loss.** Again there is much variability.

Examination of the upper limbs

- Neorological problems may be caused by lesions of the brain, spinal cord, nerve roots or peripheral nerves.
- When testing the shoulder movements ensure the scapula does not move.
- Areas of pain reflect areas of sensory innervation.
- Areas of sensory loss may be smaller than those of pain distribution.
- Two-point discrimination is impaired early in partial sensory nerve damage or peripheral neuropathy.

EXAMINATION OF THE SPINE, PELVIS AND LOWER LIMBS (I)

SPINE AND PELVIS

Look for asymmetry or deformity of chest, trunk, pelvis or hips. Confirm the normal thoracic kyphosis and lumbar lordosis, remembering that the normal spinal posture changes with age. Feel for any steps or tenderness of the spinous processes.

Localized bone pain on palpation or percussion suggests:

- osteomyelitis
- malignant deposits
- a compression fracture
- a prolapsed disc.

Assess spinal movements by standing behind the patient with your hands stabilizing the pelvis, and then ask the patient to:

- touch his toes
- arch his back

- tilt to the left
- tilt to the right
- rotate to the left
- rotate to the right.

If there is limitation of movement note whether this is caused by pain or stiffness.

Specifically test for impaired straight leg raising (unnecessary if the patient can touch his toes). With the patient on his back, lift each leg (which stretches the sciatic nerve). If positive and there is impaired straight leg raising because of pain, sciatica is the diagnosis.

Sacroiliac joint problems may be exacerbated by pelvic rotation or by pressure on the iliac crests (which 'springs' the sacroiliac joints) or by direct pressure from behind with the thumbs over the sacroiliac joints.

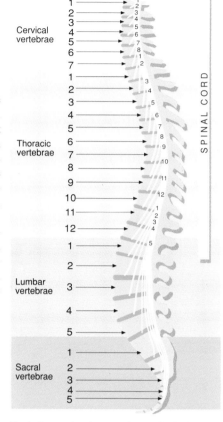

Fig. 1 **Conventional nomenclature of spinal nerve roots and their relation to the vertebrae.** Note that the root number is determined by the (vertebral) site of exit from the vertebral column, and that numbered root lesions may be caused by problems in and around vertebrae of different numbers.

LOWER LIMBS

In adults, the spinal cord terminates at the L1, L2 level, and therefore each nerve root has to travel some distance downwards in the spinal canal before exiting the spinal column (Fig. 1). Thus it may be easy to define a root *value* for a neurological abnormality, but precise localization of the *anatomical site* of the causative lesion requires further investigations.

The lower limb is innervated by the lumbar and sacral plexuses.

The lumbar plexus

The lumbar plexus is derived from L2, L3 and L4 roots (Fig. 2). All three branches of the lumbar plexus pass to the front of the leg. The lateral cutaneous nerve of the thigh passes downwards just interior to the lateral part of the inguinal ligament (where it may be trapped). The femoral nerve passes under the middle of the inguinal ligament, and in the female the obturator nerve passes adjacent to the uterus (where it is vulnerable during obstetric procedures) and exits the pelvis via the obturator foramen.

The sacral plexus

The sacral plexus (L4, L5, S1 and S2 roots) supplies the rest of the lower limb (Fig. 2). The roots form a plexus anterior to the sacro-iliac joint and leave the pelvis via the greater sciatic foramen. The main branches—the sciatic, gluteal and posterior cutaneous nerve of the thigh—lie directly behind the hip joint where they can be damaged by fractures or by misplaced intramuscular injections. The main nerve root values for various lower limb movements are detailed in Figure 3.

The sciatic nerve divides into the lateral popliteal (peroneal) and the medial popliteal (tibial) nerves. The lateral popliteal nerve is particularly vulnerable as it winds round the neck of the fibula. Motor damage at this site produces foot drop with difficulty in dorsiflexion and eversion of the foot.

SPECIFIC NERVE LESIONS

Lateral cutaneous nerve of the thigh

If the lateral cutaneous nerve of the thigh is trapped under the lateral part of the inguinal ligament there is sensory loss over the lateral aspect of the thigh. If there is pain felt in the same distribution this is called meralgia parasthetica. There is no motor loss.

Femoral nerve

Femoral nerve damage is associated with weakness of knee extension, hip flexion is only slightly impaired and hip adduction is not affected. The knee jerk may be reduced or absent.

Sciatic nerve

The sciatic nerve supplies muscles below the knee and some of the hamstrings. There will be a foot drop (a plantar flexed foot which tends to drag on walking) and weakness of knee flexion. With a profound sciatic nerve lesion the ankle jerk and plantar response will be reduced or absent, but the knee jerk will be intact.

SENSATION IN THE LOWER LIMB

The root and peripheral nerve areas of cutaneous innervation are detailed on page 90 and are also shown in Figure 4.

The femoral nerve innervates a long strip of skin which includes an area below the knee. The sciatic nerve only provides exclusive cutaneous sensation for a small area of skin on the lower leg and foot.

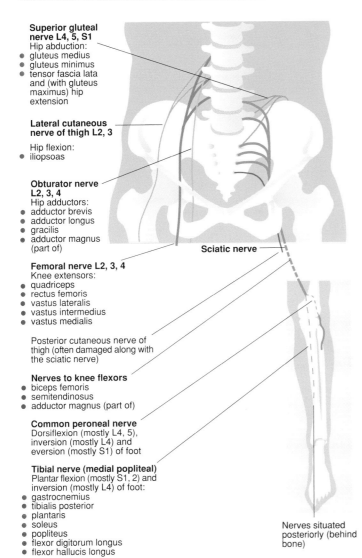

Superior gluteal nerve L4, 5, S1
Hip abduction:
• gluteus medius
• gluteus minimus
• tensor fascia lata and (with gluteus maximus) hip extension

Lateral cutaneous nerve of thigh L2, 3

Hip flexion:
• iliopsoas

Obturator nerve L2, 3, 4
Hip adductors:
• adductor brevis
• adductor longus
• gracilis
• adductor magnus (part of)

Sciatic nerve

Femoral nerve L2, 3, 4
Knee extensors:
• quadriceps
• rectus femoris
• vastus lateralis
• vastus intermedius
• vastus medialis

Posterior cutaneous nerve of thigh (often damaged along with the sciatic nerve)

Nerves to knee flexors
• biceps femoris
• semitendinosus
• adductor magnus (part of)

Common peroneal nerve
Dorsiflexion (mostly L4, 5), inversion (mostly L4) and eversion (mostly S1) of foot

Tibial nerve (medial popliteal)
Plantar flexion (mostly S1, 2) and inversion (mostly L4) of foot:
• gastrocnemius
• tibialis posterior
• plantaris
• soleus
• popliteus
• flexor digitorum longus
• flexor hallucis longus

Nerves situated posteriorly (behind bone)

Fig. 2 **The lumbar and sacral plexuses.**

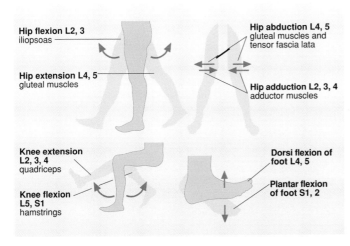

Hip flexion L2, 3
iliopsoas

Hip extension L4, 5
gluteal muscles

Hip abduction L4, 5
gluteal muscles and tensor fascia lata

Hip adduction L2, 3, 4
adductor muscles

Knee extension L2, 3, 4
quadriceps

Knee flexion L5, S1
hamstrings

Dorsi flexion of foot L4, 5

Plantar flexion of foot S1, 2

Fig. 3 **The nerve root derivation of certain lower limb movements.**

Sciatica caused by a lumbar disc should not affect the femoral nerve or posterior cutaneous nerve of the thigh. Thus, loss of sensation at the front of the thigh (femoral nerve) or at the back of the thigh (posterior cutaneous nerve) in association with sciatica demands another explanation and should not be attributed to a lumbar disc.

Lumbar disc problems are common and usually affect the L5 root and less commonly the L4 root. It is dangerous to attribute any other root lesion to a lumbar disc. The L5 pattern of pain is shown in Figure 5.

If there is bladder or bowel dysfunction, always check sensation of the perianal area (S2, 3, 4 roots) and genitalia, as this may provide evidence of a neurological lesion underlying bladder or bowel dysfunction.

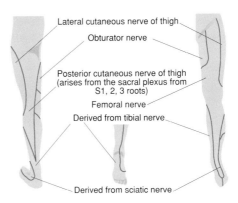

Lateral cutaneous nerve of thigh
Obturator nerve
Posterior cutaneous nerve of thigh (arises from the sacral plexus from S1, 2, 3 roots)
Femoral nerve
Derived from tibial nerve
Derived from sciatic nerve

Fig. 4 **The derivation of cutaneous innervation of the lower limb.**

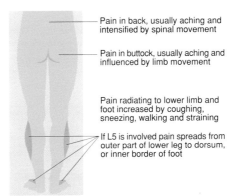

Pain in back, usually aching and intensified by spinal movement

Pain in buttock, usually aching and influenced by limb movement

Pain radiating to lower limb and foot increased by coughing, sneezing, walking and straining

If L5 is involved pain spreads from outer part of lower leg to dorsum, or inner border of foot

Fig. 5 **Sciatica with L5 pattern of pain.** Tingling or numbness may also occur.

Examination of the spine, pelvis and lower limbs (I)

• When assessing spinal and hip movements ensure the pelvis does not move.
• A nerve root value does not necessarily identify the anatomical site of a lesion.
• Lumbar disc problems usually affect the L5 root.
• If there is a bladder or bowel dysfunction always check S2, S3, S4 roots.

EXAMINATION OF THE SPINE, PELVIS AND LOWER LIMBS (II)

HIP JOINT EXAMINATION

Look for cutaneous or musculoskeletal abnormalities and note the posture of the legs. The hip is a deep joint and tenderness may be diffuse and difficult to localize to the joint.

Test for hip flexion by drawing the thigh up against the lower abdominal wall. Then flex the normal hip joint until the lumbar lordosis is obliterated (when a hand cannot be placed between the bed and lumbar spine) (Fig. 1). If the other thigh rises during this, a fixed flexion deformity is present of that hip joint which prevents its normal extension. Extension can also be tested with the patient lying face down with active and passive lifting of the straight leg being evaluated (Fig. 2).

Adduction of the hips can be tested by crossing each leg in turn (Fig. 3). Abduction can be tested by asking the patient to push outwards with both knees against resistance (Fig. 4). Prevent movement of the pelvis from interfering with these assessments by placing a hand on the iliac crest opposite to the leg being assessed.

Internal and external rotation can be assessed when the hips are flexed, in the normal 'anatomical' position, or in extension. Rotation can be tested by positioning the lower leg at right angles to the thigh and then rotating the thigh by moving the ankle in a semicircle (Fig. 5).

KNEE JOINT EXAMINATION

Look for musculoskeletal abnormalities, effusion (Fig. 6) and joint posture. Feel for joint temperature, localized tenderness and whether or not there is crepitus on movement of the joint or patella. Assess flexion, extension and rotation.

Tears of knee joint menisci are usually sustained when the knee joint is simultaneously weight bearing and being flexed. Examination shows:

- swelling (of rapid onset if there is bleeding into the joint) which subsides over a few days
- tenderness over the involved meniscus
- surrounding muscle spasm
- pain is severe initially
- loss of joint extension is common
- muscle wasting may occur later.

McMurry's sign is found in posterior meniscus tears. With the patient's knee flexed, the examiner grips the heel with one hand and, with the other hand, puts one thumb on one side of the knee

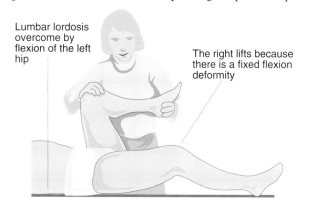

Lumbar lordosis overcome by flexion of the left hip

The right lifts because there is a fixed flexion deformity

Fig. 1 **Demonstration of a fixed flexion deformity of the hip.**

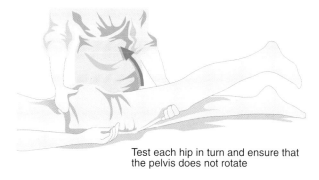

Test each hip in turn and ensure that the pelvis does not rotate

Fig. 2 **Testing extension of the hip joint.**

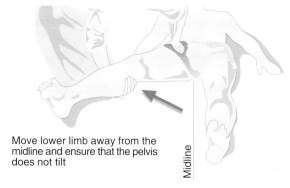

Move lower limb away from the midline and ensure that the pelvis does not tilt

Midline

Fig. 4 **Testing abduction of the hip joint.**

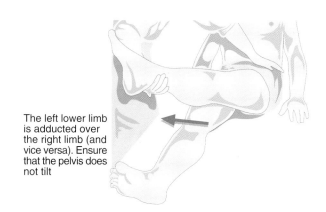

The left lower limb is adducted over the right limb (and vice versa). Ensure that the pelvis does not tilt

Fig. 3 **Testing adduction of the hip joint.**

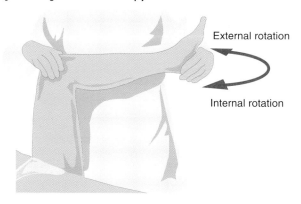

External rotation

Internal rotation

Fig. 5 **Testing internal and external rotation of the hip joint.**

joint with the middle finger on the other side (Fig. 7). Rotating the tibia on the femur whilst progressively extending the joint will then produce a click, clunk, or jump in certain positions.

Integrity of the cruciate ligaments can be assessed by gripping the lower leg with the knee at about 20° of flexion and determining the amount of movement or pain when the lower leg is moved anteriorly or posteriorly on the femur (Lachman's test). Normally, there should be neither pain nor abnormal movement (Fig. 8).

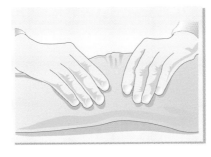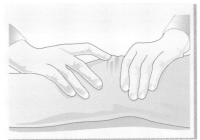

Fig. 6 **Testing for knee joint effusion.** Use one hand to press any fluid out of the bursa above the knee and then try to 'tap' the patella onto the tumour by a brisk firm pressure using the other hand. If there is a large effusion the patella will spring back.

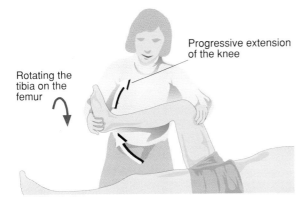

Rotating the tibia on the femur

Progressive extension of the knee

Fig. 7 **Testing for posterior meniscus tears.**

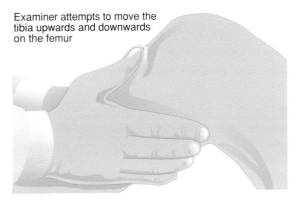

Examiner attempts to move the tibia upwards and downwards on the femur

Fig. 8 **Testing for integrity of the cruciate ligaments (Lachman's test).**

ANKLE AND FOOT EXAMINATION

Note musculoskeletal abnormality, abnormal wear of the patient's shoes or callosities (hardened thickened skin).

To test ankle dorsiflexion and plantar flexion, use one hand to steady the lower leg and one to flex and extend the ankle joint. Inversion and eversion can be assessed by gripping the heel with the hand and performing the relevant movements. The metatarsal joints can be flexed, extended and moved from side to side to a certain degree. The toes can be flexed and extended.

OBSERVATION OF THE PATIENT'S GAIT

An abnormal gait may be caused by:

- skeletal shortening
- pain
- muscle problems
- joint problems
- neurological problems (see p. 90).

In the presence of gluteal (hip abductor) weakness or a dislocated hip, standing on the leg of the affected side causes the pelvis to tilt downwards as the weak gluteal muscle cannot maintain the pelvis' relation to the femur. Normally the pelvis is tilted upwards so that the non-standing hip is elevated — Trendelenberg's sign (Fig. 9).

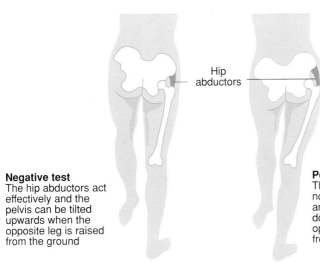

Hip abductors

Negative test
The hip abductors act effectively and the pelvis can be tilted upwards when the opposite leg is raised from the ground

Positive test
The hip abductors are not acting effectively and the pelvis thus tilts downwards when the opposite leg is raised from the ground

Fig. 9 **Trendelenberg's sign.**

Examination of the spine, pelvis and lower limbs (II)

- Movements of the hip are flexion, extension, adduction, abduction and rotation.
- Tears of knee joint menisci usually occur when the knee is simultaneously weight bearing and flexing.
- Abnormal wear on a patient's shoes may be significant.
- Abnormal gaits may be caused by bone, muscle, joint or neurological problems, or by pain.

COMMON MUSCULOSKELETAL CONDITIONS

ACUTE BACTERIAL ARTHRITIS

In acute bacterial arthritis, the history is usually brief with a rapid onset of fever and joint pain, a reluctance to move the affected joint and systemic upset. On examination the infected joint will be warm, tender, swollen, and an effusion may be detectable.

ANKYLOSING SPONDYLITIS

Ankylosing spondylitis (Fig. 1) is classically seen in males under the age of 30. They will present with insidious illness, fatigue, weight loss, low back pain and early morning stiffness, and ankylosis (abnormal immobility of a joint or joints).

The joints of the spine are affected early but peripheral, usually large, joints may be affected later. On examination there may be:

- loss of the lumbar lordosis
- difficulty in bending forwards due to muscle spasm or ankylosis
- kyphosis in advanced disease
- iritis
- heart lesions.

BACK STRAIN

Back strain usually follows bending or rotatory movements. Pain is constant ('lumbago') and muscle spasm, caused by pain, may lock the patient in a bent position. There are no leg symptoms or signs.

CAUDA EQUINA CLAUDICATION

Cauda equina claudication is caused by interruption of the blood supply to the spinal cord roots, distal to the termination of the spinal cord itself. Symptoms comprise an aching pain, usually precipitated by exertion and taking about 20 minutes to resolve.

CHARCOT'S JOINTS (NEUROPATHIC ARTHROPATHY)

Loss of pain sensation in joint tissues abolishes the protective reflexes caused by pain, leaving the joint vulnerable to repeated minor damage. Whilst there may be a history of minor pain in the joint, the major result will be joint deformity with little or no pain (Fig. 2).

On examination the joint (classically the knee joint) may be obviously disorganized with swelling caused by bony overgrowth or joint effusion, and possibly crepitus (attributable to loose bodies within the joint) may be elicited. Common causes include diabetes, syringomyelia and syphilis.

CRUSH FRACTURE OF THE SPINE

Weight-bearing vertebrae, especially those below T8, are particularly vulnerable to crush fractures. Often there is a history of trauma, but in those with osteoporosis there may be no such history. Pain if present is of abrupt onset, usually does not radiate, is worse on weight-bearing and is associated with local tenderness. A dorsal kyphosis may develop.

GOUT

The history of acute gout is often characteristic. There is acute onset severe pain, often affecting the big toe such that walking is difficult (Fig. 3). There is frequently a history of previous episodes. Attacks may be precipitated by minor trauma or surgical operations.

On examination the joint is exquisitely tender and the skin over the joint is tense, hot, shiny and red.

OSTEOARTHRITIS

The onset is usually gradual, and symptoms are often localized to one or two joints (usually spine, hips or knees), with pain being characteristically worse after exercise and relieved by rest.

On examination there is pain on movement, possibly crepitus and effusion if there has been a recent exacerbation due to external or internal trauma. Significant deformity only occurs in severe disease.

Enlarged osteophytes around terminal interphalangeal joints (Heberden's nodes) or proximal interphalangeal joints (Bouchard's nodes) may be found. Unlike rheumatoid arthritis, there are no extra-articular manifestations.

OSTEOMALACIA AND RICKETS

Osteomalacia (Fig. 4) is the adult equivalent of childhood rickets. Both are metabolic bone diseases with defective mineralization of bone resulting from vitamin D deficiency. Usually there is a history of poor dietary intake of vitamin D or lack of exposure to sunlight. There may be a history of malabsorption with steatorrhoea (fatty bowel motions) leading to vitamin D deficiency (vitamin D is fat soluble). Children with rickets may have delayed milestones and enlarged long bone cartilages and costochondral junctions, which produces a 'rachitic rosary'. Normal weight-bearing bends the leg bones, particularly in children.

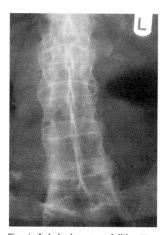

Fig. 1 **Ankylosing spondylitis.** The patient would have had a fixed 'poker' spine.

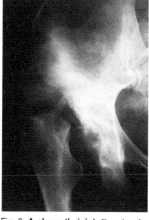

Fig. 2 **A charcot's joint.** Despite the obvious bony disruption, the pain was minimal.

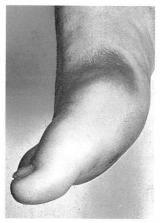

Fig. 3 **Gout.**

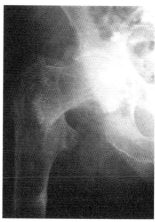

Fig. 4 **Looser zones (pseudo fractures) in osteomalacia.**

OSTEOPOROSIS

Osteoporosis is an absolute decrease in the mass of bone tissue. Crush fractures unassociated with trauma may occur.

OSTEOMYELITIS

With acute bacterial osteomyelitis there is sudden onset of bone pain and tenderness, fever and painful movement. Osteomyelitis occurring near a joint may be difficult to distinguish from acute bacterial arthritis.

POLYMYOSITIS/DERMATOMYOSITIS

The onset of polymyositis may be acute or insidious. With acute myositis there are painful muscles, fever, malaise, weight loss and loss of mobility.

The 'dermato' element, if present, comprises a dusky red rash on areas exposed to light. Periorbital oedema with heliotrope (sunburn-like) colouration is pathognomic. Skin over the knuckles may also be reddened.

PROLAPSES OF INTERVERTEBRAL DISCS

The intervertebral discs act as shock absorbers and, unfortunately, degenerate with age. Degenerative changes or trauma may cause rupture of the outer fibrous ring of the intervertebral discs, most commonly in the lumbosacral and cervical spines. The inner nucleus pulposus is forced out and 'prolapses' posteriorly or posterolaterally. Symptoms result when the herniated nucleus compresses the spinal cord or the nerve roots.

With a prolapsed lumbar disc (Fig. 5) there may have been prodromal warning twinges, but patients characteristically present with acute back pain 2–4 hours after an activity such as bending or lifting.

Lateral disc protrusion produces pain which is typically severe and exacerbated by movement or coughing, with pain down one leg. L4 and L5 are the most common discs involved and, because L4 and L5 contribute to the sciatic nerve, sciatica results. The history is of pain radiating to the back of the thigh, the calf and to the foot and toes.

Disc lesions affecting the L5 root notably cause an easily detected weakness of extension of the great toe (extensor hallucis longus). It is dangerous to attribute lumbar root symptoms or signs other than L4 and L5 to a lumbar disc.

Lumbar discs may compress the cauda equina possibly causing urinary problems.

Acute central disc prolapse is a surgical emergency. The cardinal symptoms are perineal numbness (so-called saddle anaesthesia) and incontinence of urine or faeces. The most obvious sign is inability of the patient's anal sphincter to tighten down on an examining finger during rectal examination.

PSORIASIS

Look for psoriasis (p. 118) in all patients with joint symptoms. A rheumatoid arthritis-like syndrome may result. The distal interphalangeal joints are particularly involved, and there is often pitting of the nails.

REITER'S SYNDROME

Reiter's syndrome is a disease which usually affects males. It is characterized by a combination of conditions including arthritis, urethritis and conjunctivitis.

The onset may be acute or subacute, and there may be a history of sexual contact or diarrhoeal illness. On examination there is typically an arthritis which is usually asymmetrical, especially involving feet, ankles, knees and sacroiliac joints. There may also be a rash on the soles of the feet (keratodermia blenorrhagica).

RHEUMATOID ARTHRITIS

The onset of rheumatoid arthritis may be acute or insidious. In active rheumatoid arthritis the joints involved are tender and synovial thickening may be apparent. Multiple joint involvement tends to be symmetrical. Deformities include flexion contractures (caused by spasm of muscles around inflamed joints) and ulnar deviation of the finger (see p. 9).

Unlike osteoarthritis there is:

- stiffness after inactivity ('early morning stiffness')
- rheumatoid nodules (p. 8)
- synovial or capsular swellings
- involvement of proximal interphalangeal and metacarpophalangeal joints
- sparing of the terminal interphalangeal joints.

Still's disease (juvenile rheumatoid arthritis) shares some characteristics of adult rheumatoid arthritis, but growth may also be retarded. Extra-articular manifestations, such as rash, fever, iritis, splenomegaly or lymph node enlargement, are common.

SYSTEMIC LUPUS ERYTHEMATOSUS (SLE)

About 90% of SLE patients complain of arthralgia varying from vague pains to acute arthritis which is usually initially mistaken for rheumatoid arthritis. Clues to SLE include a butterfly facial rash, light sensitive skin eruptions, alopecia and recurrent pleurisy.

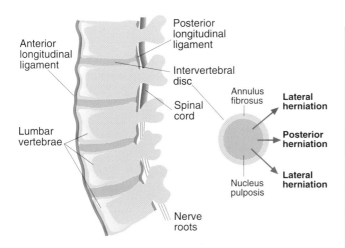

Fig. 5 **Prolapsed lumbar disc.**

Common musculoskeletal conditions

- Ankylosing spondylitis is a cause of early morning stiffness.
- Charcot's joints are often radiographically and clinicallly disorganized.
- Osteoarthritic pain is worse after exercise or weight-bearing and is relieved by rest.
- Both osteomalacia and rickets are caused by vitamin D deficiency.
- Osteomyelitis near a joint may be difficult to distinguish from a bacterial arthritis.
- Acute central disc prolapse is a surgical emergency.
- Always look for evidence of psoriasis in a patient with joint problems.
- Rheumatoid arthritis often has extra-articular manifestations.

BASIC PRINCIPLES

In a 70-kg man the skin has an area of about 1.8 sq metres which provides covering, protection and a heat regulating mechanism for the inner structures. The skin contains sweat glands, sebaceous glands, nerves, blood vessels, lymphatic vessels, and immunologically active tissues. The hair and nails are also derived from the skin.

The skin is easily examined and abnormalities are there for all to see—the patient will expect a diagnosis!

DIAGNOSIS OF SKIN LESIONS

The clinical diagnosis of skin lesions depends on recognition of patterns based on a comprehensive knowledge of numerous skin diseases. There is no infallible approach that uses a rigorous diagnostic flowchart system of classification of clinical appearances. For those without comprehensive knowledge who have to approach patients, skin lesions can be classified along sensible guidelines (Fig. 1) into those that tend to be symmetrical in distribution (suggesting a generalized or systemic disease), and those that tend to be asymmetrical (suggesting a localized and non-systemic disease). Both symmetrical and asymmetrical lesions are subdivided into those which tend to occur in well patients (suggesting a primary skin disease) or those which tend to occur in ill patients (suggesting a generalized process unless the skin abnormalities are extensive).

Often the history of the development of skin lesions and their associated features is necessary for diagnosis: recognition of patterns is essential. For example the

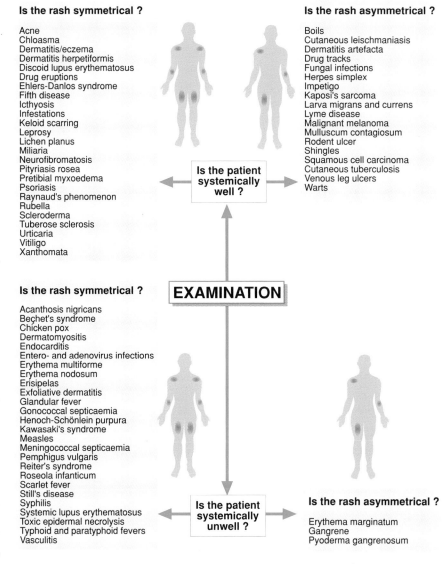

Is the rash symmetrical ?

Acne
Chloasma
Dermatitis/eczema
Dermatitis herpetiformis
Discoid lupus erythematosus
Drug eruptions
Ehlers-Danlos syndrome
Fifth disease
Icthyosis
Infestations
Keloid scarring
Leprosy
Lichen planus
Miliaria
Neurofibromatosis
Pityriasis rosea
Pretibial myxoedema
Psoriasis
Raynaud's phenomenon
Rubella
Scleroderma
Tuberose sclerosis
Urticaria
Vitiligo
Xanthomata

Is the rash asymmetrical ?

Boils
Cutaneous leischmaniasis
Dermatitis artefacta
Drug tracks
Fungal infections
Herpes simplex
Impetigo
Kaposi's sarcoma
Larva migrans and currens
Lyme disease
Malignant melanoma
Mulluscum contagiosum
Rodent ulcer
Shingles
Squamous cell carcinoma
Cutaneous tuberculosis
Venous leg ulcers
Warts

Is the patient systemically well ?

EXAMINATION

Is the rash symmetrical ?

Acanthosis nigricans
Beçhet's syndrome
Chicken pox
Dermatomyositis
Endocarditis
Entero- and adenovirus infections
Erythema multiforme
Erythema nodosum
Erisipelas
Exfoliative dermatitis
Glandular fever
Gonococcal septicaemia
Henoch-Schönlein purpura
Kawasaki's syndrome
Measles
Meningococcal septicaemia
Pemphigus vulgaris
Reiter's syndrome
Roseola infanticum
Scarlet fever
Still's disease
Syphilis
Systemic lupus erythematosus
Toxic epidermal necrolysis
Typhoid and paratyphoid fevers
Vasculitis

Is the patient systemically unwell ?

Is the rash asymmetrical ?

Erythema marginatum
Gangrene
Pyoderma gangrenosum

Fig. 1 **Guidelines for classifying skin lesions on initial presentation.**

GLOSSARY OF IMPORTANT TERMS

Abscess: a localized collection of pus.
Alopecia: absence of hair from areas which are usually hairy.
Bulla: a localized collection of fluid in the epidermis, usually greater than 5 mm in diameter.
Carbuncle: a large abscess with central necrosis (it may be considered to be a collection of furuncles).
Cellulitis: inflammation of skin and subcutaneous tissue.
Chancre: the primary lesion of certain infections that develops at the site of organism entry.
Crusting: an outer layer of solid material formed by drying of exudate or secretions.
Desquamation: peeling of the superficial skin.
Ecchymosis: a diffuse discolouration of an area of the skin or mucous membranes caused by extravasation of blood.

Enanthem: an eruption occurring on a mucous surface, usually meaning intraorally.
Erosion: a localized disintegration of outer skin layers.
Erythema (Fig. 3): a skin redness caused by vasodilation which characteristically blanches on pressure.
Exanthem: a skin rash.
Excoriation: a scratch mark.
Fissure: a linear superficial skin breach.
Herpetiform rash: composed of clusters of vesicles.
Furuncle: a boil—a painful pus-containing skin nodule often starting in a hair follicle.
Keratosis: a horn-like skin thickening.
Lichenification: skin thickening with increased skin markings.
Macule: a small circumscribed, non-elevated area of skin.

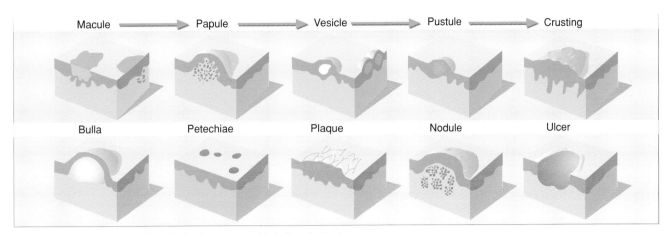

Fig. 2 **Main sequence of skin lesions (top); other common skin lesions (bottom).**

common infectious diseases of childhood (measles, chickenpox and rubella) often start on the head and work downwards.

There is a 'main sequence' of descriptive terms for skin lesions (Fig. 2).

HISTORY AND EXAMINATION OF THE SKIN

Because the patient is invariably anxious to show the rash, it is sensible for the doctor to look at the proffered rash briefly, then take a proper history and later return to examine the rash in detail.

The questions to be asked of a patient with skin lesions include:

- site of commencement?
- is the lesion itchy?
- is the lesion painful?
- pattern of spread (both anatomically and with the passage of time)
- progress of the lesion
- response to treatments given
- presence of precipitating causes including drug treatment
- presence of any symptoms suggesting an underlying disease
- a predisposing occupational history
- a predisposing family history.

To examine the skin a magnifying hand lens may be required. The skin should be gently palpated to assess the texture and blanching. It may be necessary to undress the patient to determine the extent and appearance of some rashes. Do not omit to examine the mouth, nails, hair and the genitalia, and to conduct a general examination if the diagnosis is not obviously a disease process limited to the skin.

Basic principles

- The diagnosis of skin rashes requires knowledge of numerous diseases and their pattern of skin involvement.
- Measles, chickenpox and rubella often start on the head and work downwards.
- Ask the patient to undress to determine the full extent of skin rashes.
- Examination of the skin is not complete if the genitalia have not been examined.

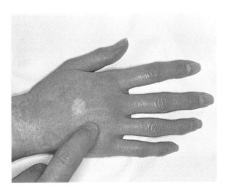

Fig. 3 **Erythema.**

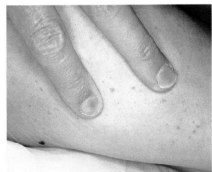

Fig. 4 **Petechiae.**

Nodule: a palpable solid or round lesion usually greater than 1 cm in diameter and deeper in the skin than a papule.

Papule: a small circumscribed, solid, palpable elevation in the skin, usually less than 5 mm in diameter.

Petechiae (Fig. 4): small spots of blood (1–2 mm in diameter) caused by small haemorrhages: they do not blanch on pressure.

Plaque: an elevated patch or flat area of skin usually more than 5 mm in diameter.

Purpura: a condition characterized by leakage of blood from blood vessels, usually either as petechiae or ecchymoses.

Pustule: a small area of skin elevation containing pus (inflammatory cells).

Telangiectasia: localized dilations of superficial small blood vessels of the skin.

Ulcer: a local defect or excavation of an organ surface, usually produced by sloughing of necrotic or inflammatory tissue.

Urticaria: a vascular reaction pattern which is usually itchy and marked by transient, smooth, slightly elevated patches which are redder or paler than surrounding skin.

Vesicle: an elevated skin lesion up to 5 mm in diameter containing fluid.

Wheal: a transient circumscribed reddish-white elevation of the skin caused by local oedema; it may be itchy.

Other useful terms to describe skin appearances include **annular** (ring-like), **centrifugal** (predominantly affecting the arms and legs), **centripetal** (predominantly affecting the head and trunk), **pleomorphic** (having different forms), **reticular** (netlike) and **symmetrical**.

SYMMETRICAL LESIONS IN SYSTEMICALLY WELL PATIENTS (I)

Symmetrical skin lesions often reflect a generalized skin or a systemic illness: systemic manifestations—if any—may provide diagnostic clues.

Acne

Acne eruptions comprise blocked hair or sebaceous ducts 'blackheads', pustules, small boils, cysts, and, in severe cases, scarring. Acne occurs predominantly on the face but may appear on the neck, chest and back. Acne rosacea, a condition rare before middle age, is a striking erythematous swelling with papules and pustules on the central areas of the face. A reddened knobbly nose (rhinophyma) may result.

Chloasma

Chloasma classically occurs in pregnancy with dark brown, well-demarcated, approximately symmetrical areas of facial pigmentation.

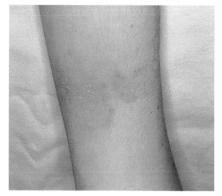

Fig. 1 **Eczema.**

Dermatitis/eczema

Dermatitis and eczema mean the same although they tend to be used in different contexts. Both indicate a superficial skin inflammation which, if acute, is associated with vesicles. Skin reddening and scaling develops with lichenification in chronic cases. Scratching of the itchy areas results in excoriations.

Eczema is often taken to refer to a bilateral approximately symmetrical eruption affecting endogenously predisposed (atopic) individuals (Fig. 1), whereas *dermatitis* is often taken to mean skin inflammation of known or unknown external (exogenous) causation. Dermatitis, depending on its causation, may be focal or bilateral. Contact dermatitis, for example, occurs on areas exposed to irritants. Dermatitis on the hands or feet may, in young adults often without a history of eczema, appear as an irritant vesicular eruption (pomphylox) which may recur especially in warm weather. An unusual distribution of a rash or an unusual shape of an eruption suggests a dermatitic aetiology (Fig. 2).

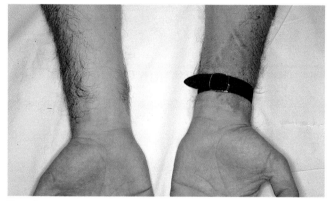

Fig. 2 **Dermatitis.** Reaction to nickel.

Eczema (as defined above) often comprises lichenified scaling areas localized to the antecubital and popliteal fossae, neck, or wrists.

Varicose eczema (Fig. 3) is distal lower leg inflammation, often with brownish discolouration which develops in patients with impaired venous return. Ulceration and secondary infection may follow. Seborrhoeic dermatitis (Fig. 4) is found in those with a greasy skin and consists of scaling of the skin or scalp, forehead, and nasolabial folds. In neonates there may be a thick yellowish crusted lesion on the scalp—'cradle cap'.

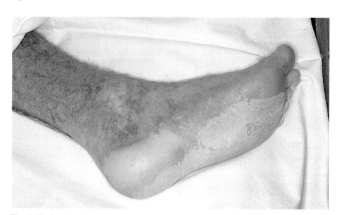

Fig. 3 **Varicose eczema.**

Dermatitis herpetiformis

There is an abrupt appearance of small patches of intensely itchy vesicles on an erythematous base, usually on extensor surfaces. They may be a marker of underlying gluten-sensitive enteropathy (coeliac disease).

Discoid lupus erythematosus

Discoid lupus gives rise to erythematous scaly disc-like eruptions which usually involve the face but occasionally affect the limbs or trunk.

Drug eruptions

Drug eruptions probably occur in about 2% of all treatment courses. Toxic erythema is the commonest manifestation followed by urticarial eruptions.

In general scarlet fever-like, rubella-like or measles-like (morbilliform) drug eruptions usually occur during or up to about

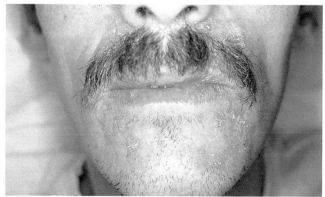

Fig. 4 **Seborrhoeic dermatitis.**

2 weeks after drug administration. There may be associated mild fever, itching, and possibly eosinophilia in the blood count. Fixed drug eruptions occur at the same site(s) each time the provoking drug is taken (commonly the cause is over the counter phenolphthalein-containing laxatives). Some drugs may precipitate photosensitivity which manifests predominantly in areas exposed to strong light.

Table 1 details some common drug eruption patterns and some possible causes. Drug eruptions usually occur abruptly, tend to be symmetrical, do not evolve from above downwards, and only occasionally stain (staining is a residual non-blanching discolouration left after the initial rash has gone: measles characteristically stains).

Fifth disease (erythema infectiosum)

Marked erythema of the cheeks (Fig. 5) gives a 'slapped cheek' appearance which may be followed by sparse macular lesions on the limbs and trunk. Typically for the next few months the cheeks become reddened again if exposed to wind or sunlight. It is caused by parvovirus infection.

Ehlers–Danlos syndrome

Velvety hyperelastic skin (with poor wound healing) and joint subluxation gives those affected an 'India-rubber man' capability (Fig. 6).

Icthyosis

Icthyosis is a fish-like scaley skin which may be an inherited condition, but if it develops in an adult it may be a marker of internal malignancy.

Infestations

Fleas may cause wheals. Lice, apart from irritation, may cause small red papular lesions, perhaps with a tiny central blood clot. Occasionally urticaria, lichenification or discolouration of the skin results from chronic infestations. Without doubt the best way to look for lice (or their eggs—nits—which are attached to hairs) is to use an ophthalmoscope. But be careful that your hair does not touch the patient's hair! Scabies causes itching with burrows usually visible in interdigital webs (Fig. 7), flexor surfaces of wrist and elbows, or breasts and genitalia.

Leprosy

In *lepromatous* leprosy there is a weak immune response and there are multiple symmetrically situated macules, nodules or plaques without impaired sensation. In *tuberculoid* leprosy there is a strong immune response in the skin and nerves leading to the development of a few raised plaques, which may be depigmented with reduced sensation. A major clue would be the presence of thickened nerves in the locality. Such lesions, unless unusually numerous, are often asymmetrical.

Systemic illness (with or without erythema nodosum) occurs when the immune status of the patient changes.

Table 1 **Eruptions seen with some commonly prescribed drugs**

Drug	Eruption
Antibiotics	Toxic erythema, urticaria, fixed drug eruption, erythema multiforme
Beta-blockers	Psoriaform, Raynaud's phenomenon
Corticosteroids	Hirsutism, acne, striae, atrophy
Non-steroidal anti-inflammatories	Toxic erythema, erythroderma, toxic epidermal necrolysis
Oral contraceptive	Chloasma, alopecia, acne, candidiasis
Phenothiazines	Photosensitivity, pigmentation
Thiazides	Toxic erythema, photosensitivity, lichenoid, vasculitis

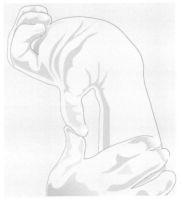
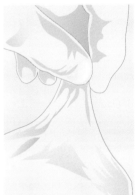

Fig. 6 **Ehlers–Danlos syndrome.**

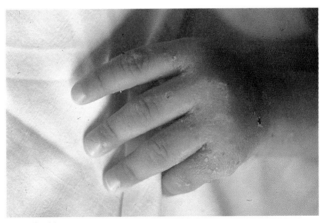

Fig. 7 **Scabies.**

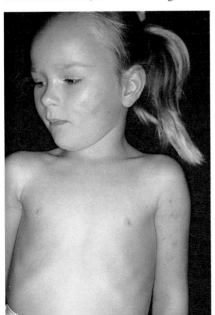

Fig. 5 **Fifth disease.**

Symmetrical lesions in systemically well patients (I)

- Symmetrical skin lesions often reflect generalized skin or systemic illness.
- The terms 'dermatitis' and 'eczema' are similar but tend to be used in differing contexts.
- Drug eruptions occur in about 2% of treatment courses.
- An ophthalmoscope is a useful and powerful magnifying device for skin examination.

SYMMETRICAL LESIONS IN SYSTEMICALLY WELL PATIENTS (II)

Lichen planus

Lichen planus is a recurring itchy papular rash occurring in adults which tends to involve the wrists and ankles, and to be symmetrical with violaceous papules which are often of rectangular or parallelogram shape. Linear lesions occur after scratching. Fine white lace-like patterns on the surface of the papules (Wickham's striae) are a useful diagnostic feature. Oral lesions are present in about 50% of those affected.

Miliaria

Small, clear, superficial vesicles develop on skin which often has been recently damaged by sunburn. They are also found in patients, particularly children, with high fevers. Miliaria rubra 'prickly heat' occurs in hot humid conditions—sweat bursts out of blocked ducts and causes irritation— hence the prickling.

Neurofibromatosis

Neurofibromatosis (Fig. 1) is usually an inherited condition often with associated cafe-au-lait spots (large brownish macules), axillary freckles and the neurofibromas emanating from nerves.

Pityriasis rosea

Pityriasis rosea is an itchy rash in which the usually eliptical lesions have a tendency to follow skin cleavage lines. Often there is an initial larger 'herald' lesion (Fig. 2).

Pretibial myxoedema

Pretibial myxoedema is reddish swellings on the anterior shin. Despite the name it occurs in thyrotoxicosis.

Psoriasis

Psoriasis is characterized by well-defined thickened salmon-pink skin plaques with superficial 'silver' scaling; plaques may be found anywhere but characteristically occur on extensor surfaces (Fig. 3). The 'rule of elbow' states that a rash affecting the flexor surface of the elbow is likely to be eczema, but a rash affecting the extensor surface is likely to be psoriasis. Guttate psoriasis resembles scattered reddish raindrops on the skin: it is often associated with an infection elsewhere (usually a throat infection in children). Psoriasis has a tendency to occur in surgical scars or other areas of skin trauma. Nail involvement may be a feature (see later).

Raynaud's phenomenon

Vascular spasm, often lasting for minutes or hours, and often caused by exposure to cold, causes pallor followed by cyanosis and, when the vascular spasm remits, a warm red flush (Fig. 4). If vasoconstriction is intense there is numbness, discomfort or pain. Causes include scleroderma, vascular disease, and connective tissue disorders.

Rubella (German measles)

Rubella can often be confused with measles but is very distinct in certain characteristics (Table 1). About 50% of patients with rubella (Fig. 5) do not have a rash and patients are usually well (patients with measles feel unwell). The rash consists of discrete delicate pink macules (unlike the coarse blotchy rash of measles). The rash starts on the face and spreads from above downwards: staining is very unusual.

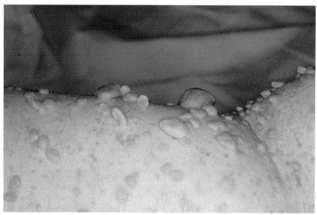

Fig. 1 **Neurofibromatosis.**

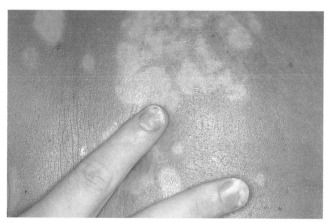

Fig. 3 **Psoriasis.**

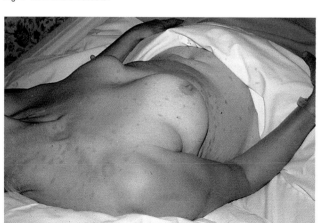

Fig. 2 **Pityriasis rosea.**

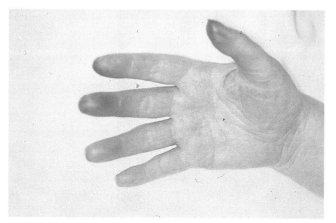

Fig. 4 **Raynaud's phenomenon.**

Table 1 **Differentiation between rubella and measles**

Rubella	Measles
Often well	'Always' unwell
No rash in 50%	'Always' a rash
Fine delicate rash	Blotchy coarse rash
Rash spreads from above downwards	Rash spreads from above downwards
Rash uniform	Rash non-uniform; early rash on face may have stained when the rash on the legs is still blanching
No Koplik's spots	Koplick's spots during prodromal illness
Minimal prodromal illness	3–4 days of fever before the rash
No staining	Characteristically stains

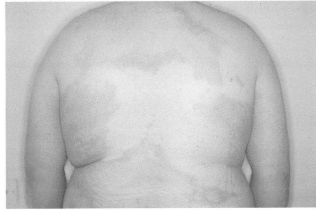

Fig. 7 **Wheal formation in urticaria.**

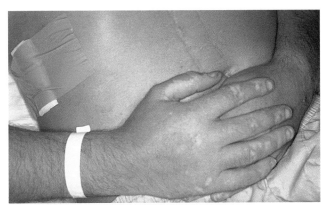

Fig. 8 **Vitiligo.**

Scleroderma

There is atrophy and tightening of face and hand skin, perhaps associated with patchy hypo- or hyperpigmentation. Scleroderma may occur in a localized form, morphoea, in which the skin is fibrotic.

Tuberous sclerosis (epiloia)

Characteristic facial angiofibromas are found, usually on the cheeks (Fig. 6). Associated epilepsy and mental retardation are common.

Urticaria

With urticaria there may be:

- intermittent transitory swelling
- wheal formations (Fig. 7)
- itching
- dermatographia (wheal development sufficient to allow large letters to be written on the skin)
- systemic illness ('serum sickness' or anaphylaxis).

Although the situation of lesions at any one time may not be symmetrical, overall it is usually obvious that, on average, the lesions occur in a symmetrical distribution.

Vitiligo

Vitiligo comprises hypopigmented areas which are often sharply demarcated from surrounding normal skin (Fig. 8). There is an association with various immune disorders including hypoadrenalism, pernicious anaemia and thyroid dysfunction.

Xanthomas / Xanthelasma

Xanthomas are lipid deposits in the skin and are often found over bony prominences or over tendons. Xanthelasma are yellowish deposits of lipid material which are usually found at the medial end of the eyelids. They may be idiopathic or caused by hyperlipidaemia.

> **Symmetrical lesions in systemically well patients (II)**
>
> - Wickham's striae are a useful diagnostic feature of lichen planus.
> - A rash on the point of the elbow is likely to be psoriasis, while one on the flexor surface on the elbow is likely to be eczema.
> - Pityriasis rosea is often preceded by a larger 'herald' lesion.

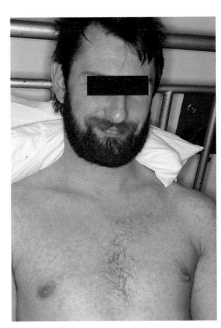

Fig. 5 **Rubella.**

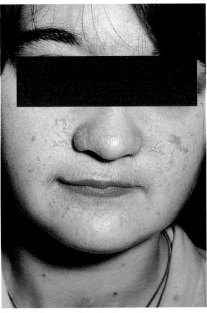

Fig. 6 **Tuberous sclerosis (epiloia).**

ASYMMETRICAL LESIONS IN SYSTEMICALLY WELL PATIENTS

Asymmetry of lesions in well patients makes systemic illness unlikely.

Boils (furuncles)
Boils are painful, reddened and hot areas of cutaneous inflammation and abscess formation, often initially based in hair follicles.

Cutaneous leishmaniasis
There are single or multiple, sharply demarcated papules which may ulcerate. They are usually found on parts of the body, particularly the face, at the site of the causative sandfly (Phlebotomus) bites. Suspect cutaneous leishmaniasis in patients returned from tropical or subtropical areas who have cutaneous lesions which fail to heal.

Dermatitis artefacta
Dermatitis artefacta lesions tend to be linear and gouged and are thus bizarre in appearance and distribution.

Drug tracks
Drug tracks are caused by injection of contaminated or caustic material by intravenous drug abusers. Patients who abuse drugs may have associated illness and infections but 'pure' drug abuse usually does not cause illness.

Fungal infections
Suspect fungal infections in any asymmetrical, well-defined, roundish, scaly inflamed area, especially if there are small vesicles or pustules at the perimeter of the area.

Tinea. There are several forms of Tinea 'ringworm'. *Tinea barbae* affects the beard area, *tinea capitis* the scalp, *tinea corporis* the body, *tinea cruris* the groin area (Fig. 1), *tinea pedis* the feet (athlete's foot) and *tinea unguium* the nails. *Tinea versicolour* (also known as *Pityriasis versicolour*) is a curious condition which, in caucasians, causes 'pale raindrop' areas in areas of suntanned skin but when the skin is pale the raindrops are darker than the surrounding skin—hence the term versicolour. In the black-skinned, the pale raindrops are very pale (Fig. 2).

Candida. Candida usually causes well-demarcated reddened patches of skin possibly with small pustules at the periphery. The white patches of candida characteristic of intraoral candida are not often seen on the skin. Candida usually involves damp areas where the skin comes into contact with opposing skin—armpits, beneath pendulous breasts, the umbilicus, and within the gluteal folds in nappy rashes (Fig. 3).

In contrast to candida nappy rash, ammoniacal or child neglect nappy rash may spare the flexures.

Herpes simplex
Clusters of vesicles erupt, typically on the lips or thereabouts 'cold sores' (Fig. 4) or on the genitals. There may be a brief prodrome of pain or tingling affecting the area to be involved. Herpes simplex complicating eczema, gives rise to eczema herpeticum (Fig. 5), a profuse widespread herpetic eruption. Herpetic whitlows give an appearance suggestive of bacterial boils (Fig. 6), but result from inoculation of the herpes virus into the skin of the hands: they are thus usually an occupational

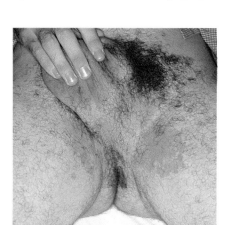
Fig. 1 **Tinea curis.**

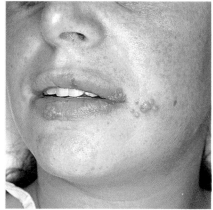
Fig. 4 **Herpes simplex 'cold sores'.**

Fig. 2 **Tinea versicolour.**

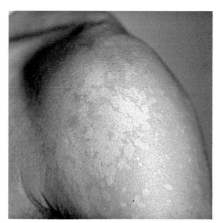
Fig. 5 **Eczema herpeticum.**

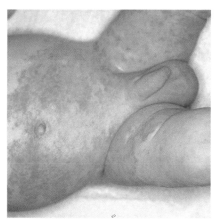
Fig. 3 **Nappy rash caused by candida.**

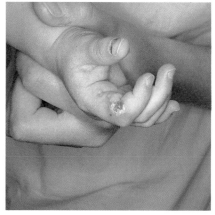
Fig. 6 **Herpetic whitlows.**

hazard for those who put their hands into patients' mouths.

Impetigo

Staphylococcal infections often produce localized lesions and in impetigo produce blisters. Streptococcal infections often spread and in impetigo cause golden yellow crusts.

Kaposi's sarcoma

In the type of Kaposi's sarcoma in Africa that is unrelated to AIDS there are multiple vascular tumours, often on the feet with plaques and nodules which may ulcerate. AIDS-related Kaposi's sarcoma has a different appearance, often with multiple brownish macules or papules anywhere on the body (Fig. 7). On presentation most patients will be well but may develop AIDS-related opportunistic infections subsequently.

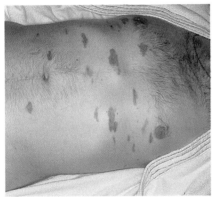

Fig. 7 **Kaposi's sarcoma.**

Keloid scarring

Keloids are the result of over-exuberant skin healing in areas of trauma. Operation scars or burns are often affected. There is swollen, non-tender, non-erythematous skin thickening.

Larva migrans and larva currens

Larva migrans is caused by the larvae of dog hookworm which penetrate human skin, usually of the feet. They fail to enter veins or lymphatics and therefore desperately meander subcutaneously until they die. The resulting urticarial rash is intensely itchy. Larva currens are the larvae of *Strongyloides stercoralis* which move more quickly. Strongyloides larvae can complete their life cycle repeatedly in humans and there may be a history of many years of transient urticarial rashes on any part of the body.

Lyme disease

Lyme disease is initiated by the bite of a tick which inoculates *Borrelia bergdorferi* into the body. There may be one or more circular or oval, reddish, macular or papular lesions which progressively expand, sometimes to a very large size (about 50 cm is possible) with central clearing. Lesions may be warm but are often painless.

Malignant melanoma

Any darkish skin lesion should be assessed by an expert if it has appeared recently or if there is spontaneous bleeding, enlargement, or satellite lesions around the periphery of the main lesion. Malignant melanomas can occur anywhere on the body.

Mulluscum contagiosum

Isolated or multiple smooth waxy umbilicated papules develop, often with a central depression on top. They are caused by a 'pox' virus and in AIDS are often profuse with multiple small papules on the face and trunk.

Rodent ulcer (basal cell carcinoma)

These are usually isolated nodular, ulcerated, or crusted lesions which persist and slowly enlarge. They are often found around the eye and nose.

Sarcoidosis

Chronic sarcoidosis may cause reddish-blue plaques, papules or nodules.

Shingles

After a prodromal period of tingling or pain, a dense, single, often confluent, crop of vesicles occurs in a dermatome pattern, either affecting single or contiguous dermatomes with a midline cut-off. Occasionally chickenpoxes occur outwith the affected dermatome(s). Ophthalmic shingles (Fig. 8) affect the first division of the trigeminal nerve. Intraocular structures may also be involved, particularly if the side of the tip of the end of the nose is involved (nasociliary nerve involvement).

Squamous cell carcinoma

Initially there is an isolated red papule which becomes nodular, perhaps with a warty surface and eventual ulceration.

Cutaneous tuberculosis (lupus vulgaris)

Brownish red papular lesions or plaques slowly develop and may later ulcerate or scar over.

Venous leg ulcers

Venous leg ulcers are almost invariably found only around the ankle. They are hyperpigmented (caused by continued minor leaking of blood from stressed blood vessels) and have associated white areas caused by scarring. They may show signs of secondary infection. Leg ulcers are often itchy, yet less painful than appearances would suggest (see Fig. 3, p. 116).

Warts

There are five main types of wart. Verruca vulgaris (the common wart) often found on the hands, verruca plana (plantar warts) often found on the face or knees, verruca plantaris (large, occasionally painful, plaques on the soles), filiform warts (horny lesions mostly found on the face), and condylomata acuminata (genital warts).

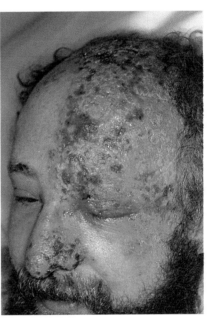

Fig. 8 **Ophthalmic shingles.**

Asymmetrical lesions in systemically well patients

- Asymmetry of lesions in systemically well patients makes systemic illness unlikely.
- Candida nappy rash often involves the skin flexures.
- A travel history must be taken if cutaneous leischmaniasis is a possibility.
- A history of a tick bite may be an important clue for a diagnosis of Lyme disease.

LESIONS IN SYSTEMICALLY UNWELL PATIENTS (I)

Systemically unwell patients tend to have multisystem processes which involve the skin and, apart from a detailed knowledge of the individual processes, some useful clues can be obtained by considering whether or not there are associated oral lesions, itchy lesions or purpuric lesions. Patients may be feverish or have constitutional symptoms.

SYMMETRICAL LESIONS

Acanthosis nigricans

Acanthosis nigricans (Fig. 1) is symmetrical pigmentation and velvet-like overgrowth of skin most marked on the sides, neck and flexures. It is often a marker of internal malignancy, and patients may have symptoms of the underlying disease.

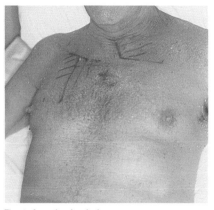

Fig. 1 **Acanthosis nigricans.** This caucasian man developed generalized pigmentation associated with a carcinoma of the lung.

Behçet's syndrome

Behçet's syndrome is a disease of uncertain causation which produces recurrent orogenital ulceration.

Chickenpox

In chickenpox there are between one and five crops of vesicles occurring over about 1 week or less. Intraoral poxes rupture to leave shallow ulcers (Fig. 2). The eruption commences on the face and works downwards, remaining in a centripetal distribution (Fig. 3).

Dermatomyositis

Dermatomyositis is characterized by purplish discolouration, resembling 'focal sunburn', of the face or eyelids, perhaps with purplish streaks on the dorsum of the fingers. There may be tenderness and weakness of the muscles.

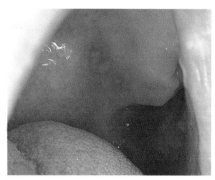

Fig. 2 **Chickenpox showing intraoral lesions.**

Endocarditis

There may be clubbing, splinter haemorrhages, Osler's nodes (bruise-like swellings on the finger tips), Janeway lesions (similar to Osler's nodes but on the feet), generalized pigmentation or purpura.

Enterovirus or adenovirus infections

These may give rise to rashes of non-diagnostic appearance—mostly rubella-like. Vesicles can occur in some infections; hand, foot, and mouth disease (with vesicles on the appropriate sites) is caused by a Coxsackie A virus infection for example.

Erythema multiforme

Erythema multiforme (Fig. 4) is a reaction pattern to certain infections or drugs. There is a multiformed erythema but the label demands the presence of concentric rings, iris or 'target lesions', sometimes with a central vesicle or purpuric lesion. If severe, there is additional involvement of mucous membranes of eyes, mouth and genitalia—the Stevens–Johnson syndrome.

Erythema nodosum

Erythema nodosum is characterized by spontaneously occurring painful reddish nodular bruise-like lesions commonly occurring on the shins as a reaction pattern to various stimuli (Fig. 5). Depending on the extent of the reaction, some patients are systemically unwell but others merely have focal symptoms relating to the

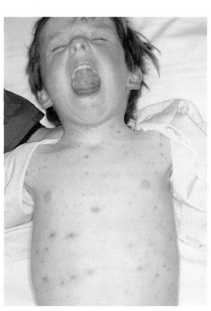

Fig. 3 **The centripetal rash of chickenpox.**

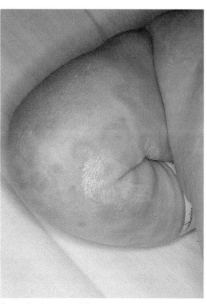

Fig. 4 **Erythema multiforme.**

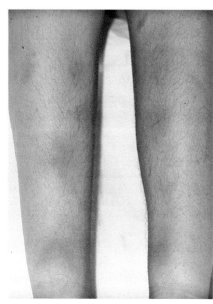

Fig. 5 **Erythema nodosum.**

lesions. The common British causes are streptococcal infection, sarcoidosis and tuberculosis.

Erysipelas

Erysipelas is a streptococcal infection of the skin. There is an acute onset of spreading erythema with well-defined borders associated with tissue swelling and local heat (Fig. 6). Erysipelas, unlike shingles, is not confined by dermatome borders. Cellulitis is a much deeper infection and usually has less well-defined borders. Facial erysipelas tends to be symmetrical but elsewhere tends to be asymmetrical.

Exfoliative dermatitis

In exfoliative dermatitis there is generalized erythema, scaling and desquamation.

Glandular fever

In glandular fever there may be a purplish maculopapular eruption (Fig. 7)—usually in patients with other manifestations of glandular fever. Nearly all patients with glandular fever who are given ampicillin (or its derivatives) develop a rash which represents only a transient hypersensitivity to ampicillin.

Gonococcal septicaemia

In gonococcal septicaemia, pustules develop which, unlike staphylococcal spots, often have a bright red halo. They typically appear on the fingers (Fig. 8).

Henoch–Schönlein purpura

Henoch–Schönlein purpura (Fig. 9) is characterized by a maculopapular purpuric eruption usually on the buttocks and extensor surfaces of the limbs. Arthritis, abdominal pains (caused by purpura in the gut) and joint pains (caused by purpura and bleeding into the joint) may be associated. It is a vasculitic reaction, usually to streptococcal infection.

Kawasaki's syndrome

After 1–3 weeks of fever, children (usually those under the age of five) develop conjunctival infection, reddened lips and tongue, lymph node enlargement and an erythematous maculopapular rash (Fig. 10). Non-pitting oedema of hands and feet is diagnostically suggestive. Characteristically the skin subsequently desquamates around the nail folds.

Measles

After a prodromal feverish period of about 3 days (during which Koplik's spots are apparent) the rash develops which comprises erythematous dusky macules and

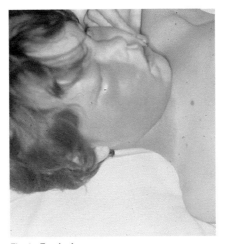

Fig. 6 **Erysipelas.**

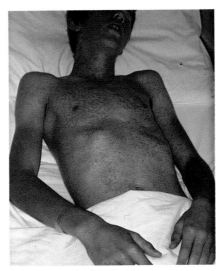

Fig. 7 **Rash in glandular fever.**

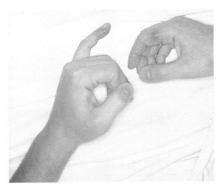

Fig. 8 **Gonococcal septicaemia.**

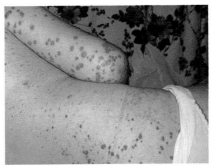

Fig. 9 **Henoch–Schönlein purpura.**

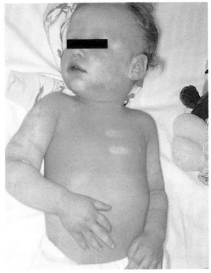

Fig. 10 **Kawasaki's syndrome.**

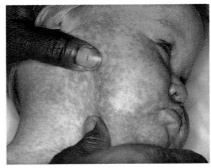

Fig. 11 **Staining in measles.**

papules which may coalesce to form blotches. The rash initially appears behind the ears, on the face and then spreads downwards. After 2 or 3 days the erythematous areas of the skin stain (again from above downwards) leaving a brownish discolouration (Fig. 11). Thus measles may be associated with a facial rash which has stained (non-blanching), but also with an erythematous (blanching) rash on the lower limbs, a sign which does not occur with drug rashes.

Lesions in systemically unwell patients (I)

- Systemically unwell patients tend to have multi-system processes which involve the skin.
- Chickenpox starts on the face and spreads downwards.
- Erythema multiforme is a reaction pattern, often caused by mycoplasma or herpes simplex infection.
- Measles rashes characteristically stain.

LESIONS IN SYSTEMICALLY UNWELL PATIENTS (II)

SYMMETRICAL LESIONS (cont.)

Meningococcal septicaemia
In meningococcal septicaemia there may be purpura or larger ecchymotic areas (Fig. 1). Initially the rash can be a non-specific erythematous rash.

Pemphigus vulgaris
In pemphigus vulgaris, crops of blisters appear in the mouth or on the skin of limbs and trunk. Lesions particularly occur on areas of traumatized skin, and superficial skin can be slid over deeper layers by lateral traction with a finger so that a blister develops at the site of traction (Nikolski's sign positive).

Reiter's syndrome
After an attack of non-specific urethritis or dysentery, a triad of urethritis, conjunctivitis and arthritis develops. This is known as Reiter's syndrome. Possible skin lesions include shallow penile erosions with a circular outline (circinate balanitis) and a pustular hyperkeratosis on the soles (keratodermia blenorrhagica).

Roseola infanticum
(exanthema subitum, sixth disease)
After 3–5 days of high fever in young children, a rubella-like rash erupts as the fever falls.

Scarlet fever
Shortly after a sore throat (streptococcal) there is a deep facial flush with circumoral pallor (Fig. 2). This is characteristic of scarlet fever. The rash, a lobster red erythema, with tiny red points superimposed (a puncate erythema), appears on the neck and trunk. As the rash fades, desquamation usually occurs. The tongue 'furs-up', then 'defurs' giving a 'white then red' strawberry-tongue appearance (Fig. 3). Pastia's sign may also be evident—areas of small haemorrhages in the skin folds, particularly of the elbow (Fig. 4).

Still's disease
(juvenile rheumatoid arthritis)
In association with high fever a characteristically flitting evanescent non-itchy rash occurs, often surrounded by zones of pallor.

Syphilis
Secondary syphilis may cause a non-irritant copper-coloured rash (Fig. 5), perhaps associated with malaise or fever.

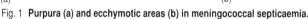

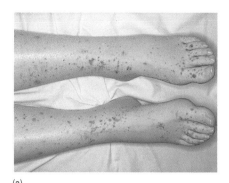

(a)

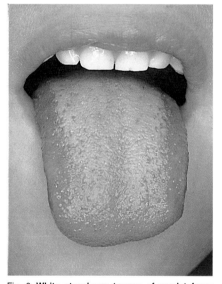

(b)

Fig. 1 **Purpura (a) and ecchymotic areas (b) in meningococcal septicaemia.**

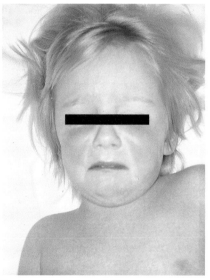

Fig. 2 **Facial flush in scarlet fever.**

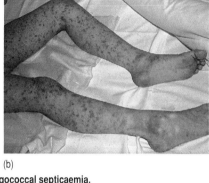

Fig. 3 **White strawberry tongue of scarlet fever.** This soon turned to red strawberry tongue.

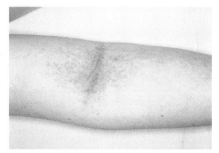

Fig. 4 **Pastia's sign in scarlet fever.**

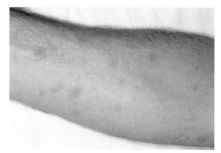

Fig. 5 **Rash of secondary syphilis.**

Systemic lupus erythematosus (SLE)
Skin rashes occur in about 85% of patients and include the classical butterfly rash across the cheeks (Fig. 6). Raynaud's phenomenon may occur. Photosensitivity may be apparent and scarring alopecia may occur; telangiectasia are also common.

Toxic epidermal necrolysis
Toxic epidermal necrolysis is usually caused by drug reactions or infection with staphylococci that produce a toxin causing

skin layers to split, allowing the skin to blister and slough and to slide and settle elsewhere. It may produce significant skin deformities.

Typhoid and paratyphoid fevers
In typhoid, rose-coloured spots may be found after careful inspection (they are easily missed, especially in dark-skinned patients) (Fig. 7). They are non-itchy macules which are usually found on the trunk.

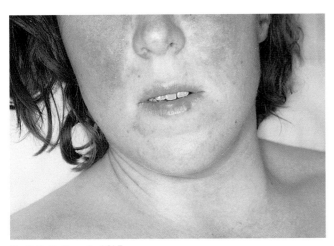

Fig. 6 **Butterfly rash of SLE.**

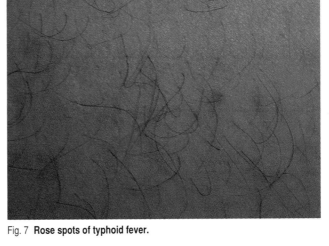

Fig. 7 **Rose spots of typhoid fever.**

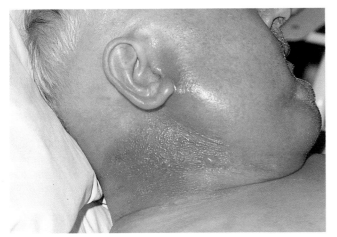

Fig. 8 **Anthrax.**

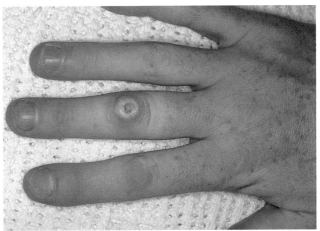

Fig. 9 **Orf.**

Vasculitis

Cutaneous vasculitis may present with palpable lesions, usually on the legs, with punched-out (well-demarcated) ulcers or haemorrhagic areas.

ASYMMETRICAL LESIONS

Erythema marginatum

Erythema marginatum is a rapidly spreading ring-like eruption, occasionally with a raised margin (resembling defibrillator burns). If of classical appearance, it is well nigh diagnostic of rheumatic fever.

Gangrene

In gangrene areas of skin and tissue death are caused by failure of the blood supply. 'Simple' tissue death causes a blackish discolouration but gangrene associated with *Clostridium perfringens* infection may result in wet gangrene with swelling and palpable crepitations on pressure over affected areas with a fingertip.

Pyoderma gangrenosum

Pyoderma gangrenosum is a necrotic ulceration of the skin, often with a

violaceous rim, which is idiopathic in about 50% of patients but recognized associations includes inflammatory bowel disease, blood disorders and rheumatoid arthritis.

OCCUPATIONAL SKIN LESIONS

Anthrax

Anthrax is a disease of animal hide and product handlers. A malignant pustule (which is neither malignant nor a pustule) develops as a tiny papule crowned by a vesicle. The lesion enlarges and becomes surrounded by a ring of vesicles (Fig. 8) and the central area ulcerates and scars. Typically, the lesion is solitary, not painful and is usually found on the forearms, head or neck.

Erysipelothrix rhusiopathiae

A disease of handlers of dead animal tissue or those bitten by animals, particularly dogs. Traumatic inoculation of the organism, usually into a finger, produces purplish-red inflammation.

Orf

Orf (Fig. 9) is a disease of those who come into contact with sheep or goats. An irritating maculopapular lesion progresses to a multiloculated vesicle which evolves into a ragged superficial ulcer.

Lesions in systemically unwell patients (II)

- Meningococcal septicaemia may feature purpura or a larger ecchymotic rash.
- Scarlet fever is characterized in the initial stages by a sore throat followed by a deep facial flush with circumoral pallor.
- Systemic lupus erythematosus (SLE) commonly produces a butterfly rash across the cheeks and photosensitivity.
- Anthrax, erysipelothrix and orf are occupation related.

OTHER SKIN LESIONS

GENERALIZED PRURITUS (ITCHINESS)

The causes of a *generalized* itchy skin include obstructive pattern jaundice, hyperthyroidism, drug reactions, uraemia and haematological malignancies. Senile pruritus is a diagnosis of exclusion as is psychogenic pruritus. Causes of *focal* itching include scabies, lice (pediculosis), insect bites, urticaria, dermatitis/eczema, fungal infection, lichen planus, miliaria and dermatitis herpetiformis.

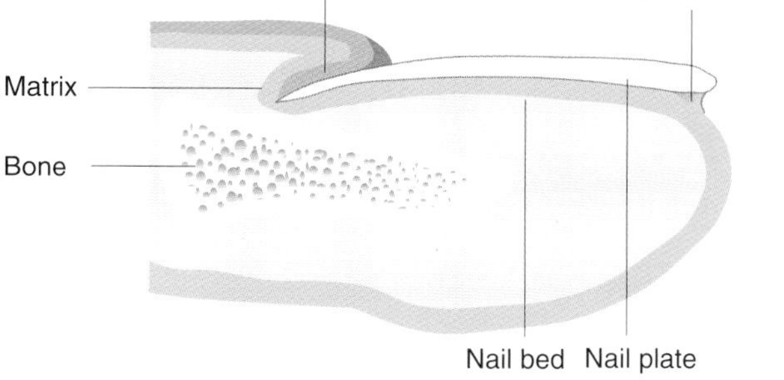

THE NAILS AND HAIR

The anatomy of the fingertip and nail is shown in Figure 1. Findings on general examination of the nails have been previously detailed on page 7.

Any disease that affects the skin will affect nail or hair growth in some way.

The nails

Systemic illness or diffuse skin diseases may cause transverse whitish areas of abnormal nail growth (Beau's lines). As the average life of a fingernail is about 6 months various illnesses can be dated.

Brittle nails may be caused by exposure to detergents, metabolic deficiency states (notably iron deficiency and thyroid dysfunction), by fungal infection or ischaemia. Koilonychia (spoon shaped indentation of the nail plate) occurs in iron deficiency anaemia and occasionally in lichen planus. Telangiectasia (dilatation of small blood vessels) affecting the nail fold may be found in connective tissue disorders. Pitting of the nailbed is notably found in psoriasis but is not specific to this condition.

The hair

Like skin lesions, the causes of hair loss can be divided into those which cause symmetrical loss (Fig. 2) and those which cause asymmetrical loss.

Balding is normal in the male and may occasionally occur in older women.

Hormonal disorders that slow down normal hair growth (such that the hair is less vigorous and may fall out) include hypothyroidism, hypopituitarism, and hypoadrenal states. Cytotoxic drugs may slow down hair growth; this slowing is usually abrupt and hair loss may start shortly after commencement of cytotoxic therapy. Severe systemic illness such as septicaemia may have a similar effect, as may exfoliative dermatitis.

Diffuse alopecia is a disease of uncertain aetiology (except when caused by syphilis) which on occasion may cause loss of all body hair—alopecia totalis.

Proximal nail fold and cuticle   Hyponychium

Matrix

Bone

Nail bed Nail plate

Fig. 1 **Anatomy of the fingertip.**

Causes of asymmetrical hair loss

Alopecia areata is not uncommon and usually presents with well-defined bald patches on the scalp. Exclamation mark hairs (which progressively thin as the scalp is approached) are characteristic. Occasionally the eyebrows and beard area can be affected.

Fungal infections including tinea (p. 120) may cause areas of reduced hair growth.

Localized hair loss can also be associated with trauma, previous shingles, burns, radiation, or localized patches of scleroderma (morphoea).

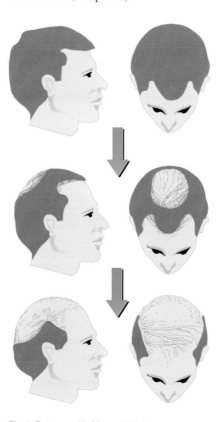

Fig. 2 **Patterns of baldness.** Hair loss can progress from bitemporal recession to severe hair loss.

Excess hair growth

Hypertrichosis (excessive hair growth of a non-male pattern) may be normal, or at least have no obvious cause. Hirsutism, in contrast, is growth of male pattern hair in a female (notably around the nipple and with the pubic hair extending upwards, pointing to the umbilicus). It may be a normal finding or may be associated with polycystic ovary disease. Some patients with hirsutism have increased sensitivity to circulating androgens. The finding of other endocrine related abnormalities (male pattern baldness, an enlarged clitoris, or a deep voice) always require further investigation.

Hypertrichosis may occur in:

- areas treated with topical steroids
- spina bifida occulta
- generalized malnutrition
- anorexia nervosa
- administration of certain drugs (e.g. phenytoin or minoxidil).

Hirsutism may occur in:

- acromegaly
- adrenal dysfunction
- polycystic ovary disease
- virilizing tumours
- exogenous androgens
- exogenous progestogens.

Other skin lesions

- Any disease that affects the skin will affect nail or hair growth.
- The average life of a fingernail is six months.
- A drug history is essential in patients with hair loss.
- Exclamation mark hairs are found in alopecia areata.

SPECIAL TOPICS

AGGRESSIVE OR POTENTIALLY VIOLENT PATIENTS

Violence is a problem in society, and doctors and their nursing colleagues are very much soft targets. They have to cope with the potentially violent behaviour without sanctions to employ if patients disregard the 'rules'.

The advice given here concerns interviews with patients in which violence is only a possibility and not a probability. Patients whose thought processes are deranged by toxic confusional states (including alcoholic intoxication) or any mental illness are not included in this account. With such patients logical argument is usually non-productive.

Most violent episodes are predictable, as those who do not deal with the realities of clinical medicine usually comment, although always in retrospect. If violence can be predicted the police are only too willing to show a presence, without taking any action, which often avoids the development of problems.

The interview with potentially violent patients (PVPs) is in essence a test of personality interaction. To achieve a moderately satisfactory outcome with PVPs demands flexibility. The exhibition of a dogmatic or authoritarian personality by doctors tends to be counterproductive.

Several ploys mentioned below contain elements of gamesmanship but these may be legitimate providing that the doctor is sincere in his ultimate wish to help the patient (Fig. 1).

THE INTERVIEW SITUATION

Prior to any interview always try to obtain background information. Has the patient recently been involved in arguments with others, has he been kept waiting for what he considers to be too long (a pre-emptive apology is often useful), or has he been drinking? Finally consider if an interview is appropriate for immediate management.

Always let others and the patient know where the interview is to be held, what you will be doing, and how long it should take. Always remain within 'shouting contact' or, if circumstances suggest, within visual contact. Potential witnesses are a deterrent for 'experienced PVPs'.

It is advantageous if the interview room used is restfully furnished. The furniture should be arranged so that a quick escape could be made with the doctor nearer the door with a desk between him and the patient.

A low comfortable armchair should be available so the PVP can be invited to sit in

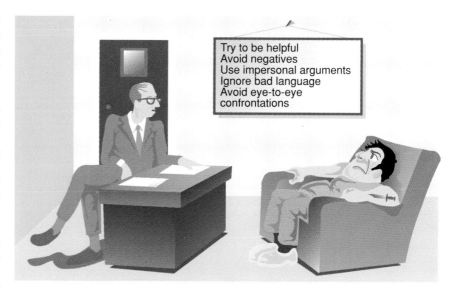

Fig. 1 **Hints on dealing with potentially violent patients in interview.**

Try to be helpful
Avoid negatives
Use impersonal arguments
Ignore bad language
Avoid eye-to-eye confrontations

the most comfortable chair in the room. The armchair should be comfortable and low because it is well nigh impossible to be aggressive whilst sitting in a low armchair.

With some PVPs listening is essential. Initially all that may be required is for the PVP to be allowed to express himself adequately and communicate his frustrations. Often doctors are able to 'run rings' round PVPs on an intellectual level but attempts to do this are likely to precipitate violence, especially if the PVP could run you around a boxing ring on a physical level!

Wearing a white coat conveys medical authority and this is an advantage, but it might also convey an establishment status.

It may be relevant to have another person in the room with you when interviewing a PVP. It is also recommended that a reason is always given to the PVP before the start of the interview. 'I hope that you do not mind if X, who is a Y, sits in because he wishes to gain experience of the medical problems of Z condition'.

CONDUCTING THE INTERVIEW (Table 1)

Open the interview with the question 'What can I do for you?'. PVPs usually need an excuse to express violence and this means trapping the doctor into a confrontation (this, I suspect, is why PVPs often undertake a complex rambling explanation, which they no doubt think is self-evidently logical, leading up to a statement of demand). Remarking 'That's all very well but what can I do for you?'

often elicits a *request* rather than a statement of *demand* and cuts short much irrelevant preamble. Often the patient's thoughts are focused by this simple question and the answer often provides distinct clarifications for both parties.

If the patient insists on continuing with his impossible demands you can diffuse by confusion: 'I'm afraid Mr X (or the current Minister of Health) would not allow me to do that' immediately begs the question 'Who is Mr X?' and once the flow of the PVP's argument is interrupted the flow can be taken over.

Have pre-arranged signs available by which you can communicate with staff (who should keep a discrete continual watch) outside the interview room. Arrange signals, such as a touch of the left ear, as an indication for a pacifying interruption: 'Would you like a cup of tea doctor?' which then allows the pressurized doctor to intercede on behalf of the PVP: 'If I'm having one then Mr PVP should have one too'. 'Do you take milk and sugar? How many?'. Few patients can carry on an aggressive stance through this pacifying onslaught.

Speak with a quiet voice and avoid eye-to-eye confrontations. Avoid aligning yourself with anything that the PVP might perceive as 'dogmatic establishment views'.

After making forthright statements ask 'Is that fair?' rather than giving the PVP no chance to put his point of view.

Try to assert a quiet dominance. Communicate and if possible show laboratory results or preferably X-rays to the patient.

Table 1 **Useful responses to provocative statements.** It is possible to use some of the responses below to 'fob off' patients with genuine grievances. *Resist this temptation.*

'Dr X [your colleague] is a fool.'

'Yes, but let's get back to the present problem.' (It is easy to use 'yes' as an acknowledgement of communication receipt rather than signifying agreement.)

'My methadone [or similar] has been stolen, lost, drunk by the dog.'

The number of explanations I have heard could fill several books. If you doubt the explanation and if you do not wish to give a repeat prescription: 'I'm sorry. What do you think the Home Office would do if they knew I had issued two prescriptions for the same patient covering the same period of time?'

For any outrageous or abusive statement

'Anyway lets concentrate on...' (You do not have to respond either negatively or positively. Use of 'anyway' enables you to put the PVP's statement on the shelf.)

'Doctor, are you just going to let them get away with it?'

(It is amazing the number of occurrences that patients think the doctor can influence.) 'What the hell' (which equivocally communicates some sympathy with the PVP position). 'However I can ...' (Again the patient's statement is put on the shelf but in this case try to follow up by offering to take action about something else.)

'Somebody has got to do something about the situation!'

'I'm sorry but there are only a few things that I can do. Can I write a letter on your behalf?' (By inviting the patient to reply 'yes' you have converted a demand into a request.)

'I think you're a lousy doctor.'

'Yes, but let me try to do my best.' It does no harm to pseudo agree in these circumstances. The main thing is to retain the initiative and move the conversation onwards.

'I want more...'

'The result of these tests [shown to and shared with the patient] show that it would be madness for you to have this.'

'I must be admitted immediately for drug withdrawal.'

(This is a very common request.) If immediate admission is not a possibility then reply 'I'm sorry there are not the facilities for immediate admission.'.

All patients are fascinated by their own X-rays and doctors can establish a self-evidently justifiable authority by showing the patient around his anatomy.

If an awkward question *has* to be asked, either because you really need to know the answer or because the patient has to be assisted to gain insights, then pre-empt a potentially violent response by asking the patient's permission to ask that question: 'Could I ask you about........?'.

Try to appreciate the PVP's point of view. Agree with as many of the patient's points as you can as this communicates willingness on your part. Obviously it is unlikely that you will able to agree with every point but do try to avoid direct confrontations and especially the word 'no'.

Whenever possible use impersonal arguments. Not 'I can't/won't do this' but rather 'I'm afraid the answer has to be no'. If the answer has to be 'no', place the reason for the refusal elsewhere. Preferably state that regulations do not allow you to do something. It is a very useful pacifying gambit to be able to say 'If left to me I would do X, but I am not allowed to do so'.

Ignore bad language. Resist the temptation to interrupt diatribes when a statement has been made which you feel you *must* contradict. Do not interrupt the patient in mid sentence as this is most irritating for anyone to experience. Rather wait until the PVP has to take a breath at the end of a sentence.

A useful technique when a PVP has expressed an outrageous opinion about some aspect of his care is to say 'That's all very well but:...'. Such pseudo-agreement is of no great import and can be followed by a gentle return to the current problem.

If a PVP claims that one of your colleagues has said something outrageous then reply 'Gosh, did he really say that?' (establishment figures of course *never* say gosh).

Whenever possible avoid personalizing conflicts. If there is an obvious conflict of opinion always try to leave the PVP a chance to retire from the argument with dignity. If you offer a PVP no verbal escape route he may resort to a non-verbal mode of expression.

Be willing to change your language. Planned lapses into the vernacular of the patient will display a willingness to be flexible, but be careful not to patronize. *Always* believe what psychopathic patients or drug abusers tell you. They are 100% sincere at the time of their statement (the only problem is that they may equally sincerely change their minds a few moments afterwards).

A warning—humour is a mixed blessing which may either reduce the chance of violence or precipitate it. Only use humour if it is part of your standard personality and *always* avoid humour if a PVP is obviously looking for an excuse to be violent.

If PVPs wish to complain then assist them. Offer paper and pen as this often helps patients to be more logical and less emotive in their demands.

If violence does occur and you are 'thumped' try to leave the situation in a non-aggressive way. 'Excuse me, I hurt.' If you are cornered and unable to extricate yourself and there is no assistance in prospect it should be remembered that it is unlikely that grievous bodily harm to yourself would be inflicted without the extra stimulus of returned aggression: therefore offer no resistance and take the punches (Field Marshall Montgomery's dictum is relevant 'Do not fight a battle unless you know that you will win').

ENDING THE INTERVIEW

Pressures on time in busy clinics may not allow for an hour or so to be spent listening. Various gambits will have to be used to bring the consultation to a close that is hopefully moderately satisfying for both PVP and doctor.

Always try to part in a friendly fashion 'Thanks, that's been useful'. If there are remaining disagreements an apology combined with a definition of the situation is often useful. 'I'm sorry, but that is the best I'm allowed to do for you.'

Aggressive or potentially violent patients

- The medical profession has a duty to provide care for all patients.
- Whenever possible anticipate and prepare for awkward interviews.
- Never let yourself be isolated.
- Try to be helpful and positive.
- Ignore bad language.
- Avoid personalizing conflicts.

PSYCHIATRIC HISTORY AND EXAMINATION (I)

INTRODUCTION

Unlike the assessment of all other systems the assessment of the mental state involves a direct interaction between the personalities of doctor and patient. The doctor must be quick thinking, flexible, and responsive to all possible situations within the limits of his or her personality. It is essential that the doctor gains the patient's confidence so that meaningful communication can occur.

'General medical' psychiatric assessments (Fig. 1) differ from formal psychiatric interviews in that there usually has been discussion about the presenting symptoms, and hopefully a route of communication set up whilst obtaining the medical history which would have included social and physical aspects. The patient's appearance, dress and demeanour may all be important clues to the presence of mental dysfunction. The background of any psychiatric history should include questions assessing all of the aspects shown in Figure 1, which is a useful classification of psychiatric symptoms and behaviour (obviously there is overlap between categories). Other

Table 1 Background information required in formal psychiatric assessment

Experience of childhood
Adolescence
Occupation(s)
Marital history
Family history
Past medical history (including head injuries)
Previous mental health
Problems with current life situation
Problems with various addictions (including alcohol and drugs)

background information that should be elicited is shown in Table 1.

Useful questions to elicit specific psychiatric symptoms include:

- **Presenting complaint**
  - 'What has been troubling you recently?'
  - 'How long have you felt these symptoms?'
  - 'Are there any precipitating or exacerbating factors?'
- **Previous psychiatric history**
  - 'Have you had any previous nervous trouble?'

- 'Have you had treatment for nerves in the past?'
- **Family history**
  - 'Did you have a good relationship with your mother and/or father and/or brothers or sisters?'
  - 'Was your family close and supportive?'
  - 'Are there any nervous problems that tend to run in your family?'
- **Personal history**
  - 'Could you tell me the main points of your life in one minute (or longer if appropriate)?'
- **Childhood**
  - 'Were there any problems when you were young?'
  - 'Did you have a happy/carefree childhood?'
- **School**
  - 'Were there any problems at school?'
  - 'Did you have a happy/carefree time at school?'
- **Adolescence**
  - 'Were there any problems during your teenage years?'
  - 'Did you have a happy/carefree time as a teenager?'

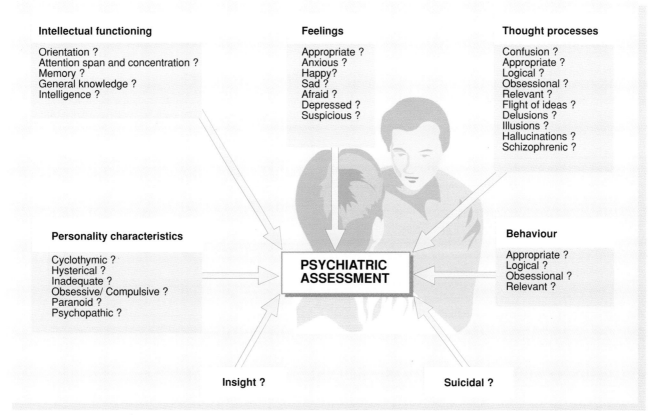

Intellectual functioning

Orientation ?
Attention span and concentration ?
Memory ?
General knowledge ?
Intelligence ?

Feelings

Appropriate ?
Anxious ?
Happy?
Sad ?
Afraid ?
Depressed ?
Suspicious ?

Thought processes

Confusion ?
Appropriate ?
Logical ?
Obsessional ?
Relevant ?
Flight of ideas ?
Delusions ?
Illusions ?
Hallucinations ?
Schizophrenic ?

Personality characteristics

Cyclothymic ?
Hysterical ?
Inadequate ?
Obsessive/ Compulsive ?
Paranoid ?
Psychopathic ?

PSYCHIATRIC ASSESSMENT

Behaviour

Appropriate ?
Logical ?
Obsessional ?
Relevant ?

Insight ?

Suicidal ?

Fig. 1 **A useful classification for history taking and presentation of psychiatric symptoms and behaviour.** Obviously there is overlap between categories.

- **Occupation**
  - 'What do you do most days?'
  - If unemployed: 'What are your job prospects?'
  - 'What training/qualifications do you have?'
- **Sexual history (see p. 5)**
  - 'Have you any problems with your sex life?'
- **Marital history (see p. 4)**
  - 'Are you single, married, separated or divorced?'
- **Head injury**
  - 'Have you ever had any serious head injury?'
- **Problems with authority**
  - 'Do you get on well with your colleagues/boss at work?'
  - 'Have you had any disagreements with the legal system?'
- **Problems with life situation**
  - 'What stresses are you under at home/work?'
  - 'Do you have any money worries?'
- **Problems with alcohol or drugs (see p. 5).**

Be aware that most psychiatric diagnoses are essentially descriptive, based on various symptom patterns that constitute recognizable syndromes. This can help the doctor to clarify his/her thoughts, and assist the identification of appropriate interventions or therapies. A psychiatric diagnosis should not be made on the basis of an isolated symptom and, in many instances, psychiatric classification and labelling oversimplifies the patient's reality and may be both inappropriate and unhelpful.

Psychiatric disturbance can present as physical symptoms. For example, pain may represent a masked depression, and anxiety and depression can present with symptoms indicating high autonomic nervous system function (including palpitations, sweating, frequent bowel movements) or muscle tension. Patients whose physical symptoms are thought to be symptoms of psychiatric disorder may have difficulty in accepting a psychiatric diagnosis as they may fear a label of mental instability.

PERSONALITY CHARACTERISTICS

The dividing line between normal and abnormal personality is often difficult to define. People with personality disorders may not present because of their personality problems (which may be a problem for others rather than themselves), but rather present because they have an incidental illness or because they want something from the doctor.

Personality disorders tend to persist and the most appropriate response for the doctor is to realize that there is no possibility of 'winning', but there is a maximum benefit for both sides if they can 'break even'. Common 'abnormal' personality types include the following:

- *Cyclothymic.* Those with a cyclothymic personality probably have a minor variant of manic depression with fluctuations of mood ranging from cheerfulness to misery. Patients can be asked:
  - 'Does your outlook vary between pessimism and optimism?'
  - 'Do you have mood swings?'
- *Hysterical.* This is a diagnosis which is often made when the doctor develops symptoms of exasperation. Such patients tend to be egocentric yet dependent, manipulative and prone to dramatic but inconsequential outbursts. They may also have coincidental genuine illness. Questions which may reveal an hysterical tendency include:
  - 'Do you find that you need to be an essential and major focus of most activities in which you are involved?'
  - 'Do other people think that you overreact?'
- *Malingering.* This probably occurs in hysterical personality types with the patient having insight and something to gain from his/her behaviour.
- *Conversion hysteria.* Signs (commonly neurological) occur which usually do not conform to any recognizable organic disease pattern. However, the diagnosis of conversion hysteria is a dangerous one because up to one-third of patients who present with physical symptoms initially diagnosed as hysteria subsequently develop signs of organic illness.
- *Inadequate personality.* This combines a lack of ability and lack of drive leading to overall lack of achievement. Having said this some people may find themselves in a life situation with which they are unable to cope and this can happen to any of us. Questions which may reveal an inadequate personality include:
  - 'Do you find it difficult to cope with the stresses and strains of everyday life?'
  - 'Do you find that you lose your temper too easily?'
- *Obsessive/compulsive.* These patients are rigidly conscientious and respond with anxiety to dynamic, uncontrollable, or unpredictable situations (if combined with high intelligence and some insight such people may even become professors!). Questions that may reveal an obsessive/compulsive personality inlcude:
  - 'Do you tend to concentrate excessively on single topics on ideas?'
  - 'Do you have checking rituals?' (Checking rituals may also occur in an attempt to combat dementia.)
- *Paranoid.* These types tend to be 'loners', and are often suspicious or frankly deluded that others are hostile. Useful questions include:
  - 'Do you get on well with most people?'
  - 'Would you describe yourself a loner?'
- *Psychopathic.* The major feature of psychopathic personality types is a failure to learn from experience. They tend to be impulsive, irresponsible and their behaviour at times may be amoral (although superficially their justification may seem reasonable). They often opt for immediate gratification, and react aggressively if this gratification is denied. There may be a history of alcoholism, drug abuse, sexual promiscuity, employment instability or imprisonment. Questions which may reveal a psychopathic tendency include:
  - 'Do you feel that you could be totally self-sufficient?'
  - 'Do you resent those who question your opinions or plans?'
  - 'Do you often act impulsively to your disadvantage?'
- *Addictive.* Drug addicts, whilst actively abusing drugs, often display psychopathic features and the truth of any of their assertions needs confirmation. Lying seems to be part of the psychopathology of active drug addiction, especially when addicts are attempting to obtain drugs.
- *Schizoid.* These personality types are introverted and withdrawn, solitary, emotionally flat, and feel themselves to be vulnerable.

Psychiatric history and examination (I)

- Patients with 'abnormal' personalities are probably no more or less likely to have 'organic' disease.
- A psychiatric diagnosis should not be made on the basis of an isolated symptom.
- Psychiatric disturbance can present with physical symptoms (somatization) and/or with signs suggestive of physical illness.

PSYCHIATRIC HISTORY AND EXAMINATION (II)

INTERPERSONAL COMMUNICATION

- Does the patient have any speech problems?
- Is there psychomotor retardation?
- Is the patient too animated?
- Is the patient superficial or incongruous?
- Does the patient have insight into his or her problems?

INTELLECTUAL FUNCTION

A patient's mental state is influenced by his/her intellectual level, thought processes, feelings, and previous experiences, all of which may influence behaviour.

Impressions of a patient's mental state gained from general medical history taking will suffice if there is clearly an exclusively medical problem, but if there may be a psychiatric component a more structured assessment of the mental state is mandatory.

It may be necessary to be tactful about asking simple questions, but it is essential that such questions are asked as it is remarkable how significant psychiatric disabilities can be concealed during social conversation. Certain 'opening-up' questions are very useful if patients are reluctant to discuss the role of mental factors in their illness:

- 'Your symptoms must make you depressed/anxious: how are you coping with this?'
- 'How much of a role do you think that your worries are playing in your illness?'
- 'Obviously your life situation is unhappy: how well are you coping?'
- 'What do you feel about...?'
- 'What can I do to help?'
- 'You obviously find this worrying – but how much do you worry?'
- 'Have you ever been so depressed that you have thought of taking your own life?'

Orientation

Orientation relates to person, time and place. Ask the patient if you can check some details for the records:

- 'What is your full name?'
- 'What is your date of birth and age?'
- 'What is today's date?'
- 'Do you know the *full* name of this place?' (Stressing the *full* name avoids offending those who are fully orientated.)

Attention span and concentration

Ask the patient:

- 'Can you subtract seven repeatedly (from a given number) 'serial sevens'?'
- 'Can you tell me the months of the year in reverse order?'

Impairment of attention span and concentration may be caused by defects in memory, specific calculating defects, or occasionally may be seen in severe anxiety or depressive states.

Memory

Questions have to be asked which test immediate, recent and remote memory. In most senile dementias memory loss is for immediate or recent events with retention of remote memories.

Short-term memory or immediate memory can be tested by asking the patient:

- 'Can you repeat a sequence of five given digits I will now give you?' (If they are successful, increase the number of given digits—a normal recall ability is about seven digits.)

Questions to detect memory loss for fairly recent events include:

- 'Can you tell me what I asked you to remember at the beginning of the interview?' (after giving the patient, at the beginning of the interview, an item of information which he is told he will have to recall at the end of the interview).
- 'What did you have for your last meal?' (if this can be checked).
- Details of current news events.
- 'How did you get here?'
- 'How long have you been here?'

Remote memory can be tested by asking the patient a series of recall questions. These questions will obviously depend on the age and background of the patient.

- 'How many world wars have there been in your lifetime?'
- 'Who was the first Prime Minister or President you can remember?'
- 'Was there colour television when you were young?'
- In the UK: 'How many shillings were there in a pound?'(The answer is 20. Decimalisation of currency occurred on 15th December 1971: anyone who was aged 20 or above in 1971 should be able to give the correct answer.)

Remote memory can also be assessed by asking about notable events in the patient's past.

Dementia is a condition associated with diminished intellect and diminished assimilation of new ideas, characterized by poor memory (particularly for recent occurrences). There may or may not be an alteration in mood. Dementia usually becomes apparent because of problems with short-term memory, and the need to make lists may be an early manifestation. Demented patients are fully conscious but, as they characteristically have defective short-term memories, a full history may not be available from the patient and so confirmation must be obtained from relatives, friends or carers. Some patients are only too aware of their declining function and depression and anxiety may result.

Do not conclude that a patient is demented without first excluding deafness and dysphasia.

As patients with dementia may be aware of their disability, you will have to enquire tactfully ('Can I check your particulars?') rather than by asking simple questions. However, if direct questions have to be asked it is appropriate to tell the patient that you want to test their memory. With some demented patients there may be a history of previous brain disease including head injury (suspect sub-dural haematomas in the elderly), alcohol abuse, or cardiovascular disease.

Beware of dementia that comes on rapidly: often there is a cause such as a toxic confusional state. Also beware of drug-induced, and therefore potentially reversible, dementia; in particular the effect of long-acting sleeping tablets may induce a demented state. A predisposition to dementia may occasionally run in families (autosomal dominant in the case Huntingdon's chorea). Figure 1 details the major causes of dementia.

Confabulation is the filling in of memory gaps with imagined occurrences. One cause is Korsakoff's syndrome which occurs in association with chronic alcoholism.

General knowledge

If memory is intact the extent of a patient's general knowledge usually becomes obvious.

Intelligence

An approximate judgement of intelligence can be made from conversation, but if there is any doubt a psychologist's assessment is necessary.

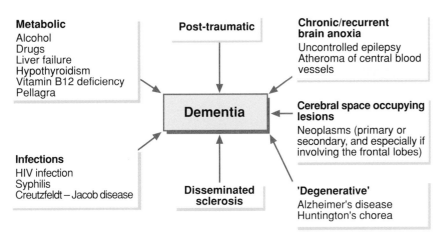

Metabolic
Alcohol
Drugs
Liver failure
Hypothyroidism
Vitamin B12 deficiency
Pellagra

Post-traumatic

Chronic/recurrent brain anoxia
Uncontrolled epilepsy
Atheroma of central blood vessels

Dementia

Cerebral space occupying lesions
Neoplasms (primary or secondary, and especially if involving the frontal lobes)

Infections
HIV infection
Syphilis
Creutzfeldt – Jacob disease

Disseminated sclerosis

'Degenerative'
Alzheimer's disease
Huntington's chorea

Fig. 1 **The major causes of dementia.**

Thought processes

Thoughts may be affected by mood, preoccupations, or confusional states. A confusional state occurs when a conscious patient has a disordered perception of reality leading to bewilderment, mingling of ideas and a consequent disturbance of comprehension and understanding. Confused patients cannot concentrate for long and later usually have an impaired memory for their episode of confusion. Aspects of abnormal conscious states are detailed on page 140. *Altered conscious states are rarely caused by psychiatric illness but are mostly caused by toxic confusional states.*

Decide whether the thoughts are appropriate, logical and relevant to the circumstances. Do repeated irrelevances constitute flight of ideas? Are recurrent thoughts obsessional?

Decide whether the patient has delusions. A delusion is having a belief that is firmly held on inadequate grounds, is not affected by rational argument or evidence to the contrary, and is not a belief that a person might be expected to hold given his or her educational and cultural background.

Questions which may reveal delusions (which may or may not indicate schizophrenia) include:
* 'How would you describe your personality?'
* 'Would other people agree with this assessment?'
* 'Is life fair to you?'
* 'Do you sometimes feel that people are plotting against you or doing you down?'
* 'Are people usually supportive of your ideas and actions?'
* 'Do you ever feel that certain external events have significance most for you?'
* 'Do you think you are treated fairly by acquaintances / police / newspapers / radio / television.'

* 'Do you see yourself as a normal person or do you have any particularly unusual qualities?'
* 'Do you feel that you are underweight/ overweight?'

Questions which may reveal illusions (incorrectly interpreted sensory stimuli), or hallucinations (erroneous visual or auditory impressions occurring without appropriate stimuli) include:
* 'Do you have unusual visual experiences that are not caused by external stimuli?'
* 'Do you have unusual hearing experiences that are not caused by external stimuli?'

Determine whether the patient has obsessions (recurrent persistent thoughts that occur despite efforts to exclude them).

Schizophrenic patients may have gradual onset of symptoms or may present with abrupt onset illness, especially if there has been a precipitating factor.

A schizophrenic's clarity of thought may be impaired with abrupt or illogical changes in the subject of conversation: 'flight of ideas' or 'knight's move' respectively. In contrast, some patients may experience blockage of their thought processes or 'thought block'. Patients may be convinced that their thoughts are being controlled by external forces or that external happenings have specific relevance for themselves ('ideas of reference'), and if such external forces are perceived as malevolent the patient may become paranoid. Schizophrenic patients may be deluded, the incongruity of their beliefs being obvious, but in some patients elaborate and internally consistent thought systems may be built on an insubstantial foundation. Some patients feel that they are alienated from their inner selves ('depersonalization').

A schizophrenic's feeling may be incongruous or blunted.

Hallucinations, usually auditory or visual, are not uncommon and questioning may have to be tactful: 'Do you have buzzing in your ears...does it sound like voices...what do they say?'.

In severe schizophrenic states patients may become catatonic (alteration in the tone of the whole body with total immobility or violent excitement) with bizarre posturing or psychomotor retardation.

Questions which may reveal schizophrenia include:
* 'Are there specific public events that have a specific significance for you alone?'
* 'Do you have insights that few others share?'
* 'Do you have unusual thoughts which seem to arise without your thinking them? How do they arise? On the other hand do you have unusual episodes in which your thought processes become blocked? Are other people aware of such thoughts even though you have not told them? Which people are aware and how do they know?'
* 'Do you have any hearing problems such that you hear noises/voices that others cannot appreciate? What do you hear/what do they say?'
* 'Do you often feel controlled by external forces or events?'
* 'Do you ever feel dissociated from reality?'
* 'Do you have any vision problems such that you see sights that others cannot appreciate? What do you see?'

Psychiatric history and examination (II)

* Use of 'opening up' questions is the key to approaching patients who might resist specific psychiatric questioning.
* Specific questions may be needed to reveal well-concealed dementia.
* Short-term memory loss is a prime feature of dementia.
* Do not diagnose dementia unless you are sure that the patient is not deaf or has dysphasia.
* Dementia that comes on rapidly is probably caused by toxic confusional state.
* Altered conscious states are rarely caused by psychiatric disorders.

PSYCHIATRIC HISTORY AND EXAMINATION (III)

FEELINGS

Is the patient's mood appropriate to his/her life situation? If mood is not blunted, is the patient inappropriately anxious, happy, sad, irritable, angry, suspicious or afraid? Formal questionnaires are available which are particularly useful as they include short simple questions which assess the presence and severity of anxiety and depression by means of numerical scores which can be used to follow the course of illness.

ANXIETY

Anxiety is often a primary complaint although some patients complain of inability to concentrate caused by their anxiety. Possible symptoms of anxiety are shown in Figure 1. Hyperventilation is often a feature of panic attacks and, once initiated, may augment anxiety to form a vicious circle (Fig. 2). Phobic states are anxiety states which only occur in specific circumstances, e.g. agoraphobia is fear of open spaces.

Table 1 **Possible symptoms of depression**

Suggestive of physical disorders	Psychological	
Sleep disorder (classically early morning waking) Loss of appetite Loss of weight Constipation Sexual difficulties Fatigue Generalized aches and pains	**Mood** Depressed **Conversation** Reduced in quantity and quality **Energy** Usually reduced (unless 'compensatory' mania) **Memory** Impaired	**Thoughts** Anxious Guilty Suicidal Worthlessness **Behaviour** Usually slow (unless 'compensatory' mania) **Hallucinations** Often auditory, accusatory, and hostile

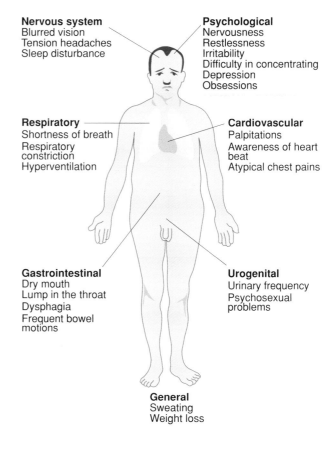

Nervous system
Blurred vision
Tension headaches
Sleep disturbance

Psychological
Nervousness
Restlessness
Irritability
Difficulty in concentrating
Depression
Obsessions

Respiratory
Shortness of breath
Respiratory constriction
Hyperventilation

Cardiovascular
Palpitations
Awareness of heart beat
Atypical chest pains

Gastrointestinal
Dry mouth
Lump in the throat
Dysphagia
Frequent bowel motions

Urogenital
Urinary frequency
Psychosexual problems

General
Sweating
Weight loss

Fig. 1 **Possible symptoms of anxiety.**

DEPRESSION

The possible symptoms of depression are shown in Table 1. Figure 3 details manifestations which lead from endogenous depression and Figure 4 the possible factors in reactive depression. Be careful not to confuse depression with dementia. In both conditions there may be manifestations of memory defect, poor orientation, or apparent confusion.

Never neglect the possibility of reversible organic causes of depression including drug therapy (steroids, methyldopa, the contraceptive pill), infections (e.g. post-influenza or after glandular fever) and organic brain disease.

When assessing any depressed patient always ascertain whether the patient has suicidal thoughts. This is very important because depressed patients do not die from depression, they die from suicide.

Although the following types of depression are useful descriptive categories, the various types of depression may exhibit overlap. Psychiatrists may adopt other classifications but the following seems to be relevant for non-specialists.

Endogenous depression

Endogenous depression is depression without extrinsic causes. A family history may be relevant because endogenous depression is thought to have a biochemical basis and to be partially genetically determined. Manifestations of endogenous depression range from profound depression to depression with episodes of mania—a manic–depressive psychosis.

Patients with endogenous depression (Fig. 3) typically give a history of progressive fatigue, loss of interest in previous activities, and a disturbed sleep

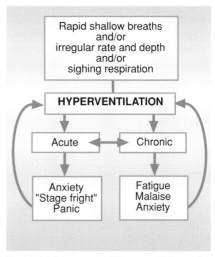

Rapid shallow breaths and/or irregular rate and depth and/or sighing respiration

HYPERVENTILATION

Acute ⟷ Chronic

Anxiety "Stage fright" Panic

Fatigue Malaise Anxiety

Fig. 2 **The vicious cycle of hyperventilation and anxiety.**

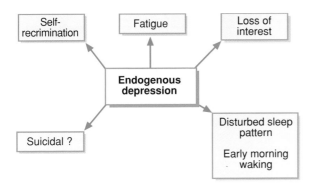

Fig. 3 **Manifestations leading from endogenous depression.**

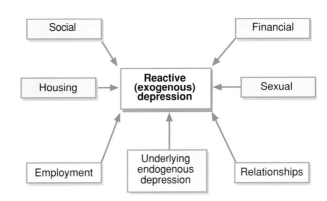

Fig. 4 **Possible factors in reactive (exogenous) depression.**

pattern with early morning waking. Patients feel emotionally flat, have impaired concentration, often express self-recrimination, may exhibit hypochondriacal features and may become paranoid if they externalize the cause for their misery. Weight loss may occur. Suicidal thoughts are common.

Neurotic depression

A specific life event often triggers off neurotic depression but symptoms persist for longer than appropriate with misery, self-pity, depression, and often anxiety. Patients may present with complaints of bodily dysfunctions such as headaches, gastrointestinal symptoms, or insomnia. Weight loss (contradicted by past medical recordings) is a common complaint of neurotically depressed patients.

Psychotic depression

Psychotic depression is profound endogenous depression with psychomotor retardation. The patient typically lacks insight into the fact that he/she is ill and suicidal thoughts are often prominent.

Reactive depression

The depth of a reactive depression may be appropriate if precipitated by a life situation (Fig. 4), but if depression is of inappropriate duration it may merge into neurotic or endogenous depression.

MANIA (Table 2)

Mania may occur as an isolated phenomenon or as part of a depressive illness. Manic patients experience elevations of mood and increased activity (which may lead to total exhaustion). Speech may be rapid, sleep may be disturbed, and appetite increased. Patients may develop ideas of self-importance and expansive ideas may verge on delusions. Questions which may reveal manic tendencies include:

- 'Are there times when you feel you have much more energy than others?'
- 'Do you ever feel 110 per cent well?'

Table 2 **Possible symptoms of mania**

Suggestive of physical disorders	Psychological		
Insomnia Weight loss Sweating Excessive thirst	**Mood** Elevated and labile **Conversation** Fast and pressurized, overanimated **Energy** Excessive, hyperdynamic	**Thoughts** Grandiose Overconfident Delusions	**Behaviour** Disinhibited Tendencies to excess **Hallucinations** Possible

SUICIDE

The risks of suicide should be considered in all psychiatrically abnormal patients, and all thoughts of suicide, no matter how superficially trivial, require serious evaluation. Questions obviously have to be personalized for each patient but in essence the doctor may have to start with questions along the lines of 'Have you ever considered doing anything foolish?' progressing to 'Have you ever thought of harming yourself?'. Always define whether or not the patient has ever actually attempted self-harm or attempted suicide.

The features of previous attempted suicide that suggest previous, and thus probably present, serious suicidal intent are shown in Table 3. Suicide attempts which are associated with an increased risk of repetition are shown in Table 4.

Table 3 **Features of serious suicidal attempts**

Made in isolated circumstances where intervention was unlikely
Precautions made to avoid intervention
Good knowledge of likely effects of tablets taken in overdose

Table 4 **Features of suicide attempts associated with increased risk of repetition**

Previous hospital admission(s) for suicide attempts
Drug or alcohol problems
Personality disorders
History of crime
Unemployment
Isolation
Low social class
Previous psychiatric treatment

Psychiatric history and examination (III)

- Always exclude organic causes of depression.
- Hyperventilation (which is treatable) may be a result of, and further exacerbate, anxiety.
- Reactive depression may complicate or initiate endogenous depression.
- Any mention of suicide requires serious evaluation.

PATIENTS TOO ILL TO GIVE A HISTORY — Initial Assessment

When patients present desperately ill, standard patterns of patient management may be inappropriate. The usual approach of history taking and examination may need to be amended so that support measures can be instituted if necessary, a rapid working diagnosis made, followed by urgent (sometimes empirical) treatment before returning to a standard pattern of management. A recommended plan of campaign is illustrated in Figure 1.

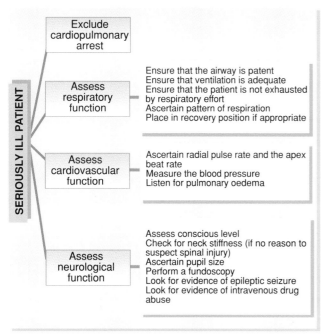

Fig. 1 **Plan of campaign for dealing with the seriously ill patient.**

EXCLUDE CARDIOPULMONARY ARREST

Ensure that the patient is not in cardiopulmonary arrest (Fig. 2). If he is, then commence cardiopulmonary resuscitation.

If the patient is not in cardiopulmonary arrest yet obviously requires urgent treatment:

- Ask the nursing staff to ensure that any relatives or friends of the patient will await your further questioning
- Perform a rapid initial assessment of the patient's respiratory, cardiovascular and nervous system function
- If indicated, establish a route for intravenous therapy
- Take blood samples before initiating any specific therapy
- Consider giving a 50 cc bolus of 50% dextrose intravenously
- Perform a secondary assessment commencing with a more detailed general examination, followed by an assessment of the various organ systems.

INITIAL ASSESSMENT

Assess respiratory function

1. *Ensure that the airway is patent and will remain so.* If necessary insert a Guedel airway (Fig. 3) or a Brook airway. Do not attempt to pass an endotracheal tube unless you have been trained in this technique. Stridor (p. 145) suggests laryngeal or tracheal obstruction and usually requires urgent attention. Intubation and/or tracheostomy may be indicated although angioneurotic oedema may respond rapidly to medical measures.

2. *Ensure that ventilation is adequate.* Observe the colour of the patient, the respiratory rate and the tidal volume.

3. *Ensure that the patient is not exhausted by respiratory effort.* If exhaustion or ventilatory failure are present or seem imminent, assisted ventilation should be considered urgently.

4. *Ascertain the pattern of respiration.* Any subsequent change in this pattern usually indicates an alteration in nervous system function.

5. *Place the patient in a semiprone 'recovery' position if the conscious level is impaired and there is no risk of spinal injuries* (Fig. 4). Rotate the head to one side, remove dentures if present, and inspect the oropharynx. Inhalation of noxious material from the oropharynx is thus made less likely.

Assess cardiovascular function

1. *Ascertain the radial pulse rate and the apex beat rate.* An electrocardiogram (ECG) should be performed as soon as is reasonable if there is:

- A fast regular heart rate, when primary cardiac dysrhythmia, heart failure, or pulmonary embolism may be responsible (if acute haemorrhage is a likely cause the ECG is less urgently required).
- A fast irregular rate. Uncontrolled atrial fibrillation, atrial flutter, or multiple ventricular ectopics may require urgent treatment.
- A slow heart rate (less than 60/min). Sinus bradycardia or complete heart block may require urgent treatment (it is usually possible to distinguish sinus bradycardia (with a normal first and second heart sound) from complete heart block (which gives rise to a varying intensity of the first heart sound).
- Pulsus alternans which suggests left ventricular failure (p. 23).

2. *Measure the blood pressure.* A very high blood pressure may suggest hypertensive encephalopathy (necessitating rapid reduction of the blood pressure) or raised intracranial pressure, whereas a low blood pressure may suggest acute fluid loss (including haemorrhage), myocardial infarction, pulmonary embolism, dehydration (including hyperglycaemic coma), hypothermia, drug overdosage and other causes of shock.

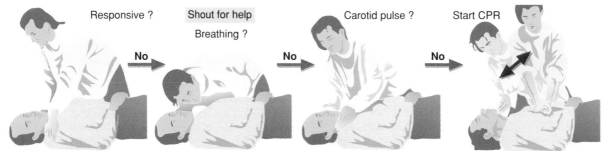

Fig. 2 **The diagnosis of cardiopulmonary arrest.**

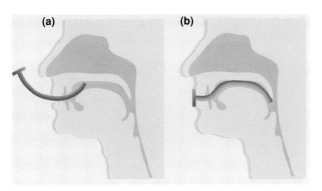

Fig. 3 **Insertion of a Guedel-type airway.** **(a)** Keep the airway patent by holding the chin up. Insert the airway with the tip pointing to the roof of the mouth. **(b)** Turn and advance the airway until it advances over the back of the tongue.

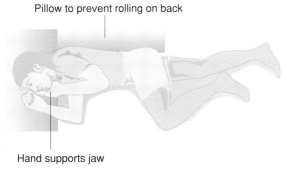

Pillow to prevent rolling on back

Hand supports jaw

Fig. 4 **The recovery position.**

3. *Listen for evidence of pulmonary oedema.* Crepitations or wheeze alone may be heard.

Assess nervous system function

After any immediately reversible abnormalities in the cardiovascular and respiratory systems have been rectified, the nervous system should be assessed.

Do not forget to examine the cranium for signs of skull fracture. If there is any suspicion of a spinal injury do not move the patient without ensuring that the position of the spine is stabilized and do not perform tests for neck stiffness.

Focal or generalized epileptic seizures should be treated with an anticonvulsant such as diazepam (a *focal* seizure implies the situation of a nervous system lesion). Then assess:

* *The conscious level.* The conscious level should be observed and recorded according to the Glasgow Coma Scales (GCS) (Table 1).
* *Neck stiffness.* Neck stiffness should be evaluated. Remember that deeply comatose patients may show no neck stiffness even if they have meningitis or a subarachnoid haemorrhage.
* *Pupil size* (p. 79). Examine briefly and record the pupil size. If the pupils are unequal, remember the possibility of a previously administered mydriatic.
* *Funduscopy* (p. 78). A brief funduscopy should be performed at this stage. Changes of long-standing diabetes, hypertension, or subhyaloid haemorrhages (in association with subarachnoid haemorrhage) may be seen. Papilloedema may be seen in raised intracranial pressure but this may be a late sign in many acute disorders causing raised intracranial pressure.
* *Evidence of tongue biting or incontinence.* Look for evidence of tongue biting or incontinence. Either or both may have occurred during a grand mal convulsion.

* *Look for intravenous drug track marks.* This provides a clue to recent intravenous drug abuse and suggests the possibility of drug overdose and the possibility that the patient may have infections such as hepatitis B or HIV.

This rapid assessment should take only a few minutes to perform.

PRELIMINARY THERAPY

A route for intravenous therapy should be established and relevant blood specimens should be taken prior to beginning any specific therapy.

Unless hyperglycaemic coma is likely, a bolus of 50 ml of 50% dextrose should be given intravenously as hypoglycaemia may be a readily reversible initiating or perpetuation factor in the dysfunction of many organ systems. However recovery from prolonged hypoglycaemia may not occur instantly after administration of intravenous dextrose. If the patient is a known alcoholic, thiamine should be given.

If the respiratory system, cardiovascular system, and nervous system do not require urgent attention, a short time should be spent in obtaining relevant diagnostic information from any readily available sources.

If further information is available, enquiries concerning the general history, previous illnesses, recent head injuries and the possibility of drug overdose should be made.

Remember to inspect the contents of wallets and pockets for diabetic and steroid cards, etc.

Table 1 **Glasgow coma scale**

Eyes	Open	Spontaneously	4
		To verbal command	3
		To pain	2
	No response		1
Best motor response	To verbal command	Obeys	6
	To painful stimulus	Localizes pain	5
		Flexion withdrawal	4
		Flexion – decerebrate	3
		Extension – decerebrate	2
		No response	1
Best verbal response		Orientated and converses	5
		Disorientated and converses	4
		Inappropriate words	3
		Incomprehensible sounds	2
		No response	1
Total			3 – 15

Patients too ill to give a history — initial assessment

* In any collapsed patient always exclude cardiac arrest.
* Always ensure that ventilation is adequate.
* Unless hyperglycaemia is likely give 50cc of 50% glucose intravenously.

PATIENTS TOO ILL TO GIVE A HISTORY — Secondary Assessment (I)

Conduct a systematic examination, starting with a more detailed general assessment and progressing to examination of each organ system in turn (Fig. 1). Obviously there are many schemes of systematic examination but in the context of the current account, a diagnostic approach to each of the bodily organ systems in turn seems sensible, emphasizing that frequently there are signs of chronic dysfunction of various systems which can produce clues to the nature of the missing history.

At each stage of the examination remember that there are three diagnoses which should be attached to every set of abnormalities found: the *anatomical*, the *functional* and the *aetiological*.

GENERAL EXAMINATION

Observe the colour of the patient

- Cyanosis suggests impaired oxygenation or methaemoglobinaemia.
- Pallor suggests anaemia or peripheral circulatory shutdown.
- A pink colour suggests carbon monoxide poisoning.
- Jaundice suggests hepatocellular dysfunction, biliary tract dysfunction, or haemolysis.
- A plethoric colouration suggests polycythaemia which may be a primary disorder or secondary to defective oxygenation of the blood, or to an underlying liver or kidney neoplasm which may present with polycythaemia.

Smell the breath

Remember that halitosis is a common finding in ill patients. Exclude the sweet odour of hyperglycaemic ketoacidosis, the fishy uraemic fetor, hepatic fetor and the odour of alcohol which may mask other olfactory clues.

Look at and feel the skin

Assess the skin turgor for evidence of dehydration. A generalized dark pigmentation may suggest hypoadrenalism, subacute infective endocarditis, haemochromatosis, or a recent holiday (usually taken abroad) which may extend the range of possible diagnoses. A purpuric rash suggests meningococcal septicaemia.

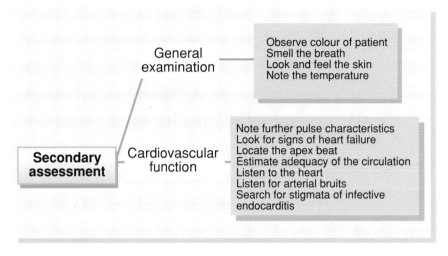

Fig. 1 **Secondary assessment.**

Note the temperature

Hyperpyrexia may be caused by heat exhaustion (usually due to a failure of the heat-regulating centre after the patient has been exposed to high temperature and high humidity). Hypothermia, which is easily missed, may be secondary to many acute illnesses, including overdoses. If hypothermia is suspected the use of a low-reading thermometer is essential.

CARDIOVASCULAR SYSTEM FUNCTION

The cardiovascular lesions that may present as an emergency with a patient too ill to give a useful history can be classified as in Table 1 and Figure 2. Approach the patient with these possibilities in mind.

Note further pulse characteristics

Detailed examination of the pulses may give immediate diagnostic information:

- *An impalpable pulse* or delay in, or asymmetry of, peripheral pulses implies either acute or chronic arterial blockage or a low blood pressure.
- *Asymmetrical pulses* should lead to measurement of the blood pressure in both arms and sometimes in the legs also. Suspect a dissecting aneurysm.

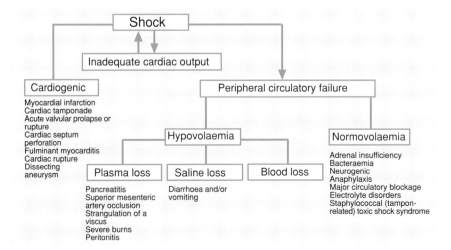

Fig. 2 **The causes of shock.**

- *A small volume pulse* may indicate circulatory obstruction which may be caused by aortic stenosis, pulmonary stenosis, hypotension, myocardial infarction or constrictive pericarditis.
- *Pulsus paradoxus* (diminution of pulse volume during inspiration) occurs in pericardial effusion and constrictive pericarditis, and on occasion in severe airways obstruction.
- *Pulsus bisferiens* (two palpable impulses in the presence of a good volume pulse) suggests mixed aortic stenosis and incompetence.
- *Pulsus alternans* (alternating strong and weak pulses) implies heart failure, usually left ventricular failure.
- A *collapsing pulse* is found in aortic incompetence, high output cardiac failure, arteriovenous fistulae, high fever and incomplete heart block.

Table 1 Cardiovascular problems which can cause patients to be too ill to give a history

Disorders which cause syncope
Vasovagal attacks
Asystolic episodes (Stokes–Adams attacks)
Aortic stenosis
Serious dysrhythmias

Disorders which cause severe pain
Myocardial infarction
Pericarditis
Dissecting aneurysms

Disorders which cause shock (see Fig. 2)

Other disorders
Acute infective endocarditis
Hypertensive encephalopathy
Acute valvular dysfunction or rupture

Look for signs of heart failure
The venous pressure should be estimated. In an ill patient, usually flat in bed, the venous pressure may be difficult to estimate as the jugular veins may be filled because of the patient's posture. However, an approximate guide to the venous pressure is obtained (in the absence of venous obstruction) by observing the height above the sternal angle at which the dorsal hand veins collapse if the straight arm is lifted slowly from the horizontal (the 'poor man's central venous pressure').

Search for oedema, ascites or pleural fluid. These are not necessarily caused by heart failure but if other signs of cardiovascular diseases are found, the likelihood of heart failure increases.

Locate the apex beat
An abnormally situated apex beat usually implies long-standing cardiovascular pathology or mediastinal displacement.

Estimate adequacy of circulation (Fig. 3)
Note the pulse rate, blood pressure and peripheral perfusion. A guide to the state of peripheral perfusion can be obtained by noting the temperature and colour of an unexposed extremity and also by observing the rate of capillary filling after exerting 'blanching' pressure on an extremity with a finger. If there is an inadequate circulation there is either 'pump' failure or peripheral circulatory failure. Acute pump failure has many causes, the most common being myocardial infarction.

Peripheral circulatory failure can be either normovolaemic (as in bacteraemic shock) or hypovolaemic due to blood, serum, or other bodily fluid loss or sequestration. Acute generalized circulatory inadequacy usually produces the clinical signs of shock:

- venous constriction
- increase in pulse rate
- decrease in pulse volume
- pallor
- cyanosis
- hypotension

- sweating (septicaemic shock may present with a warm dry skin)
- air hunger
- thirst
- pupillary dilatation
- disorientation
- coma.

Shock sufficient to prevent the patient from giving a history usually has major cardiovascular manifestations, and the final common pathway of shock, whatever the cause, is a fall in cardiac output and/or peripheral blood flow causing inadequacy of the circulation.

Listen to the heart
Listen for heart sounds, additional sounds and murmurs. Ventricular septal defect or acute mitral incompetence may occur acutely after myocardial infarction, as may the friction rub of pericarditis.

Listen for arterial bruits
In the absence of severe anaemia, arterial bruits usually signify heart or vascular disease.

Search specifically for the stigmata of infective endocarditis
Acute infective endocarditis may have few of the signs of classical subacute bacterial endocarditis.

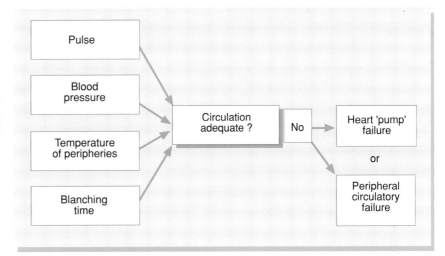

Fig. 3 **Estimating the adequacy of circulation.**

Patients too ill to give a history — secondary assessment (I)

- Look for signs of chronic disease which may provide a clue to the aetiology of acute illness.
- At each stage try to make three diagnoses for each abnormality – the anatomical, the functional and the aetiological.

PATIENTS TOO ILL TO GIVE A HISTORY — Secondary Assessment (II)

NERVOUS SYSTEM FUNCTION

It is impossible to outline an approach to nervous system abnormalities that would cover all diagnostic possibilities. The diseases which may cause diffuse dysfunction of the central nervous system are listed in Table 1.

Table 1 **Disease causing diffuse dysfunction of the central nervous system**

Metabolic dysfunctions (including drug overdoses)
Rising intracranial pressure (with coning)
Postictal states
Meningitis
Encephalitis
Subarachnoid haemorrhage
Demyelination (particularly in the brainstem)
Head injury
Pituitary infarction
Bacteraemia
Multiple microemboli (e.g. fat emboli)
Disseminated intravascular coagulation
Cerebral malaria

If there is a nervous system disorder which prevents the patient from giving a history, there must be one or more of the following:

- an altered state of consciousness
- amnesia
- dementia
- dysphasia (motor or sensory)
- dysarthria
- profound weakness such as in myasthenia gravis or severe peripheral neuropathies
- a (very rare) 'locked-in' syndrome in which there is a paralysis of all four extremities and lower cranial nerves that may or may not be associated with impaired consciousness with the patient usually being aware of himself and his environment
- akinetic mutism in which there is apparent wakefulness without awareness with a relative paucity of signs
- psychiatric conditions such as depression, mania, schizophrenia, psychopathy, malingering, or hysteria.

Ascertain the state of consciousness

There may be a state of:

- Full consciousness or clouding of consciousness. The GCS is detailed on page 137 and gives a numerical value which relates to prognosis, but which should not replace an accurate description of the patient's condition

- Coma is a state of unrousable unresponsiveness. If the patient is comatose, empty the stomach by using a nasogastric tube (which should be left in place). Emptying the stomach guards against inhalation of vomit and may reveal evidence of drug overdose. Unconscious patients must not have a stomach wash-out unless the airway is protected
- Confusion is a state in which stimuli are consistently misinterpreted and attention span is shortened
- Delirium is a state in which there is disorientation, fear, irritability, misperception of sensory stimuli, and visual hallucinations are often present
- Stupor is a state in which there is unresponsiveness from which the patient can be aroused only by vigorous and repeated stimuli.

Causes of aggressive behaviour in association with impaired consciousness include:

- hypoglycaemia
- delirium
- the presence of a painfully full bladder
- dynamic surroundings
- delusions or hallucinations.

Note the pattern of breathing

In addition to the Cheyne–Stokes respiratory pattern (p. 42), look for Biot 's breathing (periods of irregular rate and depth of respiration with periods of apnoea but lacking the periodic features of Cheyne–Stokes respiration) classically occurring in meningitis or lesions which cause profound disruption of the medullary respiratory centre. Apneustic breathing (pauses at full inspiration) usually denotes pontine infarction, hypoglycaemia, anoxia, or severe meningitis.

Look for evidence of cerebrospinal fluid otorrhoea or rhinorrhoea

Clinically obvious head injuries should have been detected during the primary assessment.

Note the resting posture

Asymmetry of posture suggests a lateralized nervous system dysfunction whereas generalized abnormality of posture is caused by deep coma of any cause, or decerebrate or decorticate rigidity (Fig. 1).

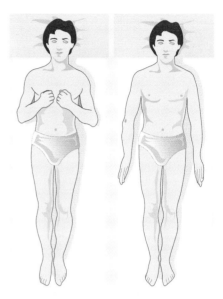

Fig. 1 **Decerebrate and decorticate postures.**

Examine the eyes

Several signs may be immediately helpful but always take great care to exclude previous administration of mydriatic drops or opiates before attempting a diagnosis.

- *Photophobia* suggests cerebral irritation
- *A unilateral dilated pupil unresponsive to bright light* suggests a third nerve lesion
- *Bilateral, unreactive, medium-sized, often irregular, pupils* suggests a midbrain lesion
- *Pin-point pupils* suggest a pontine lesion or opiate overdose
- *Bilateral pupillary dilatation on neck flexion* suggests impending tentorial herniation
- *Eyes consistently deviated to one side* suggest a homolateral cerebral lesion or a contralateral brainstem lesion.

In patients who are not fully conscious or cooperative, the doll's eye phenomenon is of diagnostic help. One must be certain that there is no danger of damage to the cervical cord before performing this test. The test is performed by rolling the patient's head to the right or left. Normally both eyes tend to lag behind the head movements, deviating to the opposite side as if they were trying to fix on the zenith (Fig. 2). Also flexion of the neck results in relative upward gaze and extension of the neck a relative downward gaze. If these responses are absent, there is damage at a site or sites within the neurological arc comprising the vestibular apparatus, their

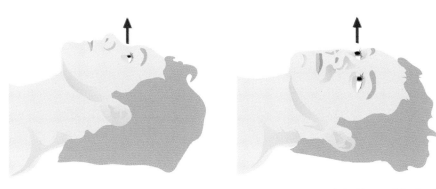

Fig. 2 **The doll's eye reflex.** On turning the head to either side, the pupils remain looking straight ahead.

afferent nerves to the brainstem, their central nervous system connections, the peripheral nerve supply to the eye, or the peripheral ocular muscles.

If the patient is in deep coma the eyes are usually fixed in the mid-position, are slightly divergent, and may not demonstrate the doll's eye phenomenon.

Eye movements can also be evoked by instillation of cold water into the external auditory meatus, whereupon the normal response is a conjugate deviation of the eyes, and nystagmus may also be elicited (before performing this test be certain that there is no tympanic membrane perforation and that there is no risk to the patient should vomiting be induced).

Marked asymmetry of eye positioning or movements in these tests usually signifies an anatomical rather than a metabolic disorder.

The pupillary light reflexes are usually preserved until the terminal stages of coma of metabolic causation unless there has been administration of drugs which affect pupil size (notably aropine, opiates, or tricyclic antidepressants).

Pupillary dilatation in response to pinching the neck (the ciliospinal reflex) implies continuity of the relevant sensory and motor nerve fibres and their brainstem connections.

Provided the patient is not unconscious it is often possible to suspect a hemianopia by observing a unilateral absence of response to a visual threat (such as waving a hand close to the face).

Pupillary inequality, especially if progressive or associated with a declining level of consciousness may indicate the need for an urgent neurosurgical opinion.

Examine the motor responses

If the patient is restless, observe spontaneous movements. Even if observations are restricted to comments such as 'patient violent, uncooperative, but moves all four limbs purposefully in response to visual,

auditory or tactile stimuli', some anatomical continuity of motor or sensory nerves, their central connections and coordinating mechanisms can be inferred.

If the conscious level is impaired, bilateral symmetrical painful stimuli or a midline painful stimulus may be used to elicit responses (the use of bilateral stimuli enables one to assess whether reactions are normal and symmetrical).

Examine muscle tone

Note particularly asymmetry, which may provide evidence of lateralized abnormal nervous system function.

Examine the tendon reflexes and plantar responses

Again note asymmetry. If the patient has only slight impairment of consciousness and the reflexes are markedly diminished, suspect a peripheral neuropathy, the aetiology of which could be related to the cause of the impaired consciousness (diabetes mellitus for example).

The diagnostic and prognostic significance of bilateral extensor plantar responses can be uncertain in the presence of impaired consciousness but asymmetrical responses are likely to signify a unilateral lesion.

Further considerations

Remember that focal anatomical disorders of the cerebral hemispheres are unlikely to produce impaired consciousness unless there is coincidental or secondary damage to other brain tissue (for example patients with unilateral 'cerebral thrombosis' rarely have an impaired conscious level). An exception is embolic infarction in the middle cerebral territory of the dominant hemisphere.

Small focal lesions sufficient to cause impaired consciousness as a primary effect are usually situated in the brainstem.

If an anatomical site for a nervous system lesion can be identified the

aetiology may be easy to suspect. However, if the nervous system is obviously involved but there are no anatomically localizing signs one would consider disorders which may cause diffuse dysfunction of the nervous system (Table 1).

Metabolic dysfunction

Metabolic dysfunctions which impair the ability to give a history are most often due to poisoning (usually self-induced), or excess or lack of various metabolic compounds consequent to specific organ failure.

In the case of specific organ failures there are often signs of chronic dysfunction which may serve as clues to diagnosis. The signs of liver, renal, thyroid, pituitary, and adrenal hormone abnormalities are detailed in the appropriate sections.

A metabolic cause is likely if there is clouding of consciousness, confusion, delirium, stupor, or coma without focal anatomical abnormality or lateralizing signs, and if there are no signs of diseases which may cause diffuse dysfunction of the nervous system.

There are three motor abnormalities characteristic of metabolic precoma states:

- Limb tremor, usually coarse and irregular at a rate of eight to ten per second
- A 'metabolic' flapping tremor (asterixis) of the hands when they are dorsiflexed at the wrist, with the arms outstretched and with the fingers extended and abducted.
- Multifocal myoclonus (unpredictable twitching of muscles or muscle groups) may be found in uraemia, carbon dioxide retention, and in Jakob–Creutzfeldt disease (a rapidly progressive dementing illness which usually occurs in the elderly).

Patients too ill to give a history — secondary assessement (II)

- If a patient is comatose, empty the stomach to prevent inhalation of vomit.
- Always exclude the possibility of prior mydriatic administration if a pupil is dilated.
- Signs are usually symmetrical in patients with metabolic coma.

PATIENTS TOO ILL TO GIVE A HISTORY — Secondary Assessment (III)

RESPIRATORY SYSTEM FUNCTION

Initially look for non-specific pointers towards the presence of respiratory pathology (Fig. 1):

- abnormally shaped chest
- abnormal respiratory rate
- cyanosis
- dyspnoea
- stridor
- wheeze.

If these are present and the patient is too dyspnoeic to give a history and a primary pulmonary pathology is likely to be a cause, suspect pneumonia, severe asthma, pneumothorax or airways obstruction.

Herpes labialis is a common accompaniment to lung infections (usually of bacterial aetiology) but may be found in any acute febrile condition. Rarely it may be a clue to underlying herpes simplex encephalitis.

Diminution of chest movement

Localized diminution may occur as a result of:

- consolidation
- collapse
- fibrosis
- pleural fluid
- pneumothorax
- chest wall deformity.

Symmetrical diminution of chest wall movements may occur in some bilateral lung lesions, emphysema, infiltrative lesions, bronchospasm, or in myasthenia gravis. *Generalized* over expansion occurs in bronchospasm and *lateralized* over expansion in partial bronchial obstruction.

Respiratory rate

If there is tachypnoea, look for evidence of:

- respiratory tract infection
- pneumothorax
- incomplete airways obstruction
- inhalation of foreign material (including vomit)
- flail chest due to fractured ribs
- painful chest lesions (such as fractured ribs or pleurisy).

Extrapulmonary initiators of tachypnoea include:

- left ventricular failure
- acute onset of severe anaemia
- central nervous system lesions
- drug overdoses
- diabetic acidosis.

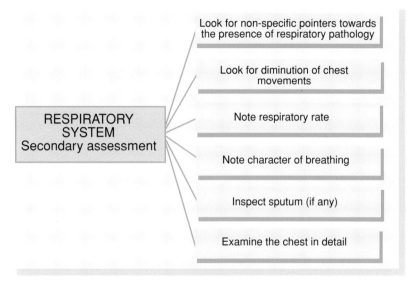

Fig. 1 **Secondary assessment of respiratory system function.**

Patients with tachypnoea due to primary lung pathology often seem to have difficulty in getting the air 'in and out' of the chest, whereas patients with tachypnoea of cardiovascular or metaboli aetiology frequently 'pant' air in and out without difficulty. Slow respirations may occur in the terminal stages of any illness, but if there are no other signs of organic dysfunction suspect drug overdose with (potentially reversible) respiratory depressing drugs.

Character of breathing

Sighing (Kussmaul's) respirations are found in ketosis or acidosis and certain drug overdoses. Cheyne–Stokes respirations (p. 43) can be a feature of severe respiratory cardiac failure, renal disease, primary cerebral disorders and drug overdosage. It is not necessarily associated with a poor prognosis.

Sputum

If sputum is being produced inspect it carefully. Mucoid sputum is found in acute pulmonary oedema, asthma, some viral pneumonias, and chronic bronchitis.

Mucopurulent sputum occurs in:

- most bacterial pneumonias (usually bronchopneumonias)
- bronchiectasis
- occasionally large numbers of eosinophils in sputum may give a false impression of infected sputum.

Frank haemoptysis may be associated with:

- various infection of the lungs (including tuberculosis)

- mitral stenosis
- bronchiectasis
- pulmonary infarction
- neoplasia (especially carcinoma of the lung)
- bleeding diatheses
- hard coughing.

Rust-coloured sputum is classically found in lobar pneumonia, and with patients who are too ill to give a history they probably have either respiratory failure or a bacteraemia.

Sputum with a foul odour should make one suspect infection with anaerobic organisms, abscess formation, or bronchiectasis.

Large amounts of sputum may be produced in:

- pulmonary cavitation
- bronchiectasis
- acute pulmonary oedema.

Chest examination

Examine the chest in detail. Use the time-honoured sequence of inspection, palpation, percussion, and auscultation. At each stage attempt to decide the anatomical lesion, its functional consequences, and its likely aetiology.

SPECIFIC ORGAN DYSFUNCTIONS

The symptoms and signs of the various organ dysfunctions have been detailed in other sections but some deserve special mention.

Deficient glucose homeostasis

Diabetes mellitus can cause coma by means of hyperglycaemia, hypoglycaemia, lactic acidosis, or hyperosmolar states. In each case there may be a precipitating factor. Hypoglycaemia may be caused by:

- oral hypoglycaemic drug accumulation
- oral hypoglycaemic drug overdosage
- excessive insulin administration
- inadequate dietary intake of glucose
- alcoholism
- liver cell failure
- intestinal malabsorption
- hypopituitary states
- hypoadrenal states
- postgastrectomy syndromes
- reactive hyperinsulinism
- consequent to an insulinoma.

Hyperglycaemia may be precipitated by inadequate pancreatic secretion of insulin which may be brought to light by intercurrent illnesses, particularly infection and myocardial infarction.

Hepatic dysfunction

Syndromes causing acute presentation include:

- hepatic coma or precoma (perhaps precipitated by gastrointestinal bleeding)
- alcoholism
- inappropriate sedatives
- infections
- excessive protein intake in those with borderline liver function
- in acute or subacute hepatic necrosis (perhaps associated with fulminant viral hepatitis or drug reactions including those to alcohol or paracetamol).

Renal dysfunction

Acute presentations may be caused by:

- rapidly progressive uraemia
- urinary tract infection (with or without bacteraemia)
- hypertensive encephalopathy
- overhydration caused by fluid overload (perhaps associated with acute tubular necrosis, dehydration, acute glomerulonephritis or urinary tract obstruction).

The presence of total anuria despite catheterization should demand the exclusion of upper urinary tract obstruction (acute cortical necrosis, complete bilateral renal infarction, and acute glomerulonephritis are possible medical causes of complete anuria to be considered).

Thyroid dysfunction

Possible signs of thyroid dysfunction are detailed on page 70.

Hypothyroidism per se rarely presents as an emergency but chronic unknown hypothyroidism may present acutely as a result of complications such as hypothermia.

Hyperthyroid crises classically used to occur in post-thyroidectomy patients who had been inadequately prepared for operation or with thyroxine overdosage. Features of thyroid crises that may render patients unable to give a history include prostration, marked tachycardia, profound muscle weakness, hyperthermia or coma.

Paradoxically hyperthyroidism may present with stupor or apathy.

Adrenal dysfunction

Hypoadrenal states may be precipitated by intercurrent illness which may produce relative cortisol deficiency. They may also occur after withdrawal from steroid therapy. Suspect a hypoadrenal state in any patient who presents with hypotension and is subsequently found to have hyponatraemia and hyperkalaemia.

Deficient calcium homeostasis

This may present with complications such as epilepsy or stridor with hypocalcaemia, or with apathy due to hypercalcaemia. Corneal calcification is the only clinical clue to hypercalcaemia.

Severe electrolyte disorders

Hypokalaemia, hyponatraemia, or hypernatraemia in children may present acutely.

Fulminant gastrointestinal disorders

Disorders which may be present with severe prostration such that a history is not available include acute gastrointestinal haemorrhage, perforation of a viscus, complications of neoplasms, severe food poisoning with vomiting and/or diarrhoea, and various surgical conditions which have not been treated in the acute stage.

Genital disorders

Do not omit to examine the genitalia of either sex as there may be evidence of primary neoplasia or, in the female, evidence of vaginal or uterine infection.

POISONING AS A CAUSE OF METABOLIC DYSFUNCTION

Self-poisoning is unfortunately a fashionable cause of presentation with impaired consciousness. The presence of blisters (often over an area of skin pressure) suggests drug overdosage but provides only a non-specific clue to the actual drug taken. More specific clues to the drug involved are detailed below.

- **Opiates:** look for vomiting, pinpoint pupils, hypoventilation or possible venepuncture marks.

- **Phenothiazines:** look for basal ganglia (Parkinsonian) features (p. 96), convulsions, hypotension, cardiac dysrhythmias.

- **Tricyclic antidepressants:** look for:
  - symmetrical hyperreflexia in a drowsy patient (an unusual combination)
  - convulsions
  - hypotension
  - cardiac dysrhythmias
  - anticholinergic effects (such as a dry mouth, dilated pupils and absent bowel sounds).

Paracetamol

If a patient who is known to have taken a paracetamol overdose presents with impaired consciousness, suspect either a mixed overdose or hepatic precoma (the latter usually develops at least 24 hours after the ingestion of the paracetamol).

Alcohol

Patients who present with alcohol on the breath without being capable of giving an account of themselves may well be drunk, but remember their 'drunkenness' may also be a presentation of:

- an additional overdose
- subdural haemorrhage
- occult head injury
- hypoglycaemia
- Korsakoff's syndrome
- hepatic precoma
- alcohol *withdrawal* syndrome.

If alcohol related illness is present always give a vitamin preparation (containing thiamine).

Aspirin

Aspirin overdosage rarely presents as coma of uncertain cause unless the patient is *in extremis*. It usually presents earlier with tinnitus, deafness, sweating, fever, tachycardia or hyperventilation.

Patients too ill to give a history — secondary assessment (III)

- Abnormal respiration may be caused by extrapulmonary illness, including drug overdose, cerebral lesions and acidosis.
- Sputum with a foul odour suggests anaerobic infection.
- Previously unsuspected hypothyroidism may be made apparent by complications such as hypothermia.

PAEDIATRIC HISTORY AND EXAMINATION (I)

HISTORY

The paediatric history is usually obtained from the parents and it is important you ensure that your understanding of the history differentiates between the facts and the parents' impressions or interpretations of the facts.

It is useful to have a mental check list of bodily systems and their relevant paediatric symptoms (Fig. 1).

The past and present 'milestone status' of the child should be ascertained (Table 1).

Table 1 **Developmental milestones in the first year**

Age	Activity
Birth	Moro and grasp reflexes active
4 weeks	Follows with eyes
6 weeks	Smiles
8 weeks	Ventral suspension – head held in plane of body
12 weeks	Turns head to sound
20 weeks	Feet in mouth
28 weeks	Sits with hands on couch
36 weeks	Sits unaided
44 weeks	Creeps
48 weeks	Crawls, walks around furniture
51 weeks	Walks alone

EXAMINATION

Ideally the child should not be aware of being scientifically assessed; indeed a lot can be learned from observation of the children as you play with them.

Although the following writing up of the examination should follow a logical sequence, the actual examination may have to be conducted in a more flexible fashion.

The principles of paediatric and adult examination are similar: here only those aspects of particular relevance to children are mentioned. Similarly, assessment of the neonate is not discussed here as this is a specialized procedure outwith the remit of this account.

Always conclude the examination with the more upsetting procedures, such as inspection of the throat or taking the blood pressure.

GENERAL ASPECTS

Always record the height and weight of children (Fig. 2) on the standard charts that are available. In babies always measure the head circumference. Even if normal, these measurements are valuable as a baseline.

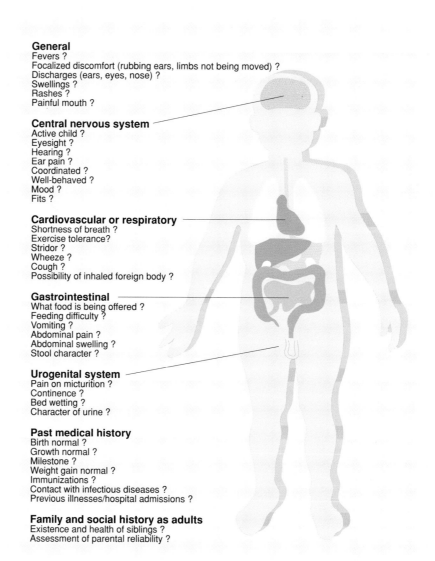

General
Fevers ?
Focalized discomfort (rubbing ears, limbs not being moved) ?
Discharges (ears, eyes, nose) ?
Swellings ?
Rashes ?
Painful mouth ?

Central nervous system
Active child ?
Eyesight ?
Hearing ?
Ear pain ?
Coordinated ?
Well-behaved ?
Mood ?
Fits ?

Cardiovascular or respiratory
Shortness of breath ?
Exercise tolerance?
Stridor ?
Wheeze ?
Cough ?
Possibility of inhaled foreign body ?

Gastrointestinal
What food is being offered ?
Feeding difficulty ?
Vomiting ?
Abdominal pain ?
Abdominal swelling ?
Stool character ?

Urogenital system
Pain on micturition ?
Continence ?
Bed wetting ?
Character of urine ?

Past medical history
Birth normal ?
Growth normal ?
Milestone ?
Weight gain normal ?
Immunizations ?
Contact with infectious diseases ?
Previous illnesses/hospital admissions ?

Family and social history as adults
Existence and health of siblings ?
Assessment of parental reliability ?

Fig. 1 **Checklist of symptoms in young children.**

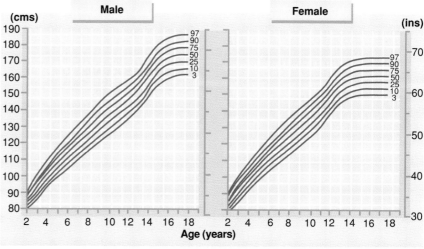

Fig. 2 **Growth charts representing normal range of developments.**

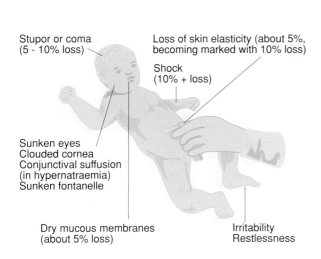

Fig. 3 **Assessment of dehydration.**

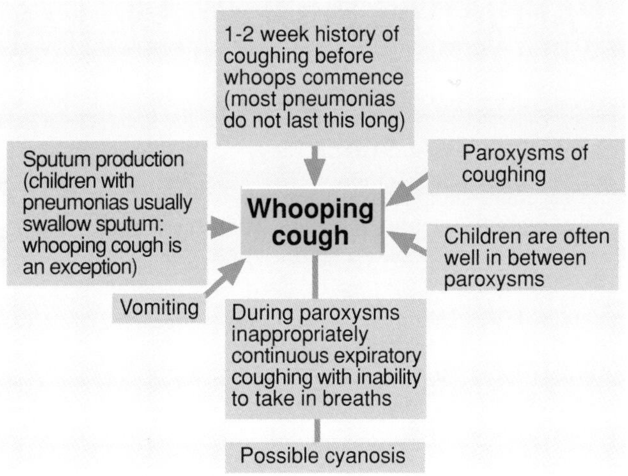

Fig. 4 **Features (other than the whoop) that suggest a diagnosis of whooping cough.**

Assessment of dehydration

Signs of dehydration (Fig. 3) in infants include irritability, sunken eyes, clouded corneas and a sunken fontanelle in those under 12 months of age. In babies and infants *less than 5% water loss* causes thirst, dry mucous membranes and loss of skin elasticity, *5–10% water loss* produces severe thirst, marked loss of skin elasticity, oliguria, and in severe cases, stupor and coma. *Water loss of 10% or more* produces circulatory inadequacy (shock).

Examination of the mouth

When examining the mouth of young children it is useful to ask to count the teeth – children are usually willing to show off their teeth allowing the examiner full access!

RESPIRATORY SYSTEM

A raised respiratory rate may be the only sign of a chest infection (or heart failure). The mean respiratory rate is 62/min in 11 week old babies, 23/min in 2–3 years old children, and 16/min in those over 12 years of age. Children with chest infection often show a short pause after inspiration rather than the normal expiration pause and, especially with bronchiolitis, there may be a grunt at the beginning of expiration.

If a child is crying, the examiner can easily assess vocal resonance, but listen for breath sound specifically in the quiet moment when the child is inspiring for the next yell. Young children often cannot take deep breaths to order, making ascultation more difficult. However they will blow out air when asked to do so, and to do this have to take the deep breaths required.

There may be chest wall deformities which can interfere with ventilation.

Harrison's sulci (see p. 46) are grooves below the nipples caused by indrawing of the lower ribs associated with excessive diaphragmatic action in long-standing respiratory obstruction.

Coughs in children

Croupy cough

A croupy cough is barking in character, and in addition there may be inspiratory stridor, intercostal indrawing and the voice may be hoarse (laryngitic).

Pneumonic or bronchitic coughs

A pneumonic or bronchitic cough may be the only obvious sign of a chest infection. Pneumonic coughs tend to be continual (not paroxysmal) and experienced clinicians can differentiate a 'chesty' cough from an upper respiratory cough because the former tends to be a lower pitch and sounds as if it has a deeper origin than whooping cough or croup.

Whooping cough

With whooping cough (Fig. 4) there is a history of 1–2 weeks of respiratory tract problems before whooping becomes predominant. Whooping cough occurs in paroxysms, between which the child is usually well. Expiratory coughing occurs in bouts during which the child may be unable to breathe in and cyanosis may occur. The whoop itself is a high pitched suction noise caused by a vast inspiration into the 'empty' lungs. Vomiting at the end of a paroxysm is very suggestive of whooping cough. Affected children usually produce mucoid sputum which is thick and tenacious: sputum production is unusual in other childhood chest infections as sputum is usually swallowed.

Epiglottitis

In epiglottitis there is usually a history of abrupt onset fever and sore throat. Early epiglottitis must be suspected if a red swollen, easily visible epiglottis is seen on inspection of a sore throat. Later stridor may occur with a predominantly inspiratory wheeze which sounds more proximal than that of laryngitis or croup. Children with established epiglottitis characteristically drool saliva. In such circumstances do *not* inspect the throat as respiratory obstruction may be precipitated. Obtain immediate ear, nose and throat (ENT) and anaesthetic advice.

Stridor

Stridor is a high pitched sound usually produced by laryngeal or tracheal obstruction. It is usually heard in both inspiration and expiration but is most prominent on inspiration and sounds like a breathy 'haaare'. Coincidental cyanosis or a marked tachycardia are danger signs: medical or surgical intervention should not be delayed.

Paediatric history and examination (I)

- Ideally children should hardly be aware that they are being examined.
- Always leave the most upsetting parts of the examination until the end.
- Use a child's cry to assess vocal resonance.
- Listen to breath sounds and for crepitations during inter-cry inspirations.
- If you suspect epiglottitis do not examine the throat.

PAEDIATRIC HISTORY AND EXAMINATION (II)

GASTROINTESTINAL SYSTEM

The examiner should have warm hands and do his best to relax the child. With babies it may be best to examine the child lying on the mother's lap or even to examine during bathtime: this assists the baby to relax and the water allows your palpating fingers to slide along the abdomen thereby assisting identification of abnormal organ edges.

Gentle rotatory movements of the examiner's finger tips assist the definition of organ edges. If a child is crying one may have to postpone the examination, but brief episodes of palpation can be achieved by 'dipping' the palpating fingers into the abdomen when crying ceases during inspiration.

The abdomen usually moves freely on respiration in infants: if it does not, suspect peritonitis.

Detection of an enlarged liver is important as this may be the only signs of heart failure. In children who cannot regulate their breathing to order, a gentle rippling of the examining fingers of the right hand can be useful: successive gentle pressing in with the tips of the little finger, then ring finger, then middle finger and then the index finger in a line at right angles to the expected liver edge (Fig. 1). Percussion can confirm the liver edge. In most normal children the liver edge can be felt.

In children it is not abnormal for the kidneys to be palpable and a just palpable spleen is not necessarily abnormal.

In male children always ensure that the testes can be felt in the scrotum.

Infantile pyloric stenosis

There may be visible gastric peristalsis proceeding from left to right across the upper abdomen. The swelling of the thickened contracted pylorus is perhaps best felt by placing the tips of the fingers of the left hand just inferior to the right rib cage and external to the rectus sheath, and gently rippling the fingers from left to right (little, ring, middle, index fingers successively; Fig. 2). Feeding the baby (classically a first-born male about 6 weeks of age) during the examination will elicit peristalsis and make the pylorus become prominent. The walnut-like pyloric swelling may be intermittently palpable and so palpation must be continued for up to 15 minutes.

Intussusception

Intussusception is an invagination of the gut into itself resulting in a soft sausage-shaped swelling which may be palpable. Symptoms may be intermittent with abrupt bouts of pain in which infants go pale and draw up their legs. Fresh blood may be seen in and on the stool – 'redcurrant jelly stools'.

CENTRAL NERVOUS SYSTEM

In children who can speak the examination can proceed as in the adult, but otherwise assessment has to rely on observation of posture and movements, either spontaneous or elicited by the examiner.

The anterior fontanelle (the triangular shaped gap between the cranial bones) (Fig. 3) is usually closed by 12 months of age.

Cries of significance

A high-pitched 'cerebral' cry suggests meningitis or significant brain damage at birth whilst an abnormally articulated cry may suggest cerebral palsy.

Some specific paediatric reflexes

Early reflexes include the following:

- *The sucking and swallowing reflexes* are initially automatic.
- *The rooting reflex* is movement of the head towards a soft stimulus delivered to the cheek – 'in search of the nipple'.
- *Plantar responses* (p. 93) are extensor until about 12 months of age.
- *Pupillary light reflexes* are present from birth. Infants cannot be requested to move their eyes to order and so eye movement assessment depends on observation. At about 4 weeks infants will watch their mother and at about 8 weeks the baby will be fixing on objects.

Reflexes that normally have disappeared by 2–3 months of age include:

- *The grasp reflex* is an automatic clutching of the examiner's finger.
- *The Moro reflex* is a response to sudden 'threats' such as a loud noise. To elicit the Moro reflex the baby should be held on its back. With one hand of the examiner supporting the trunk and the other

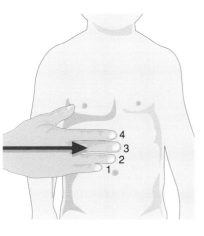

Fig. 1 **Palpating for a liver edge if a child cannot breathe regularly.**

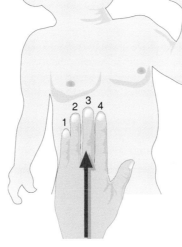

Fig. 2 **Palpating for infantile pyloric stenosis.**

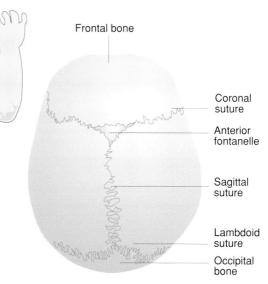

Frontal bone

Coronal suture

Anterior fontanelle

Sagittal suture

Lambdoid suture

Occipital bone

Fig. 3 **The position of the anterior fontanelle.**

hand the head and neck. The hand supporting the head is abruptly lowered a few centimetres. A normal response comprises abduction and extension of the arms followed by flexion (Fig. 4). A diminished or absent response implies cerebral abnormality, and a unilateral absence of response implies a predominantly unilateral abnormality.

- *The tonic neck reflex* is elicited with the baby on its back: rotation of the head to one side produces increased tone and partial extension of the arm and leg of that side, perhaps with flexion of the contralateral arm and leg. A strong tonic neck reflex after the first week suggests cerebral palsy.

These three reflexes may be absent with severe cerebral birth damage but in cerebral palsy they may be slow to disappear.

Meningitis
In babies signs of meningitis may be:
- non-specific with fever in 60%
- lethargy in 50 %
- irritability in 30%
- anorexia or vomiting in 50%
- respiratory distress in 50%
- convulsions in 40%
- a bulging fontanelle in 30%
- diarrhoea in 20%
- neck stiffness in only 15%.

The message is clear: a lumbar puncture must be performed if you think there is a chance of meningitis. In older children a useful test for neck and back stiffness is to ask them to kiss their knees.

Hearing
It is important to detect deafness as early as possible, otherwise there will be 'knock-on' speech problems and impaired intellectual progress. With babies any impairment of response to sounds provides the initial clue. Any suspicion of deafness necessitates referral for specialist assessment.

Musculoskeletal system
Examination should proceed along the same lines as adult examination.

CHILD ABUSE
There are five types of abuse:
- *physical injury* which may have been deliberately inflicted or caused by parental neglect permitting the child to become injured
- *neglect* by failing to provide a suitable environment
- *emotional neglect* may impair both mental and physical development of the child
- *sexual abuse*
- *potential abuse* if there is known or suspected abuse of another child in the family or if a large number of risk factors are present.

Physical injury (child battering, non-accidental injury)
Musculoskeletal injuries range from petechiae, bruises (particularly those that could be caused by finger-tip pressure) and lacerations to burns and scalds. Fractures and visceral damage, subdural effusions and retinal haemorrhages may be caused by vigorous shaking. Battered children may show evidence of previous neglect or deprivation including stunted growth.

Either or both of the parents may show evidence of immaturity, depression, psychopathic personality, or may appear superficially normal; guilt may cause parents to present the child for medical advice and help for no immediately obvious reason, so a lack of obvious reason for a consultation may be an important clue.

The first step in diagnosis is to think of the diagnosis: accordingly every childhood injury should be viewed with suspicion. Children should always be undressed completely to allow a full inspection. Suspicious features include:
- inadequate or vague explanations of injuries
- too facile explanations of injury
- a previous history of child neglect or abuse in the child or its siblings
- inappropriate delay in the presentation of the child to the medical services after injury
- multiple injuries
- injuries sustained at night
- a torn lip frenulum
- a history of failure to thrive
- multiple fractures of long bones
- circular blisters (which may result from cigarette burns)
- bruises of differing ages.

Suspicion of child battering should necessitate removal of the child to a place of safety, usually to hospital in the first instance. It is not necessary and indeed may be unproductive to accuse the parents on the spot (you might be wrong); the child can be admitted for 'medical observation'. Never forget that 'Mongolian blue spots' (naturally occurring bluish or dark areas, often more than 2 cm in diameter, usually on the buttock) which resemble bruising may give rise to false suspicions of non-accidental injury.

It is essential that all findings are carefully recorded and that photographs of visible injuries are taken as part of the medical record.

SEXUAL ABUSE
Sexual abuse of children is more common than is realized: before the age of 16 years at least one in ten girls and one in 15 boys have been sexually assaulted, often by adults known to them. Clues may include:
- injuries to genitalia or anus
- recurrent urinary tract infections in girls
- unusual sexual awareness
- sudden changes in behaviour.

If sexual abuse is suspected a consultant should be involved *ab initio*. Interpretation of some of the signs usually requires much experience.

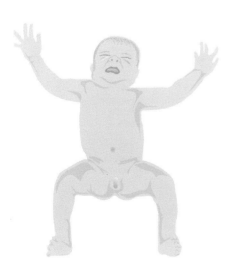

Fig. 4 **The Moro response.**

Paediatric history and examination (II)

- The abdomen usually moves freely on respiration in infants; if it does not then suspect peritonitis.
- Plantar responses are extensor until about 12 months of age.
- Pupillary light reflexes are present from birth.
- In babies with meningitis, signs may be minimal.
- Always think about non-accidental injury if any circumstance of injury is not straightforward.

GERIATRIC HISTORY AND EXAMINATION

The general principles of history and examination also apply to the elderly, but here common geriatric problems are dealt with specifically.

MULTIPLE PATHOLOGY

Although not exclusively the province of the elderly, multiple pathology is common, possibly caused by a lifetime's accumulation of chronic diseases. Multiple pathology also implies a 'limiting factor' phenomenon: patients can cope with multiple disabilities, but eventually a relatively minor deterioration in any one disability may provide 'the last straw' causing 'snowballing decompensation' of accumulated disabilities: thus early identification of all such 'limiting factors', particularly those that may be reversible, is essential and this is one reason why any assessment of the elderly must be comprehensive.

NON-SPECIFIC SYMPTOMS

Both elderly patients and their medical advisors may have a low expectation of good health in the elderly, and may dismiss vague symptoms as 'due to age'. Classical symptoms of certain illnesses may be non-existent or vague.

- Infections may not cause fever but may present with hypothermia.
- Pneumonias may present without fever or cough.
- Thyroid dysfunction may present as heart failure or apathy.
- Myxoedema may present as constipation.
- Depression may simulate myxoedema.
- Myocardial infarction or pneumonia may cause confusion.
- Strokes may be caused by a drop in cerebral perfusion secondary to silent myocardial infarction.

MISLEADING SYMPTOMS

Diseases in one system may cause symptoms in another. Almost any disorder may present with acute confusion, falls, incontinence, diarrhoea or vomiting, or non-specific deterioration in health.

COMMUNICATION DIFFICULTIES

Ensure that 'demented' patients are not deaf, dysphasic or partially sighted. Great patience may be required to elicit the history and later confirmation of relevant historical points may be appropriate.

MEMORY IMPAIRMENT

Useful information may be provided by relatives, previous medical notes, the patient's general practitioners, health visitors, or neighbours. The cheapest investigation is often a telephone call.

DRUGS

Always check that a patient's drug history is correct, especially when the elderly may be on complex multiple medications. Always ensure that the drugs were being taken; 'increasing' the dosage of a diuretic in a patient who was not actually taking them can have disastrous circulatory effects. Likewise always consider the possibility that adverse effects of drugs may be a limiting factor. For example immobility may be a basal ganglia manifestation of phenothiazine therapy.

SOME SPECIFIC ASPECTS OF GERIATRIC EXAMINATION

- A complete examination is essential because disorders may present illogically – a septic foot may present at the other end of the body with confusion.
- If there is a suspicion of hypothermia use a low-reading thermometer.
- The back of the chest should be examined immediately after helping the patient to undress as the patient will then not have to sit up a second time for you to examine the back of the chest.
- Most students seem to know how to undress patients, but show no skill at helping them to replace their nightgowns (Fig. 1). To do this the examiner should put his arms into the sleeves of the discarded nightgown and gather up the bottom of the gown with his hands, then grip the patient's hands and slide the sleeves onto the patient's arms, and assist the patient to put her head through the nightgown collar. If a patient has a hemiparesis always put the sleeve of the nightgown or pyjamas onto the paralysed arm first so that the patient can assist in placing the more mobile second arm into its sleeve.
- The commonest cause of diarrhoea in the elderly is faecal impaction and thus a rectal examination is mandatory in elderly patients with diarrhoea.

- Patients with unilateral cerebral infarction and a normal mental state are not normally incontinent of urine: if they are, then the cause may be urological.
- Some reflexes, including the abdominal reflexes and ankle jerks, may be absent in the elderly. Joint position sense and vibration sense may be absent at the ankle.
- Never forget Parkinson's disease as a cause of immobility or apparent apathy.
- Especially in the elderly a diagnosis must comprise three aspects, the anatomical, the aetiological, and the functional. Of these three the last is often neglected: what a patient can or cannot do, especially in terms of mobility, is often of paramount importance.

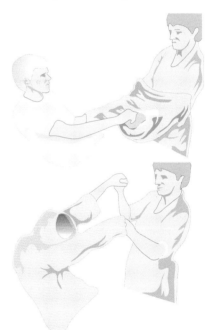

Fig. 1 **Replacing an elderly patient's nightgown after examination.** This patient's left arm is paralysed and is dealt with first, allowing the (good) right arm to be of assistance.

Geriatric history and examination

- Classical symptoms or signs of certain pathologies may be absent in the elderly.
- Diseases in one body system may cause symptoms in another.
- Always obtain an accurate and confirmed drug history.
- If hypothermia is a possibility use a low–reading thermometer.

WRITING UP

It is best to write up the history and examination as soon as possible after the interview. In general practice a few relevant notes are usually all that is required, but in hospital practice or with new complex problems the notes should be structured so that any omission becomes obvious. The history should form a coherent story and, if written at the conclusion of the clerking, will obviously be influenced by the findings on examination.

Never omit to read the letter of referral and never omit to scan through previous notes when they arrive, usually later, on the ward.

STRUCTURE (Table 1)

The presenting complaint(s) and their development should be at the top of the clerking after the patient's identification details. With illness of well-defined onset it is often useful to preface the presenting complaint with an introductory statement such as 'Previously well until (date)...' or 'Against a background of long standing chest problems [which would be detailed later] this man developed acute shortness of breath on [date]'. The principle symptom(s) of the current illness must be identified and put in a defined time sequence, along with all relevant circumstances. Use dates whenever possible: on 2/6/92 defines precisely the day of onset whereas 'last Thursday' means little to someone reading the notes years later.

When writing up the history either record the patient's own words in inverted commas (especially if the patient has provided a poetic, yet scientifically interpretable, statement of his/her problem). Alternatively translate, with precision, the symptoms as given into medical terms.

Simple 'routine surgical' clerkings can be written up as the history is recounted by the patient, but more complex histories usually cannot. To give the patient maximum attention only write down numerical information of relevance that you might otherwise fail to remember. For example: 'dyspnoea 2/6/94, purulent sputum 4/6/94, haemoptysis 9/6/94, pulmonary TB 1946, thoracoplasty 1948, bronchiectasis diagnosed 1960'. The rest of the time you can spend communicating with the patient (p. 150). In busy clinics, arrows can usefully replace words. For example:

'Pain on micturition for 3 days commencing on (date)→General Practitioner →ampicillin for 3 days→no better→ cotrimoxazole for 2 days→ rash→given chlorpheniramine →rash worsening →admission requested.'

Resist the tendency to record snide comments no matter how truly these may reflect your feelings. Always presume that your notes will be read critically by others and this, in the United Kingdom at least, might well include the patient.

Avoid the use of acronyms. Does NAD mean 'no abnormality detected' or 'not actually done'? Often it means both. Does PRN (pro re nata) mean 'as the situation requires' or per rectum nocte?

Before writing up the history and examination always take a metaphorical step backwards from the situation and (before making a diagnosis) ask the more basic question 'What is going on here?'. This often assists an overall conception of the problems and allows a more lucid written account.

Providing a one paragraph summary at the end of the clerking often helps to focus your thoughts and assist those who may need to use the notes subsequently.

Always conclude writing up of the history and examination by recording the:

- differential diagnoses or diagnosis
- immediate investigations requested
- elective investigations requested
- immediate treatment
- follow-on treatment
- information or advice you have told the patient
- information or advice you have told the relatives
- information or advice you have told anyone else
- who else needs to be informed of the patient's progress (e.g. the GP).

LEAVING THE PATIENT

Never leave, or allow the patient to leave, without explaining what (you should have discovered) the patient *wants* to know about his condition. If there are findings that the patient *needs* to know these should be communicated appropriately at the time or later. Always explain what investigations are planned and why (after all the patient has the right to refuse any intervention). Always explain in terms that the patient will understand, using a minimum of medical jargon. Be aware that you may have to return later when the patient has had time to think and may have further questions for you to answer.

Table 1 **Headings for writing up.** Some need not be covered depending on circumstances.

Date of clerking

History
  Patient's name
  Date of birth (age)
  Occupation
  Time of admission

History of presenting complaint(s)
  Cardiovascular system
  Respiratory system
  Gastrointestinal system
  Nervous system
  Locomotor system
  Urinary system
  Gynaecological system
  Family history
  Social history
  Psychiatric history
  Past medical history

Examination
  General comments
  Specific findings relevant to presenting complaint
  Cardiovascular system
  Respiratory system
  Gastrointestinal system
  Nervous system
  Locomotor system
  Urinary system
  Gynaecological system

Diagnosis or differential diagnosis

Investigations (immediate and elective)

Treatment (immediate and follow-on)

Information given (to patient, relatives, anyone else)

Information to be given

Your signature

Your status

Writing up

- Never accept anyone else's diagnosis: make up your own mind!
- Always tell a story when writing up the history.
- Accentuate positive aspects of the findings.
- Relegate routine or irrelevant negative findings to the systematic questioning section.

DOCTOR – PATIENT COMMUNICATION

There have been many papers and articles written on communication with patients. Almost all are based on a mixture of experimentally proven techniques and personal opinion. What follows is no exception.

The satisfaction that both doctor and patient feel after an interview is often a reflection of the interpersonal interaction: on occasion the interpersonal interaction is the treatment.

When interviewing patients it is necessary to develop confidence and rapport quickly so that mutual trust can be established (Fig. 1).

Talking with patients requires various skills (Fig. 2). Most people cannot remember more than about a third of what they have been told. The more complex the information, the less will be the proportion that will be remembered. Therefore make specific efforts to help the patient increase recall (Fig. 3).

Whenever possible try to accentuate the positive. *Not* 'the risks of smoking are' *but* rather 'the benefits of not smoking are a reduced incidence of...'.

ASKING QUESTIONS

Open-ended questions are particularly useful to reassure patients that you are interested and need to know more:

- 'How did that affect you...?'
- 'That must have been very worrying...'
- 'Do tell me more about this...'.

On the other hand if you are short of time questions should be more specific in nature.

Escalating questions can be useful to pursue historical points of importance (Table 1).

Leading questions sometimes help patients to confess poor compliance. Non-compliance with advice or with drug treatment may be as high as 40-50%. Non-compliance is financially costly and jeopardizes your professional standing with the patient: 'If the doctor can't tell I am not taking the drugs then he/she obviously thought that they wouldn't have been very helpful.' Useful questions to help patients admit poor compliance are shown in Table 2.

When asking questions that may offend patients always explain why you have to ask.

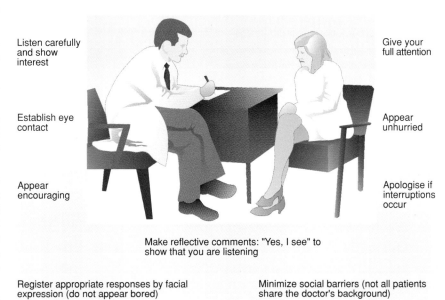

Adopt a warm friendly manner

Make clarifying comments : "So you mean that........"

Listen carefully and show interest

Give your full attention

Establish eye contact

Appear unhurried

Appear encouraging

Apologise if interruptions occur

Make reflective comments: "Yes, I see" to show that you are listening

Register appropriate responses by facial expression (do not appear bored)

Minimize social barriers (not all patients share the doctor's background)

Fig. 1 **Establishing rapport and mutual trust.**

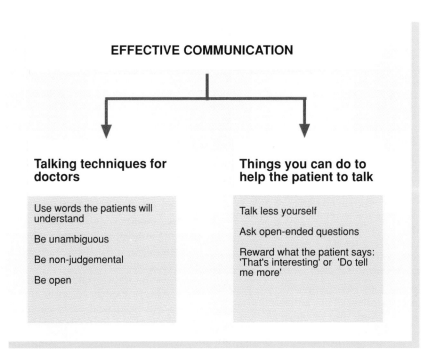

EFFECTIVE COMMUNICATION

Talking techniques for doctors

Use words the patients will understand

Be unambiguous

Be non-judgemental

Be open

Things you can do to help the patient to talk

Talk less yourself

Ask open-ended questions

Reward what the patient says: 'That's interesting' or 'Do tell me more'

Fig. 2 **Communication skills required for talking with patients.**

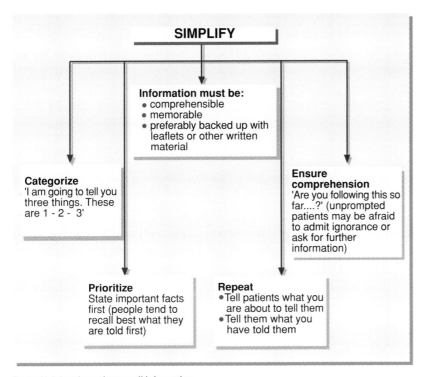

Fig. 3 **Helping the patient recall information.**

Table 1 **Use of escalating question**

'Is there anything else you wish to tell me?'
'Is there anything else you ought to tell me?'
'What else is there I ought to know?'
'But I suspect that there is more to this than what you have told me...'
An expectant silence following such questions often acts as a powerful evoker of information

Table 2 **Questions to help patients admit non-compliance**

'Do you find it difficult to take the tablets?'
'Do you ever forget to take your tablets?'
'What proportion of the tablets do you miss?'
'When you feel better do you sometimes stop taking the tablets?'
'If you feel worse do you sometimes stop taking the tablets?'

EXAMINING PATIENTS

Whilst examining patients explain what you are doing and why. I once examined a lady in the presence of a chaperone yet her sister wrote to complain about my normal examination: 'He held her hand, then his hand moved up her arms, he looked in her eyes, caressed her neck etc...' An explanation at the time would have avoided this: 'I'm taking your pulse, seeing if you are anaemic, feeling for lymph glands in your neck' etc. Such explanations also involve patients in their own care.

ENDING INTERVIEWS

It is often helpful to summarize the results of discussions to assist the patient's understanding and recall.

If, at the end of the interview, you feel that something is still being held back, confess that you have not been able to get to grips with the problem and ask if the interview could be resumed later. This may usefully be combined with a request for the patient to write out his/her story for your records.

When an interview does not end naturally or have an obvious conclusion, yet must be concluded, always be polite, friendly, yet firm and do not let the patient think he/she is being rejected. Different individuals will have to evolve their own techniques so that a positive atmosphere is retained whilst the interview is being (negatively) brought to a close. One useful technique is to smile in a friendly fashion whilst asking a question: 'Is that all right?' or 'That seems to be the best we can do' whilst intimating with body language (perhaps an open gesture with the hands?) that you are about to rise to open the door for the patient.

Whatever you may feel about various groups of patients, your job is to look after individuals to the best of your ability and this demands a wide repertoire of communication skills. Verbal communication skills are essential but do not forget other aspects of communication. A flexible voice intonation suggests interest and non-verbal signs (body language) can be used to reinforce verbal communication. Most people are unaware of their body language and obtaining feedback from observers can be valuable. However the quintessential problem is that useful feedback regarding your communication skills is hardly ever forthcoming from the patients. Role play enables valuable feedback without the need to learn (often by mistakes) whilst dealing with actual patients (see box on this page).

The technique of role play

Take the history from a student colleague who should, after relevant study, role-play a patient with a condition he/she has chosen whilst adopting a personality trait (garrulous, taciturn, uncommunicative, or aggressive). There are three potential gains. Your student colleague learns about his/her chosen condition, the history-taker gains experience and the student colleague (or other observers) can give feedback on the effectiveness of the history taking (similar role-play techniques can also be used to practise communication skills).

Doctor–patient communication

- Do not assume that patient compliance with drug treatment will be 100%.
- Always explain to patients why you have to examine parts of the body not obviously relevant to the symptoms.
- Obtain feedback concerning your history taking and examination skills: patients can rarely provide this, therefore use role play techniques.

EXAM TAKING TECHNIQUES

In most examinations the examiners are looking for confident and safe doctoring with evidence that the candidate can use his or her initiative to good effect, rather than provide brilliant expositions of 'state of the art medicine'. Examiners usually examine in pairs and most examiners are fair markers. The generous markers 'doves' are usually matched with harsh markers 'hawks' so that fair treatment of candidates is assured.

Sad though it may be to relate, the ability to take a competent history and perform a competent examination is not sufficient to pass examinations: you have to convince examiners that you have these abilities and the realities are that certain examination techniques are helpful in this endeavour.

Many of the techniques described below are useful in that grand continuous assessment examination called life.

PRESENTATION OF HISTORY

Use of certain words, *by themselves*, may earn extra marks: therefore include them in your remarks. 'Interesting' (i.e. you have a lively enquiring mind), 'fascinating' (you are very interested in clinical medicine), and 'thought-provoking'. It helps to have a small list of key words in your mind to include almost as a reflex:

'I think X *because*'
'Causes of Y *include*'
'The *major* complications are'
'*Important* causes of Z are'
'*Notwithstanding* the finding of Z, I think that...'.

Always qualify a diagnosis: 'I think this patient has X disease *because*...'. If however you are uncertain of the diagnosis, the approach can be altered: 'I am happy that this is *not* X because...'.

Take and keep the initiative. If you are talking sense in an interesting fashion then it is difficult for an examiner to interrupt or fail you. Try to avoid sudden silences or stumblings in your presentation because then the initiative passes to the examiner and, if this occurs suddenly, the examiner may then have to improvise unplanned questions which may be difficult to answer.

Make incidental comments which show powers of observation and deduction. Draw obvious conclusions and state them confidently. Oil beneath the tips of the finger-nails and a copy of the motor trade journal on the bedside locker: 'Obviously a worker in the motor trade'. Tar stains on the right hand: 'Obviously a smoker and also right handed'. Diabetic orange juice on the locker: 'This diabetic patient....'. In short cases such simple deductions can be very impressive especially if the examiner is surprised enough to ask you, 'How did you know that?'. The similar deductive abilities of the fictional Sherlock Holmes were based upon those possessed by a doctor who had taught the then medical student Conan Doyle.

If a diagnosis is elusive and the examiners have not given any helpful leads then you can either give a list of differential diagnoses or proceed straightaway to the investigations: 'To make a definite diagnosis I would need to know the results of ....'.

When preparing for examinations in which you will be shown short cases have a brief but eloquent speech relevant to common clinical signs that you might be shown: 'This is pitting oedema because it is ... and the most common cause would be... and in this patient almost certainly the cause is ....'. Even if you were wrong and it was non-pitting oedema the examiner would be impressed with your knowledge. Your prepared repertoire should included topics like:

- a raised jugular venous pressure
- a displaced apex beat
- an irregular pulse
- dullness on percussion of the chest.

If the answer to a question is controversial then say so as this suggests that you have read the relevant literature widely and realize there is more than one opinion (the statement that your reply is controversial will also protect you against potential clashes of opinion with examiners).

If you are totally at a loss for a diagnosis admit your ignorance (this stops examiners pestering) and start to discuss the possibilities.

If you are cautiously optimistic that a diagnosis is correct you can always ask the examiner: 'Could this be...?'. If you are correct the examiner will be pleased that you gave a considered suggestion. If you are incorrect examiners will hardly ever say no and not also give you some help.

If you are presenting a patient by the bedside and are discussing the differential diagnosis in front of the patient, it creates a good impression to take a few seconds to reassure the patient that he does not have the majority of the conditions mentioned. This is also a useful ploy for bringing to an end your list of differential diagnoses.

If you are uncertain as to the presence of certain clinical signs use the scientific-sounding euphemism for 'I have no idea' by saying instead: 'There is an equivocal....'. If the examiner indicates that he/she thought it should have been easy to elicit the abnormality in question, you can always say that it was difficult to detect — this flatters the examiner who presumably had detected it!

In long cases the examiner will either ask you to present the patient or, less likely, will ask you if you have made a diagnosis or diagnoses. In either case you can retain the initiative (Fig. 1) and either present the history, examination and diagnosis in classical fashion, or present your diagnosis initially. In either case it is beneficial to indicate that you established a friendly rapport with the patient, 'Mr X is a cheerful/rather depressed/garrulous/worried man.' If the patient is a poor historian, say so at the start of your presentation but then show that you have the ability to cope with such situations: 'Mr X is a worried man with a multitude of complaints. Nevertheless there are three complaints of immediate relevance.'

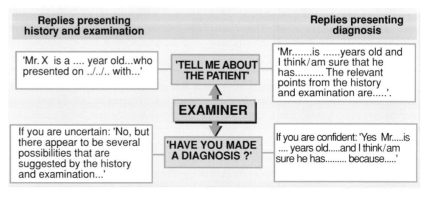

Fig. 1 **Retaining the initiative.**

EXAMINATION

Always approach the patient from the left-hand side of the bed and always be friendly. The patient's name is often easily visible (or has been told to you). Always introduce yourself and mention the patient's name: 'Good morning Mr Blank. I'm Dr X. Could I examine you please?'.

When requested to examine a specific part of a patient always take a brief look at the patient and his surroundings. When asked to examine the abdomen a failure to note that the patient is mildly jaundiced is putting yourself at a grave disadvantage. Never omit to notice the patient's observation charts (Table 1). If the patient has an infusion in situ always note what is being infused; if a patient is receiving an antibiotic then at least you can assume that the doctors think the patient has an infection. With cardiac short cases in which you are unable to characterize murmurs it is a good ploy to state that you would like to take the blood pressure. A sphygmomanometer is rarely instantly available in short cases and the examiner almost inevitably will ask why you want to take the blood pressure and you can then give a prepared and eloquent reply.

Table 1 **The patient's observation chart**
This contains a large amount of information and is usually neglected by doctors!

- Is the patient febrile? (making uncomplicated metabolic disorders unlikely)
- Is the respiratory rate raised? (making respiratory or cardiac pathology likely)
- Is the blood pressure raised? (making certain heart valve abnormalities unlikely)
- Is the apex rate being recorded as well as the usual pulse rate? (making atrial fibrillation almost certain)
- Is the drug therapy the patient is receiving entered on the observation chart? (a chest problem and three or four drugs on the chart imply tuberculosis)
- Is there a diabetic urine testing chart attached? (implying that diabetes is the likely cause of retinal abnormalities).

Even if asked specifically to examine a certain part of a patient you can reasonably ask the patient one or two questions provided that they are brief, elicit a one-word answer, and show the examiner that you are thinking along usual clinical lines: 'Has your urine been dark?' to a jaundiced patient or (even more impressively) remark that a male patient obviously has obstructive pattern jaundice because of scratch marks on his skin (haemolytic jaundice does not cause itching).

Opinions differ as to whether candidates should give commentary on their activities as they examine a patient.

Probably a running commentary is useful in the vast majority of cases. There are three reasons for this opinion:

- The examiner will realize that you have approached the problem in a knowledgeable fashion even if you derive an incorrect diagnosis.
- Words can substitute for actual examination and thereby save time. For example if asked to *examine* the abdomen of a jaundiced patient it is reasonable to remark 'this patient has no *obvious* signs of chronic liver disease' — the 'obvious' is an important word to include as it tells the examiners you would normally have made a detailed search but in the circumstances you are not doing this.
- Examiners have often examined on each patient several times and become bored if a succession of candidates go about their task in silence.

ANSWERING QUESTIONS

If you know the simple answer to a simple question answer clearly without equivocation. There are probably so many things that you are uncertain about that it is a tragedy to preface what you *do* know by seeming hesitant or saying 'Probably ....'. Whenever possible put positives before negatives and put the most important positive first: 'I would perform X investigation and then Y.'.

If you do not know the answer to a specific question a useful gambit is to state: 'Apart from the fact that (very important or basic fact that you do know) I do not know many other details about X.'.

Develop techniques for bringing failing replies to an end. To avoid awkward silences at the end of your answers learn to use non-verbal ways of intimating that your reply has come to an end.

Answering questions requires practice. A useful practice technique is to open any medical text book at the index and put your finger randomly on an entry: think for 5 seconds and then start talking. It is very helpful if you do this with a small number of your contemporaries, each talking on his or her randomly chosen topic in turn, so that you all have the benefit of experiencing how others handle awkward questions. Often it is surprising how much can be recalled about a subject by sensible free-association talking.

Practise answering questions in front of a mirror or on video — you will be surprised how much hand waving and gesturing occurs. In particular resist the tendency to illustrate your answers' by

clutching the appropriate part of your anatomy: this is a very common practice and looks extremely gauche.

If you do not understand a question say so. Do not guess, and do not try to reply because your answer may be totally inappropriate. If you do not understand the question in most cases the examiner will rephrase the question or provide clarification (after all it may be the examiner's fault that you cannot understand the question).

When asked a question you do not have to answer that question: you can answer a *slightly* different question — listen to politicians answering awkward questions for copious examples of this art form.

If asked for a list of causes of a condition or a differential diagnosis list, *never* say there are a defined number of causes unless you know you are correct and can finish the list (if you say that there are six causes of X and can only give three causes, then the examiner can only give you half marks). If you know you cannot provide a comprehensive list start off by saying: 'The most important (or major) causes are ....' (if you do not know the important causes then you probably do not deserve to pass!). This technique can be combined, once the important causes have finished, with: 'Other causes include ....'. This does not commit you to a defined number of answers and such prioritizing sounds very impressive.

All the above are simple points, attention to which can be worth a disproportionate number of marks (Table 2).

Table 2 **Pitfalls in oral exam taking**

Sudden silences

Hesitancy when you can be confident

Boring the examiners

Declaring a definite diagnosis (which might be wrong) without explaining why you reached that diagnosis

Spending too much time examining parts of the patient that are peripheral to the examiner's request

Asking the patient open–ended questions when the examiner asked you to examine the patient

Exam taking techniques

- Always take a brief look at the patient's surroundings.
- Always inspect the patient's observation charts.
- Do not illustrate your answers by clutching the relevant part of your anatomy.
- Try to retain the initiative.

INDEX

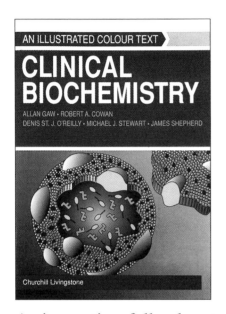

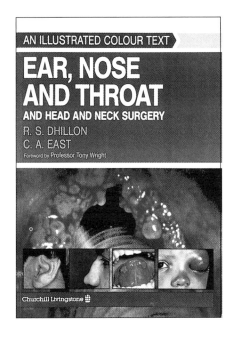

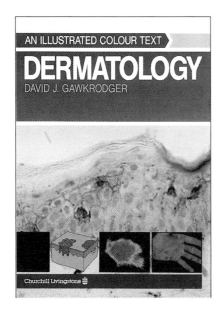